RESPIRATORY PHYSIOLOGY

Look for these other volumes in the *Mosby Physiology Series:*

Blaustein, Kao, & Matteson: *CELLULAR PHYSIOLOGY AND NEUROPHYSIOLOGY*

Johnson: *GASTROINTESTINAL PHYSIOLOGY*

Koeppen & Stanton: *RENAL PHYSIOLOGY*

Pappano & Wier: *CARDIOVASCULAR PHYSIOLOGY*

White, Harrison, & Mehlmann: *ENDOCRINE AND REPRODUCTIVE PHYSIOLOGY*

Hudnall: *HEMATOLOGY: A PATHOPHYSIOLOGIC APPROACH*

RESPIRATORY PHYSIOLOGY

2ND EDITION

Michelle M. Cloutier, MD

Professor Emerita Pediatrics and Medicine
UCONN Health
Farmington, Connecticut

ELSEVIER

ELSEVIER

1600 John F. Kennedy Blvd.
Ste 1800
Philadelphia, PA 19103-2899

RESPIRATORY PHYSIOLOGY, SECOND EDITION

ISBN: 978-0-323-59578-0

Library of Congress Control Number: 2018943593

Content Strategist: Marybeth Thiel
Content Development Specialist: Marybeth Thiel
Publishing Services Manager: Shereen Jameel
Senior Project Manager: Kamatchi Madhavan
Design Direction: Ryan Cook

Printed in the United States of America

Last digit is the print number: 9 8 7 6 5 4 3 2 1

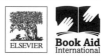

To my husband, John B. Morris,
who grounds, supports, and challenges me
and to my three stepchildren who are amazing.
Thank you all.

PREFACE

I wrote this book to help teach medical students and other students of medicine. I have been gratified by the many positive responses from students about how they have used this book to learn respiratory physiology, and also by how many pulmonary fellows and new pulmonologists have used this book to prepare for certification and recertification—in particular, in pulmonary medicine. In this revised edition, I have included many more clinical vignettes to help students fill the gaps between respiratory physiology and its application to respiratory disease. The vignettes were chosen to demonstrate how respiratory physiology is used in medicine to guide diagnosis and treatment.

I hope students will find this book especially useful in understanding difficult concepts. I encourage your feedback and comments.

Michelle M. Cloutier

CONTENTS

Overview of the Respiratory System: Function and Structure

OBJECTIVES

1. Introduce the major functions of respiration.
2. Describe the components of the upper and lower airways.
3. Outline and briefly describe the components of the respiratory system including:
   - The conducting airways
   - The alveolar–capillary unit
   - The alveolar surface
   - The pulmonary circulation
   - The cells of the airway
   - The muscles of respiration
   - The central nervous system and neural pathways regulating respiration
4. Relate lung structure to lung function.

The principal function of the respiratory system is to bring oxygen from the external environment to the tissues in the body and to remove from the body the carbon dioxide produced by cell metabolism. In addition, respiration functions in acid–base balance (see Chapter 9), in host defense, in metabolism, and in the handling of bioactive materials (see Chapter 11).

The **respiratory system** is composed of the lungs; the upper and lower airways, including the nose; the chest wall, including the muscles of respiration (diaphragm, intercostal muscles, and abdominal muscles) and the rib cage; the pulmonary circulation; and those parts of the central nervous system that regulate respiration (Fig. 1.1).

BASIC STRUCTURE OF THE RESPIRATORY SYSTEM

The airways are divided into upper and lower airways. The **upper airway** consists of all structures from the nose to the vocal cords, whereas the **lower airway** consists of the trachea and the bronchial structures to the alveolus.

Air flows to the lower airways through either the mouth or the nose. Nasal breathing is the preferred route for two reasons: first, the nose filters particulate matter and plays a major role in lung defense (see Chapter 11); second, the nose humidifies inspired air as a result of the large surface area created by the nasal septum and the nasal turbinates. The nose also offers a higher resistance to airflow than the mouth, however, and this resistance is increased in the

presence of nasal congestion, large adenoids, or nasal polyps. Increasing airflow as occurs during exercise results in increasing resistance in the nose, with a switch from nasal to mouth breathing during exercise around inspiratory flow rates of 35 L/min.

The tracheobronchial tree is an arrangement of branching tubes that begins at the larynx and ends in the alveoli. The trachea begins at the larynx and in the tracheobronchial tree nomenclature has been designated Generation 0. The trachea divides at the carina, or "keel" (so named because it looks like the keel of a boat), into the right and left main-stem bronchi (Generation 1) that penetrate the lung **parenchyma** (tissue of the lung). The right main-stem bronchus is larger than the left, and the angle of the take-off is less acute. This has implications for aspiration of foreign bodies, which most often enter the right rather than the left main-stem bronchus. Main-stem bronchi branch into lobar bronchi (three on the right and two on the left) (Generation 2) that in turn branch into segmental bronchi (Generation 3) and an extensive system of subsegmental and smaller bronchi. As a rough rule, in the first six airway generations, the number of airways in each generation is double that in the previous generation and the number of airways in each generation is equal to the number 2 raised to the generation number. Airway branching beyond the sixth generation is asymmetric in branching angle, size, number of branches, and number of subsequent generations. As a result, although in general there are between 15 and 20 generations of airways from the trachea to the level of the

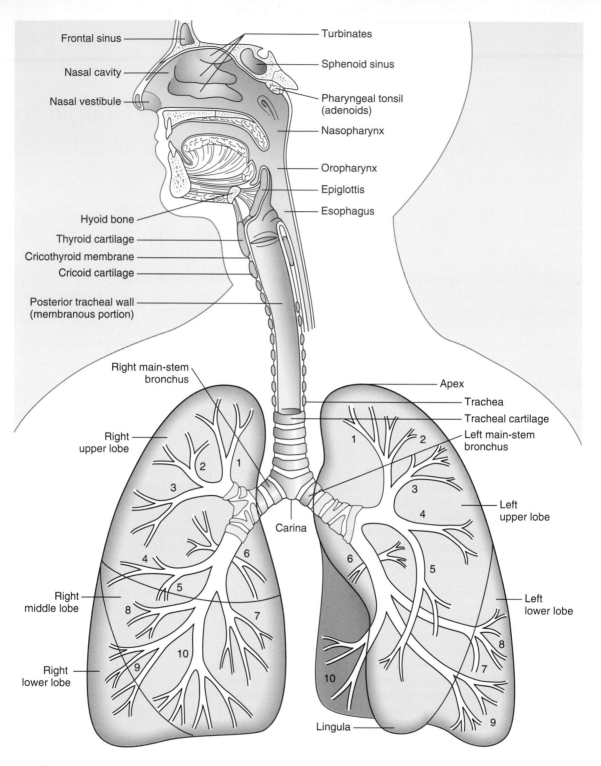

Fig. 1.1 Schematic diagram of the respiratory system including the bronchopulmonary segments; anterior view. Numbers refer to bronchopulmonary segments: 1, apical; 2, posterior; 3, anterior; 4, lateral (superior on the left); 5, medial (inferior on the left); 6, superior; 7, medial basal; 8, anterior basal; 9, lateral basal; 10, posterior basal (see Fig. 1.13).

	Generation			Diameter, cm	Length, cm	Number	Total cross sectional area, cm²
Conducting zone	Trachea		0	1.80	12.0	1	2.54
	Bronchi		1	1.22	4.8	2	2.33
			2	0.83	1.9	4	2.13
			3	0.56	0.8	8	2.00
	Bronchioles		4	0.45	1.3	16	2.48
			5	0.35	1.07	32	3.11
	Terminal bronchioles		16	0.06	0.17	6×10^4	180.0
Transitional and respiratory zones	Respiratory bronchioles		17				
			18				
			19	0.05	0.10	5×10^5	10^3
	Alveolar ducts	T_3	20				
		T_2	21				
		T_1	22				
	Alveolar sacs	T	23	0.04	0.05	8×10^6	10^4

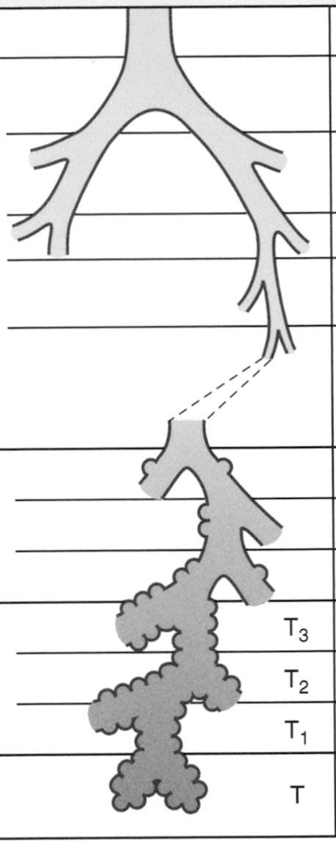

Fig. 1.2 Airway generations and approximate dimensions in the human lung. In the adult, alveoli can be found as early as the 10th airway generation and as late as the 23rd generation. (Redrawn from Weibel ER. *Morphometry of the Human Lung*. Berlin: Springer Verlag; 1963. Data from Bouhuys A. *The Physiology of Breathing*. New York: Grune & Stratton; 1977.)

terminal bronchioles, there can be as few as 10 or as many as 20 generations (Fig. 1.2). With each airway generation, the airways become smaller and more numerous (Fig. 1.3) as they penetrate deeper into the lung parenchyma.

Both the right and the left lung are encased by two membranes—the **visceral pleura** and the **parietal pleura**. The visceral pleural membrane completely envelops the lung except at the hilum where the bronchus, pulmonary vessels, and nerves enter the lung parenchyma. The parietal pleural membrane lines the inner surface of the chest wall, mediastinum, and diaphragm and becomes continuous with the visceral pleura at the hilum. Under normal conditions, the space between the two pleuras contains a small amount of clear, serous fluid that is produced by filtration from the parietal pleural capillaries and is resorbed by the visceral pleural capillaries. This fluid facilitates the smooth gliding of the lung as it expands in the chest and creates a potential space that can be involved in disease. Air can

enter this potential space between the visceral and parietal pleuras because of trauma, rupture of a weakened area at the surface of the lung, or surgery producing a **pneumothorax**. Fluid can also enter this space, creating a **pleural effusion**. Because the pleuras of the right and left lung are separate, a pneumothorax involves only the right or the left hemithorax.

Structurally, the trachea is supported by C-shaped (sometimes referred to as U-shaped) cartilage anteriorly and laterally that prevents tracheal collapse and by smooth muscle posteriorly, which can invaginate and markedly decrease the cross-sectional area of the trachea. Like the trachea, cartilage in large bronchi is also semicircular, but as the bronchi enter the lung parenchyma, the cartilage rings disappear and are replaced by plates of cartilage. As the airways further divide, these plates of cartilage decrease in size and eventually disappear around the 11th airway generation. Airways beyond the 11th generation are imbedded in

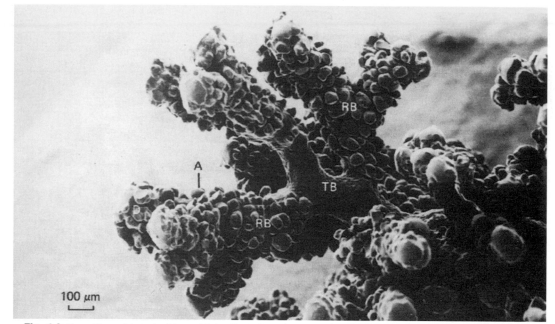

Fig. 1.3 Transition of terminal bronchiole. Scanning electron micrograph of airway branches peripheral to terminal bronchiole in a silicon-rubber cast of cat lung. Note multiple, smaller branches from respiratory to terminal bronchioles. A, alveolus; RB, respiratory bronchiole; TB, terminal bronchiole. Note absence of alveoli in terminal bronchiole (From Berne RM, Levy ML, Koeppen BM, Stanton BA (eds.). *Physiology*, 7th ed. St. Louis: Mosby; 2018.)

TABLE 1.1   Anatomic Features of Bronchi and Bronchioles

	Cartilage Present	Size	Epithelium	Blood Supply	Alveoli	Volume
Bronchi	Yes	>1 mm	Pseudostratified columnar	Bronchial	No	~675 mL
Terminal bronchioles	No	<1 mm	Cuboidal	Bronchial	No	>150 mL
Respiratory bronchioles	No	<1 mm	Cuboidal/alveolar	Pulmonary	Yes	2500 mL

the lung parenchyma, and the caliber of their lumen is regulated by the elastic recoil of the lung and lung volume. In addition, the number of bronchioles increases beyond the 11th generation more rapidly than the diameter decreases. As a result the cross-sectional area increases rapidly at this point and is 30 times the cross-sectional area of the mainstem bronchi. This results in a marked decrease in airway resistance to approximately one-tenth of the resistance of the entire respiratory system (see Chapter 3).

The airways can thus be divided into two types: cartilaginous airways, or bronchi; and noncartilaginous airways, or bronchioles (Table 1.1). Bronchi contain cartilage and are the conductors of air between the external environment

and the distal sites of gas exchange. They do not participate in gas exchange. Bronchioles do not contain cartilage and are subdivided into terminal bronchioles, which do not participate in gas exchange; and respiratory bronchioles, which contain alveoli and alveolar ducts and function as sites of gas exchange.

The airways from the nose to and including the terminal bronchioles are known as the **conducting airways** because they bring (conduct) gas to the gas-exchanging units but do not actually participate in gas exchange. The conducting airways (primarily the nose) also function to warm and humidify inspired air. Because the conducting airways contain no alveoli and therefore take no part in gas

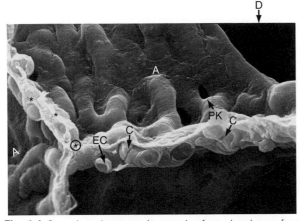

Fig. 1.4 Scanning electron micrograph of an alveolar surface demonstrating the alveolar septum. Capillaries (C) are seen in cross section in the foreground with erythrocytes (EC) in their lumen. At the circled asterisk, three septae come together. The septae are held together by connective tissue fibers (uncircled asterisks). A, alveolus; D, alveolar duct; PK, pores of Kohn. (Micrograph courtesy of Weibel ER, Institute of Anatomy, University of Berne, Switzerland.)

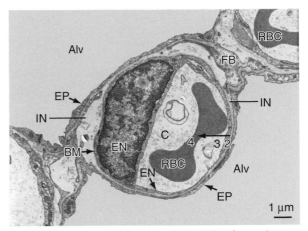

Fig. 1.5 Transmission electron micrograph of a pulmonary capillary in cross section. Alveoli (Alv) are on either side of the capillary that is shown with a red blood cell (RBC). The diffusion pathway for oxygen and carbon dioxide (arrow) consists of the areas numbered 2, 3, and 4, which are the alveolar–capillary barrier, plasma, and erythrocyte, respectively. BM, basement membrane; C, capillary; EN, capillary endothelial cell (note its large nucleus); EP, alveolar epithelial cell; FB, fibroblast process; IN, interstitial space. (Reproduced with permission from Weibel ER. Morphometric estimation of pulmonary diffusion capacity, I. Model & method. *Respir Physiol.* 1970;11:54–75.)

exchange, they constitute the **anatomic dead space** (see Chapter 5). In normal individuals, the first 16 generations of airway branchings, with a volume of 150 mL, constitute the anatomic dead space, whereas the next 7 generations contain an increasing number of alveoli and constitute the gas exchange unit.

Alveolar–Capillary Unit

The terminal bronchioles divide into respiratory bronchioles, which contain alveolar ducts and alveoli and constitute the last three to five generations of the respiratory system. Gas exchange occurs in the alveoli through a dense meshlike network of capillaries and alveoli called the **alveolar–capillary network** (Fig. 1.4). The alveolar–capillary unit consists of the respiratory bronchioles, the alveolar ducts, the alveoli, and the pulmonary capillary bed. It is the basic **physiologic unit of the lung** and is characterized by a large surface area and a blood supply that originates from the pulmonary arteries. In the adult, there are approximately 300 million alveoli, which are 250 μm in size and are entirely surrounded by capillaries. In addition, there are 280 billion capillaries in the lung or almost 1000 capillaries for each alveolus. The result is a large surface area for gas exchange—approximately 50 to 100 m², which occurs in a space that is only 5 mm in length. It is one of the most remarkable engineering feats in the body. The portion of the lung supplied by respiratory bronchioles is called an **acinus**. Each acinus contains in excess of 10,000 alveoli; gas movement in the acinus is by diffusion rather than tidal ventilation.

The barrier between the gas in the alveoli and the red blood cells is only 1 to 2 μm in thickness and consists of type I alveolar epithelial cells, capillary endothelial cells, and their respective basement membranes (Fig. 1.5). O_2 diffuses across this barrier into plasma and red blood cells, whereas the reverse occurs for CO_2 (see Chapter 8). Red blood cells pass through the pulmonary network in less than 1 second, which is sufficient time for CO_2 and O_2 gas exchange to occur.

In some regions of the alveolar wall there is nothing between the airway epithelial cells and the capillary endothelial cells other than their fused basement membranes. In other regions there is a space between the epithelial and endothelial cells called the **interstitial space** or **interstitium** (see Fig. 1.5). The interstitium is composed of collagen, elastin, proteoglycans, a variety of macromolecules involved with cell–cell and cell–matrix interactions, some nerve endings, and some fibroblast-like cells. The alveolar septum creates a fiber scaffold through which pulmonary capillaries are threaded and is supported by the basement membrane. There are also small numbers of lymphocytes that have migrated out of the circulation in the interstitium and capillary endothelial cells. The basement membrane is capable of withstanding high transmural pressures and sometimes is the only remaining separation between blood and gas.

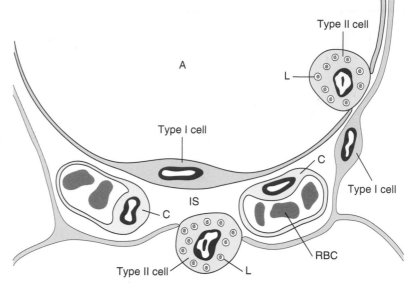

Fig. 1.6 Structure of the normal alveolus. The type I cell, with its long thin cytoplasmic processes, lines most of the alveolar surface, whereas the cuboidal type II cell, which is more numerous, occupies only about 7% of the alveolar surface. Capillaries (C) with red blood cells (RBC) are also shown. A, alveolar surface; IS, interstitial space; L, lamellar body, source of surfactant. (Modified from Weinberger S, Cockrill, BA, Mandel J. *Principles of Pulmonary Medicine*, 5th ed. Philadelphia: W.B. Saunders; 2008.)

Alveolar Surface

The alveolar epithelium is a continuous layer of tissue composed primarily of **type I cells** or squamous pneumocytes. These cells have broad, thin extensions that cover approximately 93% of the alveolar surface (Fig. 1.6). They are highly differentiated cells that do not divide, which makes them particularly susceptible to injury from inhaled or aspirated toxins and from high concentrations of oxygen (see Chapter 11). They are joined into a continuous sheet by tight junctions that prevent large molecules such as albumin from entering the alveoli, resulting in pulmonary edema. The thin cytoplasm of the type I cell is ideal for optimal gas diffusion.

Type II cells, or granular pneumocytes, are more numerous than type I cells; however, because of their cuboidal shape, they occupy only approximately 7% of the alveolar surface and are located in the corners of the alveolus (see Fig. 1.6). The hallmarks of the type II cell are their microvilli and their osmiophilic lamellar inclusion bodies that contain **surfactant**, a compound with a high lipid content that acts as a detergent to reduce the surface tension of the alveoli (Fig. 1.7; also see Chapter 2). The type II cell is the progenitor cell of the alveolar epithelium. When there is injury to the type I cell, the type II cell multiplies and eventually differentiates into a type I cell. In a group of diseases that result in pulmonary fibrosis, the type I cell is injured and the alveolar epithelium is now lined entirely by type II cells, a condition that is not conducive to optimal

gas exchange. This repair system is an example of **phylogeny recapitulating ontogeny**, because the epithelium of the alveolus is composed entirely of type II cells until late in gestation.

The lumen of the alveolus is covered by a thin layer of fluid composed of a water phase immediately adjacent to the alveolar epithelial cell and covered by surfactant. Within the alveolar epithelium there are also a small number of **macrophages**, a type of phagocytic cell that patrols the alveolar surface and ingests (phagocytizes) bacteria and inhaled particles (see Chapter 11).

Pulmonary Circulation

The lung has two separate blood supplies (see Chapter 6). The **pulmonary circulation** brings deoxygenated blood from the right ventricle to the gas-exchanging units (alveoli). **Pulmonary perfusion** ($\dot{Q}$) refers to pulmonary blood flow, which equals the heart rate multiplied by the right ventricular stroke volume. The lungs receive the entire right ventricular cardiac output and are the only organ in the body that functions in this manner. The **bronchial (or lesser) circulation** arises from the aorta and provides nourishment to the lung parenchyma. The dual circulation to the lung is another of the unique features of the lung.

The pulmonary capillary bed is the largest vascular bed in the body, with a surface area of 70 to 80 m². It is best

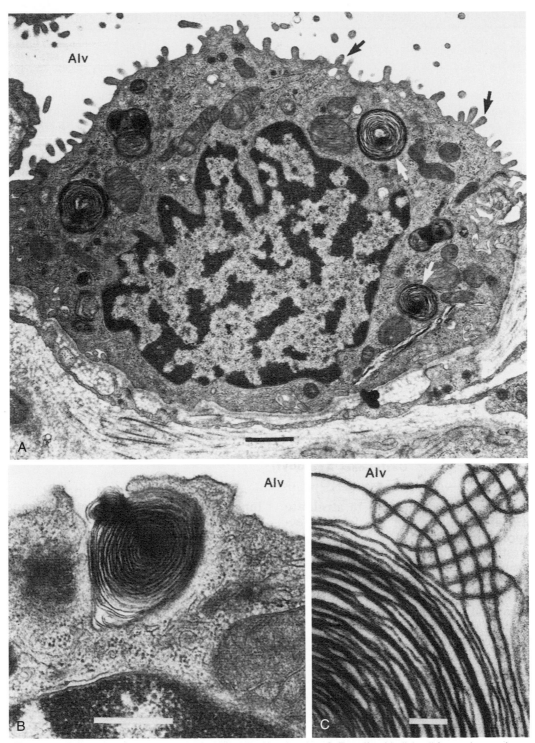

Fig. 1.7 Surfactant release by type II epithelial cells. Alv, alveolus. **A,** Type II epithelial cell from a human lung showing characteristic lamellar inclusion bodies (white arrows) within the cell and microvilli (black arrows) projecting into the alveolus. Bar = 0.5 μm. **B,** Early exocytosis of lamellar body into the alveolar space in a human lung. Bar = 0.5 μm. **C,** Secreted lamellar body and newly formed tubular myelin in alveolar liquid in a fetal rat lung. Membrane continuities between outer lamellae and adjacent tubular myelin provide evidence of intraalveolar tubular myelin formation. Bar = 0.1 μm. (Courtesy Dr. Mary C. Williams.)

viewed as a sheet of blood interrupted by small vertical supporting posts (Fig. 1.8). When the capillaries are filled with blood, about 75% of the surface area of the alveoli overlies the red blood cells. The capillaries allow red blood cells to flow through in single file only; this greatly facilitates gas exchange between the alveoli and the red blood cells. Once gas exchange is complete, the oxygenated blood returns to the left side of the heart through pulmonary venules and veins and is ready for pumping to the systemic circulation. In contrast to the systemic circulation, the pulmonary circulation is a highly distensible, low-pressure system capable of accommodating large volumes of blood at low pressure. This is another unique feature of the lung.

Pulmonary arteries that contain deoxygenated blood follow the bronchi in connective tissue sheaths, whereas pulmonary veins cross segments on their way to the left atrium (Fig. 1.9). Bronchial arteries also follow the bronchi and divide with them. In contrast, one-third of the blood

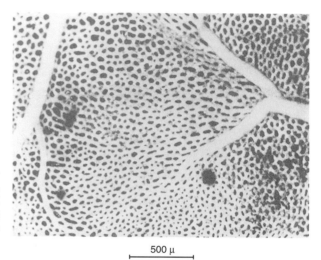

500 μ

Fig. 1.8 Pulmonary capillary surface of the lung. View of alveolar wall (in a frog) demonstrating the dense network of capillaries. A small artery (left) and vein (right) can also be seen. The individual capillary segments are so short that the blood forms an almost continuous sheet. (From Maloney JE, Castle BL. Pressure-diameter relations of capillaries and small blood vessels in frog lung. *Respir Physiol.* 1969;7:150–162.)

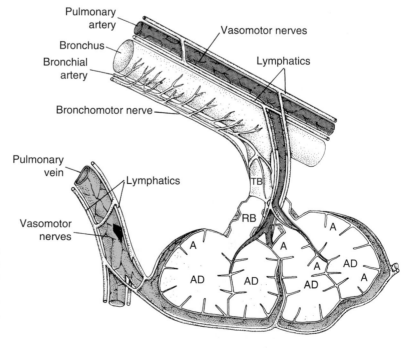

Fig. 1.9 The anatomic relation between the pulmonary artery, the bronchial artery, the airways, and the lymphatics. A, alveoli; AD, alveolar ducts; RB, respiratory bronchioles; TB, terminal bronchioles. (From Berne RM, Levy ML, Koeppen BM, Stanton BA (eds.). *Physiology*, 7th ed. St. Louis: Mosby; 2018.)

from the bronchial veins (deoxygenated blood) drains into the right atrium, and the remainder drains into pulmonary veins that drain into the left atrium. Thus a small amount of deoxygenated blood that has nourished the lung parenchyma mixes with oxygenated blood in the left atrium. Pulmonary capillaries, on the other hand, are not confined to a single alveolus but pass from one to another as well as to adjacent alveolar septae before emptying into a venule. This improves the efficiency of gas exchange and minimizes the effect of alveolar disease on gas exchange.

Cells of the Airways

The respiratory tract (with the exception of the pharynx, the anterior one-third of the nose, and the area distal to the terminal bronchioles) is lined by a pseudostratified, ciliated, columnar epithelium interspersed with mucus-secreting goblet cells and other secretory cells (Fig. 1.10; also see Chapter 11). In the distal airways, the columnar epithelium gives way to a more cuboidal epithelium. The airway epithelial cells are responsible for maintaining a thin, aqueous layer of fluid adjacent to the cells (periciliary fluid) in which the cilia can function. The depth of this periciliary fluid is maintained by the movement of ions across the epithelium.

Interspersed among the epithelial cells are **surface secretory cells**, which are also known as goblet cells. In general, there is one goblet cell per five to six ciliated cells. Goblet cells decrease in number between the 5th and 12th lung generation and in normal individuals disappear beyond the 12th tracheobronchial generation. Both goblet cell number and secretions increase in many diseases including asthma and cystic fibrosis. Secretions also increase by rapid exocytosis in response to chemical irritation, inflammatory cytokines, and neuronal stimulation. In the bronchioles, goblet cells are replaced by **Clara cells**, another type of secretory cell.

Basal cells are located underneath the columnar epithelium and are responsible for the pseudostratified appearance of the epithelial surface. They are absent in the bronchioles and beyond. Although their function is not clear, they appear to be the stem cells for the airway epithelium and the goblet cells.

Submucosal tracheobronchial glands are present wherever there is cartilage in the tracheobronchial tree. These glands empty to the surface epithelium through a ciliated duct and are lined by mucous and serous cells. Submucosal tracheobronchial glands increase in number and size in **chronic bronchitis**, a chronic lung disease primarily occurring in smokers, and extend down to the bronchioles in disease.

The ciliated epithelium, goblet cell, Clara cell, and tracheobronchial glands are important in host defense and are discussed in Chapter 11.

The Muscles of Respiration

The chest wall encases the lung, and normally the two structures move together. The lungs do not self-inflate. The force for lung inflation is supplied by the muscles of respiration, which are skeletal muscles. Like all skeletal muscles, their force of contraction increases when they are stretched and decreases when they are shortened. Thus the force of contraction of the respiratory muscles increases with increasing lung volume.

Dividing the thoracic cavity from the abdominal cavity is the **diaphragm**, the major muscle of respiration (Fig. 1.11). The diaphragm is a thin, musculotendinous, dome-shaped sheet of muscle that is inserted into the lower ribs and separates the thoracic from the abdominal cavity. It is supplied by the phrenic nerve that arises from the second cervical vertebra. When it contracts, the abdominal contents are forced downward and forward and the vertical dimension of the chest cavity is increased. In addition, the rib margins are lifted and moved out, causing an increase in the transverse diameter of the thorax. In adults, the diaphragm is capable of generating airway pressures of 150 to 200 cm H_2O during a maximal inspiratory effort. During quiet breathing (known as **tidal volume breathing**), the diaphragm moves approximately 1 cm, but during large-volume breathing, the diaphragm can move as much as 10 cm. If the diaphragm is paralyzed, it moves higher up in the thoracic cavity during inspiration because of the fall in intrathoracic pressure. This **paradoxical movement of the diaphragm** can be demonstrated using the radiographic technique called **fluoroscopy**.

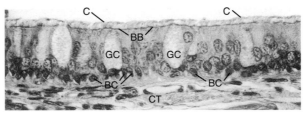

Fig. 1.10 Scanning electron micrograph of airway, showing the ciliated, pseudostratified, columnar epithelium of a bronchus. Each cilium is connected to a basal body (BB), which collectively appears at the base of the cilia (C) as a dark band. Goblet cells (GC) and basal cells (BC), the potential precursors of the ciliated cells, are shown. CT, connective tissue. (From Berne RM, Levy ML, Koeppen BM, Stanton BA (eds). *Physiology*, 5th ed. St. Louis: Mosby; 2004.)

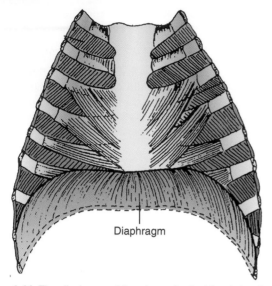

Fig. 1.11 The diaphragm. View from the inside of the thorax illustrates the position of the diaphragm in the thorax. (From Grippi MS, Elias JA, Fishman JA, et al. *Fishman's Pulmonary Diseases and Disorders*, 5th ed. New York: McGraw-Hill; 2015.)

The other significant muscles of inspiration are the external intercostal muscles that pull the ribs upward and forward during inspiration, causing an increase in both the side-to-side and front-to-back diameters of the thorax (Fig. 1.12). Innervation of these muscles originates from intercostal nerves that originate from the spinal cord at the same level. Paralysis of these muscles has no significant effect on respiration because of the dominance of the diaphragm as the major muscle of respiration. Accessory muscles of inspiration (scalene muscles, which elevate the sternocleidomastoid; the alae nasi, which cause nasal flaring; and small muscles in the neck and head) are quiet during quiet breathing but contract vigorously during exercise and with significant airway obstruction.

The upper airway must remain patent during inspiration; therefore the pharyngeal wall muscles, the genioglossus, and the arytenoid muscles are also considered muscles of inspiration.

Exhalation during quiet breathing is passive but becomes active during exercise and hyperventilation. The most important muscles of exhalation are those of the abdominal wall (rectus abdominis, internal and external oblique, and transversus abdominis) and the internal intercostal muscles that oppose the activity of the external intercostal muscles (i.e., pull the ribs downward and inward).

The Central Nervous System and Neural Pathways

The central nervous system (CNS), and in particular the brainstem, functions as the main control center for respiration (see Chapter 10). Breathing is both voluntary and automatic. Each breath begins in the brain, where the signal to breathe is carried to the respiratory muscles through the spinal cord and the nerves that innervate the respiratory muscles. It is remarkable that despite widely varying demands for O_2 uptake and CO_2 removal, the arterial levels of O_2 and CO_2 are normally maintained within tight limits. Regulation of respiration requires three components (see Chapter 10):

1. Generation and maintenance of a respiratory rhythm (**respiratory control center**)
2. Modulation of the respiratory rhythm by sensory feedback loops and reflexes that allow adaptation to various situations and minimize energy costs
3. Recruitment of respiratory muscles that can contract appropriately for effective gas exchange.

Unlike the heart, which begins beating at approximately 6 weeks' gestation, rhythmic respirations do not begin until birth.

ANATOMIC AND PHYSIOLOGIC CORRELATES

Lung structure is closely correlated with lung function in health and disease. Because lung disease is described in anatomic terms (e.g., right middle lobe pneumonia), knowledge of lung anatomy is essential. The **bronchopulmonary segment** is the region of the lung supplied by a segmental bronchus. It is the **functional anatomic unit of the lung**, so named because disease usually involves one segment at a time and because surgical resection follows along segments. When using a stethoscope (auscultation), all of the bronchopulmonary segments can be examined with one exception, namely the hilar segments of the lower lobes (Fig. 1.13). The **hilum** is the area of the lung where the main-stem bronchi and pulmonary arteries and veins enter and leave the right and left lung. These segments have no topographic relationship to the chest.

The various lobes of the lung (three on the right and two on the left) are subdivided by **fissures**. The division into the lobes, however, is incomplete, which allows for collateral ventilation. **Collateral ventilation** is an accessory pathway that connects airspaces supplied by other airways. There are two types of accessory pathways in the lung: (1) **canals of Lambert**, which connect respiratory bronchioles and terminal bronchioles to airspaces supplied by other airways; and (2) **pores of Kohn**, which are openings in the alveolar walls that connect adjacent alveoli. These accessory pathways help prevent collapse of terminal respiratory units (**atelectasis**) when their supplying airway becomes obstructed and are particularly important in individuals with lung diseases such as **emphysema**.

MUSCLES OF RESPIRATION

**Muscles
of inspiration**

**Muscles
of expiration**

Accessory

Sterno-
cleidomastoid
(elevates
sternum)

Scalenes
  Anterior
  Middle
  Posterior
(elevate
and fix
upper ribs)

Principal

External
intercostals
(elevate ribs,
thus
increasing
width of
thoracic
cavity)

Interchondral
part of
internal
intercostals
(also elevates
ribs)

Diaphragm
(domes
descend,
thus
increasing
vertical
dimension
of thoracic
cavity;
also elevates
lower ribs)

**Quiet
breathing**

Expiration
results
from
passive
recoil
of lungs
and rib
cage

**Active
breathing**

Internal
intercostals,
except
interchondral
part

Abdominals
(depress
lower ribs,
compress
abdominal
contents,
thus pushing
up diaphragm)

Rectus
abdominis

External
oblique

Internal
oblique

Transversus
abdominis

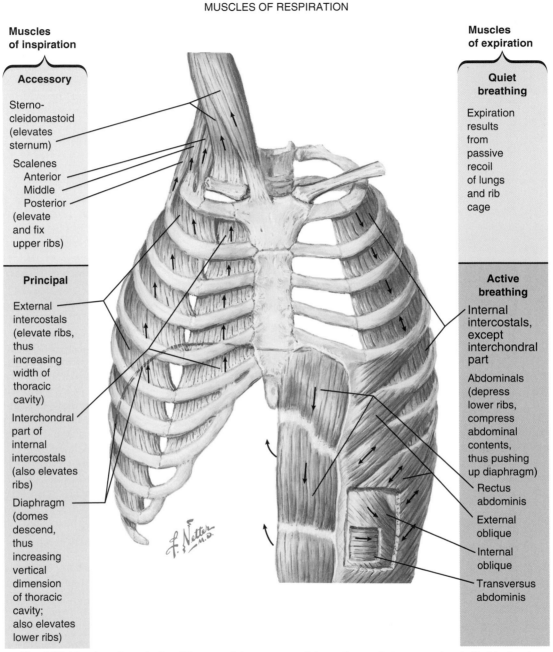

Fig. 1.12 Muscles of respiration. Diagram of the anatomy of the major respiratory muscles. Left side, inspiratory muscles; right side, expiratory muscles. (Kaminsky D. *The Netter Collection of Medical Illustrations: Respiratory System*, vol. 3, 2nd ed. Philadelphia: Elsevier; 2011.)

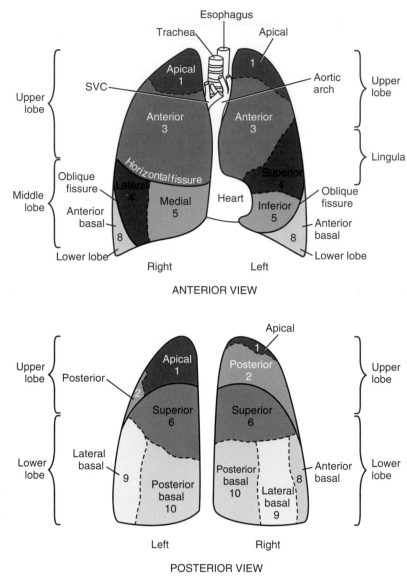

Fig. 1.13 Topography of the lung demonstrating the lobes, segments, and fissures. Numbers refer to specific bronchopulmonary segments that are also shown in Fig. 1.1. SVC, superior vena cava. (From Berne RM, Levy ML, Koeppen BM, Stanton BA (eds.). *Physiology*, 7th ed. St. Louis: Mosby; 2018.)

Physiologically, the lung demonstrates functional unity; that is, every alveolar unit has the same structure and the same function as every other alveolar unit. This is in contrast to the heart, in which the various chambers have both a different structure and a different function. The significance of functional unity is that a large portion of the lung can be removed without significantly compromising overall lung function (i.e., gas exchange).

CLINICAL BOX

Understanding lung topography is useful in both diagnosing and localizing disease. For example, a 2-year-old boy presents with a 2-day history of fever, cough, and recent onset of tachypnea (an increased respiratory rate). On examination, there are intercostal muscle retractions and nasal flaring, and the child appears ill. On auscultation, breath sounds are decreased over the right upper lobe anteriorly.

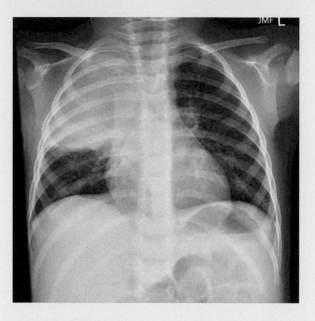

A chest x-ray reveals opacification (known as consolidation) over the right upper lobe anteriorly consistent with lobar (specifically right upper lobe) pneumonia.

SUMMARY

1. The principal function of the respiratory system is gas exchange. Other functions include acid–base balance, host defense and metabolism, and the handling of bioactive materials.
2. Gas exchange occurs in the alveolar–capillary unit, the basic physiologic unit of the lung.
3. The bronchopulmonary segment is the segment of the lung supplied by a segmental bronchus. It is the functional anatomic unit of the lung.
4. The alveolar surface is lined by type I and type II cells. The thin cytoplasm of the type I cell is ideal for optimal gas diffusion, whereas the type II cell is important for the production of surfactant, which decreases the surface tension of the alveolus.
5. The lung has two separate circulations. The pulmonary circulation brings deoxygenated blood from the right ventricle to the gas-exchanging units. The bronchial circulation arises from the aorta and nourishes the lung parenchyma.
6. The circulation to the lung is unique in its dual circulation and in its ability to accommodate large volumes of blood at low pressure.
7. The anatomic dead space is composed of all of the airways that do not participate in gas exchange—that is, the airways to the level of the respiratory bronchioles.
8. The cells of the conducting airways include the pseudostratified, ciliated, columnar epithelial cells, surface secretory cells, Clara cells, and submucosal tracheobronchial gland cells.
9. The diaphragm is the major muscle of respiration.
10. Breathing is both voluntary and automatic.
11. The lung demonstrates both anatomic and physiologic unity—that is, each unit is structurally identical and functions just like every other unit.

KEY WORDS AND CONCEPTS

Alveolar macrophage
Alveolar–capillary unit
Alveolus
Anatomic dead space
Atelectasis
Bronchial circulation
Bronchiole
Bronchopulmonary segment
Bronchus
Canals of Lambert
Chemoreceptor
Clara cell
Collateral ventilation
Diaphragm
Emphysema
Fissure
Functional unity
Glottis
Hilum

Interstitium/interstitial space
Lower airway
Parenchyma
Parietal pleura
Partial pressure
Periciliary fluid
Pleural effusion
Pneumothorax
Pores of Kohn
Respiratory control center
Surface secretory cells (goblet cells)
Surfactant
Tracheobronchial glands
Turbinates
Type I cell
Type II cell
Upper airway
Visceral pleura

SELF-STUDY PROBLEMS

1. What anatomic features of the alveolar–capillary unit make it appropriate to function as the gas-exchanging unit?
2. How can you distinguish type I cells from type II cells?
3. If the pulmonary artery that supplies the left lung was occluded for a short period of time and the cardiac output remained unchanged (that is, all of the blood from the right ventricle now goes to the right lung), what would be the effect on the pressure inside the right pulmonary artery?
4. What are the components of the blood–gas barrier?
5. What are the anatomic features that make the lung ideally suited for its principal function?

ADDITIONAL READINGS

Baile EM. The anatomy and physiology of the bronchial circulation. *J Aerosol Med.* 1996;9:1–6.

Boggs DS, Kinasewitz GT. Review: pathophysiology of the pleural space. *Am J Med.* 1995;309:53–59.

Broaddus VC, Mason RJ, JD Ernst, et al., eds. *Murray & Nadel's Textbook of Respiratory Medicine.* 6th ed. Philadelphia: WB Saunders; 2016.

Fehrenbach H. Alveolar epithelial type II cell: defender of the alveolus revisited. *Respir Res.* 2001;2:33–46.

Gandevia SC, Allen GM, Butler J, et al. Human respiratory muscles: sensations, reflexes and fatigability. *Clin Exp Pharm Physiol.* 1998;25:757–763.

Grippi MA, Elias JA, Fishman JA, et al. *Fishman's Pulmonary Diseases and Disorders.* 5th ed. New York: McGraw Hill; 2015.

Hlastala MP, Berger AJ. *Physiology of Respiration.* 2nd ed. New York: Oxford University Press; 2001.

Horsfield K, Cumming G. Morphology of the bronchial tree in man. *J Appl Physiol.* 1968;24:373–383.

Leff AR. Schumacker PT. *Respiratory Physiology: Basics and Applications.* Philadelphia: WB Saunders; 1993.

Lumb AB. *Nunn's Applied Respiratory Physiology.* 8th ed. Philadelphia: Elsevier; 2017.

Massaro D, Massaro GD. Invited review: pulmonary alveoli: Formation, the "call for oxygen," and other regulators. *Am J Physiol Lung Cell Mol Physiol.* 2002;282:L345–L358.

Nettesheim P, Koo JS, Gray T. Regulation of differentiation of the tracheobronchial epithelium. *J Aerosol Med.* 2000;13:207–218.

Poole DC, Sexton WL, Farkas GA. Diaphragm structure and function in health and disease. *Med Sci Sports Exerc.* 1997;29:738–754.

Rogers DE. Airway goblet cells: Responsive and adaptable front-line defenders. *Eur Respir J.* 1994;7:1690–1706.

Weibel ER. *The Pathway for Oxygen: Structure and Function of the Mammalian Respiratory System.* Cambridge, MA: Harvard University Press; 1984.

Mechanical Properties of the Lung and Chest Wall

OBJECTIVES

1. Describe static lung mechanics and the measurement of lung volumes.
2. Define lung compliance and its measurement.
3. Relate lung and chest wall compliance to lung volumes.
4. Characterize lung and chest wall interactions in terms of pressure gradients and pressure volume relationships.
5. Describe surfactant and its role in altering surface tension.

STATIC LUNG MECHANICS

Air movement in and out of the lung is controlled by the mechanical properties of the lung and chest wall. Static lung mechanics is the study of the mechanical properties of the lung and chest wall whose volume is not changing with time and is discussed in this chapter. Dynamic lung mechanics, which is the study of the lung and chest wall in motion (i.e., changing volume), is discussed in Chapter 3.

The mechanics of the **lung** are composed of the combined mechanical properties of the airways, lung parenchyma, interstitial matrix (composed of fibrin, collagen, and a few cells), alveolar surface, and pulmonary circulation. The mechanical properties of the **chest wall** include the properties of all of the structures outside of the lungs that move during breathing, including the rib cage, diaphragm, abdominal cavity, and anterior abdominal muscles. The interaction between the lung and the chest wall determines lung volumes, and static lung volumes play a major role in gas exchange and in the work of breathing. They can be measured and are abnormal in many lung diseases.

LUNG VOLUMES

The static volumes of the lungs are shown in Fig. 2.1. All lung volumes are subdivisions of the total lung capacity (TLC) and are measured in liters. They are reported either as volumes (e.g., residual volume) or capacities (e.g., vital capacity). A capacity is composed of two or more volumes.

The total volume of air that is contained in the lung is called the TLC. It is composed of the volume of air that an individual can exhale from a maximum inspiration to a maximum exhalation, known as the vital capacity (VC), and the volume of air that is left in the lung after a maximal exhalation, known as the residual volume (RV). Two other important lung volumes are the tidal volume (TV, or V_T) and the functional residual capacity (FRC). The TV is the volume of air that is breathed into and out of the lung during quiet breathing. The FRC is the volume of air contained in the lung after a normal exhalation. The FRC is composed of the residual volume and the volume of air that can be exhaled from the end of a normal exhalation to residual volume. This latter volume is called the expiratory reserve volume (ERV). The FRC represents the resting volume of the respiratory system, in which the forces of the chest wall to increase in size and the forces of the lung to decrease in size are equal but opposite (see later in this chapter).

To get a sense of the importance of lung volumes in respiration, breathe quietly close to TLC (take a deep breath in, and breathe at this high lung volume for a few minutes). Now breathe out until you cannot force any more air out, and try breathing at this volume, which is close to your RV. Both of these maneuvers should be uncomfortable and associated with increased work; both increases and decreases in lung volume occur in lung disease as a result of a change in lung mechanics. The measurement of lung volumes is used to detect and follow the progression of lung disease and is discussed in Chapter 4.

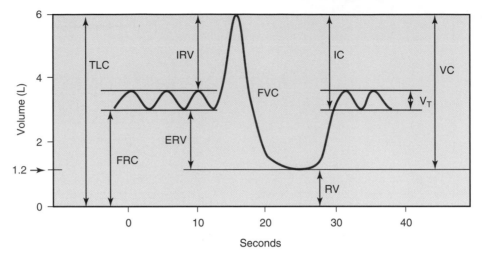

Fig. 2.1 The various lung volumes and capacities. ERV, expiratory reserve volume; FRC, functional residual capacity; FVC, forced vital capacity; IC, inspiratory capacity; IRV, inspiratory reserve volume; RV, residual volume; TLC, total lung capacity; VC, vital capacity; V_T, tidal volume. (From Koeppen BM, Stanton BA, eds. *Berne and Levy's Physiology*, 7th ed. Philadelphia: Elsevier; 2018.)

USING AND INTERPRETING RESULTS OF LUNG VOLUME MEASUREMENTS

Two major types of pathophysiologic abnormalities involving the lung and chest wall can be described using lung volumes. One group of diseases is called **obstructive pulmonary disease (OPD)**. In OPD, during exhalation the airways close (premature airway closure, the hallmark of OPD) trapping air behind them (see Chapter 3). This results in an increase in TLC, RV, and FRC. In contrast, in **restrictive pulmonary disease**, the other major pathophysiologic abnormality involving the lung and chest wall, lung volumes are reduced.

One of the most useful tests for distinguishing obstructive and restrictive types of lung disease is the measurement of the RV/TLC ratio. In normal individuals, the RV/TLC ratio is less than 0.25, that is, approximately 25% of the air in the lungs is trapped and cannot be exhaled. An elevated RV/TLC ratio, characterized by an increase in RV out of proportion to any increase in TLC, is due to air trapping secondary to airway obstruction and is seen in individuals with OPD. An elevated RV/TLC ratio due to a decrease in TLC out of proportion to any change in RV is seen in individuals with restrictive types of pulmonary disease.

LUNG COMPLIANCE AND LUNG ELASTIC PROPERTIES

Lung compliance (C_L) is a measure of the elastic properties of the lung and is a reflection of lung distensibility. These distensibility properties of the lung are seen in the pressure volume relaxation curve for the lung that is called the **compliance curve of the lung**. **Compliance** of the lungs is defined as the change in lung volume resulting from a change in the distending pressure of the lung equal to 1 cm H_2O. The units of compliance are mL (or L)/cm H_2O. A lung with high lung compliance refers to a lung that is easily distended. A lung with low compliance or a "stiff" lung is the one that is not easily distended. Thus the compliance of the lung (C_L) is:

$$C_L = \Delta V/\Delta P$$

where ΔV is the change in volume and ΔP is the change in pressure.

The compliance of the isolated lung is measured in animals by removing the lung and measuring the changes in lung volume that occur with each change in the pressure between the inside of the lung and the outside (also known as **transpulmonary or translung pressure**). As transpulmonary pressure increases, lung volume increases (Fig. 2.2A). The line that is generated, however, is curvilinear, not linear. That is, at low lung volumes, the lung distends easily, but at high lung volumes, larger increases in transpulmonary pressure are needed to produce only small changes in lung volume. This is in part because at high lung volumes all of the elastic fibers in the alveolar units and airways have been maximally stretched. More important than elastic recoil in the determination of compliance is the surface tension at the air–water interface lining the alveoli due to surfactant (see later in this chapter).

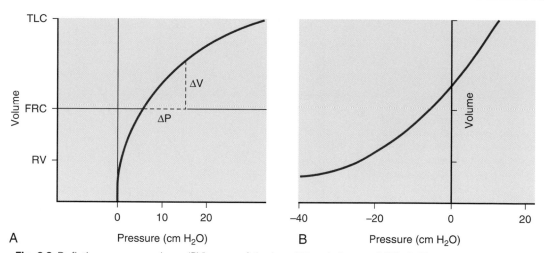

Fig. 2.2 Deflation pressure volume (PV) curve of the lung **(A)** and chest wall **(B)**. **A,** The compliance of the lung at any point along the curve is the change in volume (ΔV) per the change in pressure (ΔP). From the curve, it is apparent that the compliance of the lung changes with lung volume. By convention, the deflation pressure volume curve is used, and lung compliance is the change in pressure when going from functional residual capacity (FRC) to FRC + 1 L. RV, residual volume; TLC, total lung capacity. **B,** PV curve of the chest wall demonstrating a change in compliance with change in lung volume. Note that at volumes greater than 60% of the TLC, the pressure needed to expand the chest wall is positive (inward recoil), whereas at lower lung volumes, the chest wall pressure is negative (outward recoil).

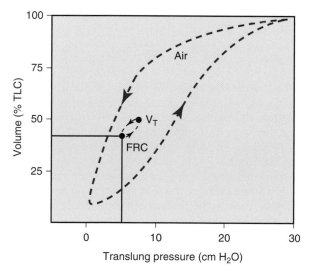

Fig. 2.3 Inflation: deflation pressure–volume curve of the lung. The direction of inspiration and exhalation is shown by the arrows. The difference between the inflation and deflation pressure-volume curves is due to surface tension variation with changes in lung volume. FRC, functional residual capacity; TLC, total lung capacity; VT, tidal volume. (From Koeppen BM, Stanton BA, eds. *Berne and Levy's Physiology*, 7th ed. Philadelphia: Elsevier; 2018.)

Lungs that are highly compliant will have a steeper slope than lungs with a low compliance. Lung compliance or distensibility is the inverse of elasticity or **lung elastic recoil** (PEL). Compliance is the ease with which something is stretched, whereas elastic recoil is the tendency to resist or oppose stretching and return to its previous configuration when the distorting force is removed.

By convention, the compliance of the lung is measured as the slope of the line between any two points on the deflation limb of the pressure volume loop. The compliance of the lung is greater when measured from TLC to RV (deflation) than from RV to TLC (inflation) (Fig. 2.3). This is due in large part to the changes in surface tension with changing lung volume and is discussed later in this chapter. This difference between the inflation and exhalation curve is called **hysteresis.** As we

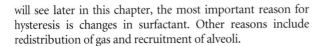

Fig. 2.4 The relaxation pressure–volume curve of the lung, chest wall, and respiratory system. The curve for the respiratory system is the sum of the individual curves ($P_{RS} = P_L + P_W$). The curve for the lung is the same as in Fig. 2.2A, and the curve for the chest wall is the same as in Fig. 2.2B. FRC, functional residual capacity; Pw, chest wall pressure; PL, transpulmonary pressure; PRS, respiratory system pressure; TLC, total lung capacity. (Koeppen BM, Stanton BA, eds. *Berne and Levy's Physiology*, 7th ed. Philadelphia: Elsevier; 2018.)

will see later in this chapter, the most important reason for hysteresis is changes in surfactant. Other reasons include redistribution of gas and recruitment of alveoli.

COMPLIANCE OF THE CHEST WALL

When the lungs are removed, the chest wall has a springlike character with a relatively high resting volume. In much the same way as the lung, the compliance curve of the chest wall relates the volume of gas enclosed by the chest wall to the pressure across the chest wall. The curve (see Fig. 2.2B) is relatively flat at low volumes; that is, the chest wall is stiff with the shortened respiratory muscles maximally contracted. The curve is also flat at high lung volumes where the respiratory muscles are maximally stretched. At both high and low lung volumes, large changes in pressure across the chest wall result in small changes in the volume enclosed by the chest wall.

COMPLIANCE OF THE RESPIRATORY SYSTEM

Both the lungs and the chest wall contribute to the compliance of the respiratory system (Fig. 2.4). The lung and chest wall are held together by the thin layer of pleural fluid that functions like a liquid film holding two pieces of glass together. The glass pieces slide easily relative to each other, but it is difficult to pull them apart. The compliance of the respiratory system is also analogous to electrical capacitance, and in the respiratory system the compliances of the lung and chest wall are in parallel. Thus their individual compliances

add as reciprocals; that is, 1/compliance of the respiratory system = 1/compliance of the lung + 1/compliance of the chest wall or

$$1/C_{RS} = 1/C_L + 1/C_W$$

In contrast, the reciprocal of compliance is elastance, and the elastance of the lung and chest wall add directly. In addition, compliances in series add directly. For example, the compliance of the lungs in the two hemithoraces that are in series is the sum of the compliances of the lung in each hemithorax.

As noted previously, lung compliance varies with lung volume (see Fig. 2.2). It is greater at lower lung volumes than at higher lung volumes. For this reason, specific compliance, or compliance divided by the lung volume at which it is measured (usually FRC), is used (Fig. 2.5). As an example, consider the individual with chronic bronchitis in whom FRC is increased. As a result, pulmonary compliance, which is now being measured at this higher lung volume, would also be increased. However, when corrected for the FRC (specific compliance), the compliance is normal. In individuals with normal FRC, the compliance of the lung is about 0.2 L/cm H_2O, of the chest wall is 0.2 L/cm H_2O, and of the respiratory system is 0.1 L/cm H_2O. Note that the compliance of the respiratory system is lower than the compliance of either the lung or the chest wall. Lung compliance is not affected by age.

CLINICAL BOX: CLINICAL USE OF COMPLIANCE

The compliance of the lung is not altered by airflow per se, but the compliance of the lung and chest wall is affected by a number of respiratory disorders. In *emphysema*, the lung is more compliant because of destruction of lung elastic tissue; that is, for every 1 cm of H_2O pressure increase, there is a larger increase in volume than in the normal lung. In contrast, a proliferation of connective tissue in the lung called *pulmonary fibrosis* can be seen in lung diseases such as interstitial pneumonitis and sarcoidosis or in association with chemical or thermal lung injury. The lungs in these diseases are "stiff," or noncompliant; that is, for every 1 cm H_2O pressure change, there is a smaller change in volume. Similarly, in diseases associated with increased fluid in the interstitial spaces such as *pulmonary edema* or in diseases associated with fluid, blood, or infection in the intrapleural space (*pleural effusion, hemothorax,* or *empyema,* respectively), lung compliance is reduced.

The compliance of the chest wall is decreased in individuals with obesity in whom adipose tissue results in an additional load on the chest wall muscles and the diaphragm.

Individuals with decreased mobility of the rib cage such as in *kyphoscoliosis* or other types of musculoskeletal diseases that affect chest wall movement also have decreased chest wall compliance.

Individuals with decreased compliance must generate greater transpulmonary pressures to produce changes in lung volume than individuals with normal compliance. This results in increased work associated with breathing (see Chapter 3).

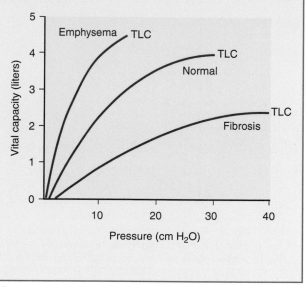

Fibrosis/emphysema pressure–volume curve. TLC, total lung capacity.
From Koeppen BM, Stanton BA, eds. *Berne and Levy's Physiology,* 7th ed. Philadelphia: Elsevier; 2018.

FACTORS DETERMINING LUNG VOLUME

Why can't we inspire above TLC or exhale beyond RV? The answers lie in the properties of the lung parenchyma and in the interaction between the lungs and the chest wall. Both the lungs and the chest wall have elastic properties. Both have a resting volume (or size) that they would assume if there were no external forces or pressures exerted on them. Both expand when stresses are applied and recoil passively when stresses are released. If the lungs were removed from the chest and no external forces were applied, they would become almost airless. To expand, these lungs would require either the exertion of a positive pressure on the alveoli and airways or the application of a negative pressure from outside the lungs. Either would result in a positive transpulmonary pressure. These situations are analogous to the balloon and the vacuum canister. A balloon is airless until positive pressure is exerted at the opening to distend the balloon walls (positive-pressure "ventilation"). In the case of the vacuum, negative external pressure is applied and results in sucking materials (air) into the canister (negative-pressure "ventilation").

The lungs are enclosed by the chest wall, which expands during inspiration. The lungs and chest wall always move together in healthy individuals. Lung volumes are determined by the balance between the lung's elastic recoil properties and the properties of the muscles of the chest wall. TLC occurs when the forces of inspiration decrease because of chest wall muscle lengthening and are insufficient to overcome the increasing force required to distend the lung and chest wall (see Fig. 2.4). Thus TLC is limited by the distensibility of both the lungs and the chest wall and the amount of force that the inspiratory muscles can generate. Disease that affects any of these three components will affect TLC.

At RV, a significant amount of gas remains within the lung. As RV is approached, the chest wall becomes so stiff that additional effort by the expiratory chest wall muscles to contract is unable to further reduce the volume. Thus RV occurs when the expiratory muscle force is insufficient to cause a further reduction in chest wall volume (see Fig. 2.4). As the chest wall is squeezed by the expiratory muscles, the recoil pressure of the chest wall (the chest wall wanting to increase in size) increases. The expiratory muscles

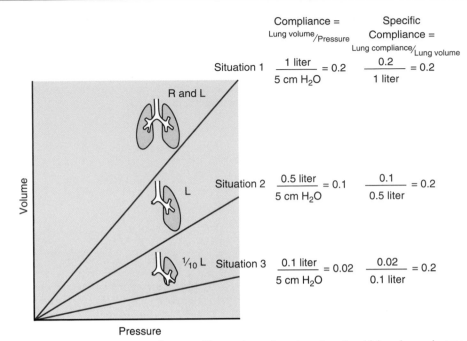

Fig. 2.5 Relationship between compliance and lung volume. Imagine a lung in which a change in pressure of 5 cm H_2O results in a change in volume of 1 liter. If half of the lung is removed (Situation 2), the compliance will decrease, but when corrected for the volume of the lung, there is no change (specific compliance). Even when the lung is reduced by 90% (Situation 3), the specific compliance is unchanged. R, right lung; L, left lung. (From Koeppen BM, Stanton BA, eds. *Berne and Levy's Physiology*, 7th ed. Philadelphia: Elsevier; 2018.)

shorten, and their capacity to generate force decreases; the point at which the force generated by the expiratory muscles is insufficient to overcome the outward recoil of the chest wall determines the RV. This simple model of RV applies to (young) individuals with normal lungs. In older individuals and in individuals with lung disease, premature airway closure, a property of the lung (see Chapter 3), becomes the major determinant of RV rather than outward chest wall recoil.

The FRC is the volume of the lung at the end of a normal exhalation and is determined by the balance between the elastic recoil pressure generated by the lung parenchyma to become smaller and the pressure generated by the chest wall to become larger (see Fig. 2.4). FRC occurs when these two forces are equal and opposite. In the presence of chest wall weakness, the FRC decreases (lung elastic recoil is greater than chest wall muscle force). In the presence of airway obstruction, the FRC increases because of premature airway closure that traps air in the lung. Always, however, the FRC occurs at the lung volume at which the outward recoil of the chest wall is equal to the inward recoil of the lung.

LUNG–CHEST WALL INTERACTIONS

The lung and chest wall move together in healthy people. The pleural space that separates the lung and the chest wall is best thought of as a "potential" space because of its small volume. Because the lung and chest wall move together, changes in their respective volumes are the same. The pressure changes across the lung and across the chest wall are defined as the **transmural pressures**. Transmural pressure refers to any pressure difference across a wall and by convention represents the inside of the wall pressure minus the outside of the wall pressure. For the lung, this transmural pressure is called the **transpulmonary pressure** (P_L; also called the translung pressure) and is defined as the pressure difference between the airspaces (alveolar pressure [P_A]) and the pressure surrounding the lung (pleural pressure [P_{PL}]); that is,

$$P_L = P_A - P_{PL}$$

The lung requires a positive P_L to increase its volume and lung volume increases with increasing P_L. The lung assumes its smallest size when the transpulmonary pressure is zero. The lung, however, is not airless when the P_L is zero because of the surface tension–lowering properties of surfactant (discussed later). The transmural pressure across the chest wall (Pw) is the difference between the pleural pressure and the pressure surrounding the chest wall (inside pressure minus outside pressure), which is the barometric pressure (P_B) or body surface pressure. That is,

$$P_W = P_{PL} - P_B$$

During the inspiratory phase of quiet breathing, the chest wall expands to a larger volume. Because the pleural pressure is negative relative to atmospheric pressure during quiet breathing, the transmural pressure across the chest wall is negative. The pressure then across the respiratory system (P_{RS}) is the sum of the pressure across the lung and the pressure across the chest wall; that is,

$$P_{RS} = P_L + P_W$$
$$= (P_A - P_{PL}) + (P_{PL} - P_B)$$
$$= P_A - P_B$$

A number of important observations can be made by examining the pressure volume curves of the lung, chest wall, and respiratory system (see Fig. 2.4). First, the lung volume at which the pressure across the respiratory system is 0 is the FRC. The resting volume of the chest wall is approximately 60% of the VC. Thus in the absence of the lungs, the resting volume of the chest wall would be approximately 60% of the VC. At less than 60% of the VC, the chest wall has outward elastic recoil. At lung volumes greater than 60% of the VC, the chest wall, like the lung, has inward elastic recoil.

The transmural distending pressure for the normal lung alone flattens at pressures greater than 20 cm H_2O because the elastic limits of the lung have been reached. Thus further increases in transmural pressure produce no change in volume, and compliance is low. Further distention is limited by the connective tissue of the lung (collagen, elastin) and surfactant. If further pressure is applied, the alveoli close to the lung surface can rupture and air can escape into the pleural space. This is called a *pneumothorax.*

As lung volume increases above FRC, the pressure across the respiratory system becomes positive because of two factors: the increased elastic recoil of the lung and the decreased outward elastic recoil of the chest wall. Below FRC, the relaxation pressure at the mouth is negative because the outward recoil of the chest wall is now greater than the reduced inward recoil of the lungs.

This relationship between pleural, alveolar, and elastic recoil pressure is shown in Fig. 2.6. The alveolar pressure is the sum of the elastic recoil pressure P_{EL} and the pleural pressure of the lung:

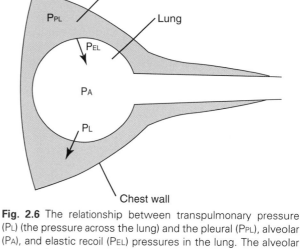

Fig. 2.6 The relationship between transpulmonary pressure (P_L) (the pressure across the lung) and the pleural (P_{PL}), alveolar (P_A), and elastic recoil (P_{EL}) pressures in the lung. The alveolar pressure is the sum of the pleural and the elastic recoil pressures; that is, $P_A = P_{PL} + P_{EL}$. (From Koeppen BM, Stanton BA, eds. *Berne and Levy's Physiology*, 7th ed. Philadelphia: Elsevier; 2018.)

$$P_A = P_{EL} + P_{PL}$$

Because

$$P_L = P_A - P_{PL}$$

Then

$$P_L = (P_{EL} + P_{PL}) - P_{PL}$$

Therefore

$$P_L = P_{EL}$$

In general, P_L is the pressure distending the lung and P_{EL} is the pressure tending to collapse the lung. As shown later, P_{EL} is the driving pressure for expiratory gas flow.

If the seal between the chest wall and the lung is broken, such as by a penetrating knife injury, the inward elastic recoil of the lung is no longer opposed by the outward recoil of the chest wall, and their interdependence ceases. As a result, lung volume will decrease and airways and alveoli will collapse. At the same time, the chest wall will expand because its outward recoil is no longer opposed by the inward recoil of the lung. When the chest is opened, as during thoracic surgery, the lung recoils until the transpulmonary pressure is zero and the chest wall increases in size (to approximately 60% of the VC). The lungs do not, however, become totally airless but retain approximately 10% of their total lung capacity.

What happens in the supine position? The supine position has no effect on lung elastic recoil. However, when an individual is supine, the position of the diaphragm is changed due to gravitational effects, and the result is that the recoil pressures for the chest wall, and as a consequence for the respiratory system, are shifted to the right. Upright, the diaphragm is pulled down by gravity; supine, the abdominal contents push inward against the relaxed diaphragm. The displacement of the diaphragm into the chest decreases the overall outward recoil of the chest wall and displaces the chest wall elastic recoil pressure to the right. This change from the upright to the supine position results in a decrease in FRC.

CLINICAL BOX

This important relationship between the lung and chest wall is illustrated in the static pressure volume curves for the lung and the chest wall (see Fig. 2.4). These curves are obtained by asking participants to breathe into a spirometer (see Chapter 4) to measure lung volumes. An esophageal balloon is placed in the distal one-third of the esophagus to measure intrapleural pressure. In addition, pressure at the mouth is measured. Participants then inspire to a specific lung volume; a stopcock in the spirometer tubing near the mouth is closed, and the participant is instructed to relax the respiratory muscles. The pressure at the mouth is equal to alveolar pressure because there is no airflow, and this is equal to the recoil pressure of the lungs (P_L) and the chest wall (P_W). This is the pressure of the respiratory system ($P_{RS} = P_L + P_W$). Because the intrapleural pressure is known, the individual recoil pressure of the lungs and the chest wall can be calculated.

If the esophageal pressure is -5 cm H_2O and the pressure at the mouth in the absence of airflow is -5 cm H_2O what is the transpulmonary pressure?

$$P_L - P_A - P_{PL}$$
$$= -5\ cm\ H_2O - (-5\ cm\ H_2O)$$
$$= 0\ cm\ H_2O$$

That is, this transpulmonary pressure would result in no airflow into the lung and would represent either end inspiration or end exhalation.

PRESSURE–VOLUME RELATIONSHIPS

Both pressure and volume change during respiration. Before the start of inspiration, the pressure in the pleural space in normal individuals is slightly negative (approximately

-5 cm H_2O). That is, pleural pressure is less than atmospheric pressure. This negative pressure is created by the elastic recoil pressure of the lung, which acts to pull the lung away from the chest wall. Alveolar pressure at this point is zero because there is no airflow, and at points of no airflow alveolar and atmospheric pressures must be equal. As inspiration begins, the diaphragm contracts and moves into the abdominal cavity and the rib cage moves out and upward. The volume of the thoracic cavity increases and because of Boyle's law (see Appendix C), the pressure inside the alveoli decreases.

As alveolar pressure decreases below atmospheric pressure, the glottis opens and air rushes into the airways. The decrease in alveolar pressure is small during tidal volume breathing in normal individuals (1–3 cm H_2O) but is much larger in individuals with airway obstruction who must generate larger inspiratory pressures to overcome the obstructed airways.

As alveolar pressure falls during inspiration, intrapleural pressure also falls. The decrease in intrapleural pressure is equal to the sum of the elastic recoil pressure, which increases as the lung inflates and the pressure drops along the airways as gas flows into the lung from higher (atmospheric or 0 pressure) to lower pressure (alveolar, subatmospheric pressure). Airflow stops when alveolar pressure and atmospheric pressure become equal.

On exhalation, the diaphragm moves back into the chest, intrapleural pressure increases (i.e., becomes less negative), alveolar pressure rises, the glottis opens, and gas again flows from higher to lower pressure. In the alveoli, the driving pressure for expiratory gas flow is the sum of the elastic recoil of the lung and the intrapleural pressure. The pressure volume events that occur during inspiration and exhalation are shown in Fig. 2.7; Fig. 2.8 shows the relationship between transpulmonary, intrapleural, and elastic recoil at end exhalation and during inspiration.

SURFACE TENSION

The elastic properties of the lung, including elastin, collagen, and other constituents of the lung tissue, are responsible for some but not all of the elastic recoil of the lung. The other important factor that contributes to lung elastic recoil is the **surface tension** at the air–liquid interface in the alveoli. Surface tension is a measure of the attractive force of the surface molecules per unit length of the material to which they are attached. The units of surface tension are those of a force applied per unit length (dynes/cm).

The role of surface tension forces in lung elastic recoil can be illustrated by comparing the volume pressure curves of saline-filled and air-filled lungs (Fig. 2.9). Similar to

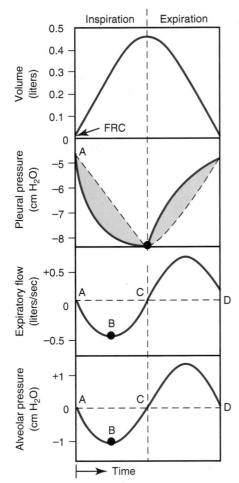

Fig. 2.7 Changes in alveolar and pleural pressure, expiratory flow, and lung volume during a tidal volume breath. Inspiration is to the left of the vertical dotted line, and exhalation is to the right. Positive (relative to atmosphere) pressures are above the horizontal dotted line, and negative pressures are below. At points of no airflow (A, C, and D), alveolar pressure is zero. Point B represents the midpoint of inspiration. IPleural pressure has two courses noted by the solid and the dotted lines. The dotted line represents the pleural pressure changes needed to overcome the elastic recoil of the alveoli; the solid line includes the additional pressure changes required to overcome tissue and airflow resistance. Thus the dotted line is a more accurate representation of intrapleural pressure. FRC, functional residual capacity. (From Koeppen BM, Stanton BA, eds. *Berne and Levy's Physiology*, 7th ed. Philadelphia: Elsevier; 2018.)

Fig. 2.3, in this experiment a pressure volume curve is generated using an excised lung. When the lung is inflated with air, an air–liquid interface is present in the lung and surface tension contributes to alveolar elastic recoil. After all the gas is removed, the lung is inflated again, but this time

saline instead of air is used. In this situation, surface tension forces are absent because there is no air–liquid interface. The difference between the two curves is the recoil due to surface tension forces.

For a sphere such as an alveolus, the relationship between the pressure within the sphere (Ps) and the tension in the wall is described by **Laplace's law:**

$$Ps = \frac{2T}{r}$$

Or
$$T = \frac{Ps \times r}{2}$$

where T is the wall tension (dynes/cm) and r is the radius of the sphere.

Consider what would happen in the alveolus with changes in volume. Note here that the surface of most liquids (such as water) is constant and is not dependent on the area of the air–liquid interface. Imagine two alveoli of different sizes connected by a common airway (Fig. 2.10A). If the surface tension in both of these alveoli is equal, Laplace's law states that the pressure in the smaller alveolus must be greater than the pressure in the larger alveolus, and because gas always flows from higher to lower pressure, the smaller alveolus will empty into the larger alveolus.

Alveoli in the lung are of variable sizes. With a constant surface tension, these interconnected alveoli would be unstable—that is, the smaller alveoli would empty into the larger alveoli. The collapsed alveoli would have significant cohesive forces at their liquid–liquid interface and would therefore require a high distending pressure to open. The result would be a marked increase in the distending pressures and in the work of breathing due to "stiff" alveoli. Two major factors cause the alveoli to be more stable than would be expected based on a constant surface tension. The first factor is **pulmonary surfactant;** the second is the **structural interdependence** of the alveoli.

SURFACTANT

Surfactant is a surface–active component of the alveolar surface fluid that lowers the elastic recoil due to surface tension even at high lung volumes. It increases the compliance of the lungs above that predicted by an air–water interface, and as a result, it decreases the work of breathing.

Surfactants are generally considered to be soaps or detergents. Pulmonary surfactant is a complex mixture of phospholipids, neutral lipids, fatty acids, and proteins. This

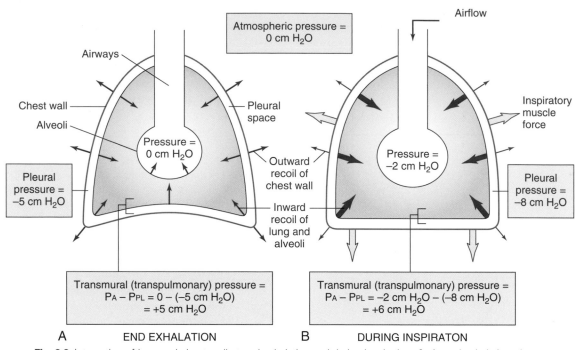

Fig. 2.8 Interaction of lung and chest wall at end exhalation and during inspiration. **A,** At end exhalation, the respiratory muscles are relaxed, the diaphragm sits high in the thoracic cavity, and there is no airflow because there is no difference between atmospheric and alveolar pressure. Lung elastic recoil pulls the lung inward, whereas chest wall elastic recoil pulls the chest wall outward. The tension created by the two opposing forces creates a negative pleural pressure. **B,** During inspiration, the diaphragm and other muscles of inspiration contract, resulting in a further decrease in pleural pressure. This negative pleural pressure is transmitted to the alveoli, causing a drop in alveolar pressure. Gas flows into the lung along the pressure gradient. Note that as lung volume increases, lung elastic recoil increases (solid arrows) and the outward recoil of the chest wall (open arrows) decreases.

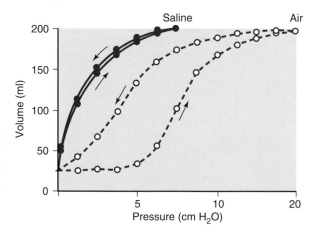

Fig. 2.9 Volume–pressure curves of lungs filled with saline and with air. The arrows indicate whether the lung is being inflated or deflated; note that when using saline, hysteresis (i.e., the difference between inflation and deflation limbs of the curve) is virtually eliminated. (From Clements JA, Tierney DF. In: Fenn WO, Rahn H, eds. *Handbook of Physiology, Section 3: Respiration*, vol. II. Washington, DC: American Physiological Society; 1964.)

substance constitutes a thin film that lines the surface of the alveoli. The fatty acids are hydrophobic and lie parallel to each other projecting into the gas phase, whereas a hydrophilic end lies within the alveolar lining fluid. In addition to its surface tension–lowering properties, surfactant has "antistick" properties, and it acts as a barrier at the air–liquid interface.

Surfactant stabilizes the inflation of alveoli because it allows the surface tension to increase as the alveoli become larger and to decrease as the alveoli become smaller (see

Fig. 2.10B). As a result, the transmural pressure required to keep an alveolus inflated increases as lung volume (and transpulmonary pressure) increases, and it decreases as lung volume decreases. In the absence of surfactant, the surface tension at the air–liquid interface would remain constant and the transmural (transalveolar) pressure needed to keep it at that volume would be greater at lower lung (alveolar) volumes. Thus it requires a greater transmural pressure to produce a given increase in alveolar volume at lower lung volumes than at higher lung volumes. Stated another way, in the absence of surfactant, the transmural pressure necessary to keep an alveolus inflated would decrease as the transpulmonary pressure (i.e., lung volume) increases; conversely, the transmural pressure necessary to keep an alveolus inflated would increase as the transpulmonary pressure (i.e., lung volume) decreases. This would create instability of alveolar inflation and alveolar collapse.

Surfactant contains 85% to 90% lipids (of which 85% are phospholipids and 5% are neutral lipids) and 10% to 15% protein (Table 2.1). The major phospholipid in surfactant is **phosphatidylcholine**, of which approximately 75% is present as **dipalmitoyl phosphatidylcholine (DPPC)**. DPPC is the major active component in surfactant, and it readily decreases surface tension. The second most abundant phospholipid is phosphatidylglycerol (PG), which constitutes 7% to 10% of total surfactant. Both of these lipids are important in the formation of the

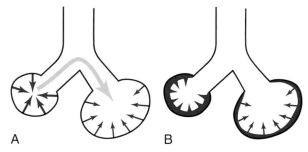

A   B

Fig. 2.10 Surface tension in a sphere. Surface forces in a sphere attempt to reduce the area of the surface and generate a pressure within the sphere. By Laplace's law, the pressure generated is inversely proportional to the radius of the sphere. A. Surface forces (Ps [surface pressure]) in the smaller sphere generate a higher pressure (heavier arrows) than the forces (PL [transpulmonary pressure]) in the larger sphere (lighter arrows). As a result, air moves from the smaller sphere (higher pressure) to the larger sphere (lower pressure); see large shaded arrow. This causes the smaller sphere to collapse and the larger sphere to become over- distended. B. Surfactant (dark areas) lowers surface tension, decreasing it more in the smaller sphere than in the larger sphere. The net result is that Ps is approximately equal to PL, and the spheres are stabilized. (From Koeppen BM, Stanton BA (eds): *Berne and Levy's Physiology*, 7th ed. Philadelphia, Elsevier; 2018.)

TABLE 2.1 Composition of Mature Surfactant	
Component	**Weight(%)**
Total lipids	85–90
Protein	10–15
Specific lipids	
Phospholipids	85–90
Neutral lipids	5
Glycolipids	5–10
Specific phospholipids	
Phosphatidylcholine	70–80
Dipalmitoyl phosphatidylcholine	45–50
Phosphatidylglycerol	7–10
Phosphatidylethanolamine	3–5

liquid monolayer on the alveolar–air interface, and PG is important in the spreading of surfactant over a large surface area.

Pulmonary surfactant is secreted from the small cuboidal type II cells, which occupy only about 2% to 7% of the surface area of the alveoli; once released, the surfactant must spread over the remaining surface area. This is accomplished with the aid of surfactant components such as PG, with spreading properties. Cholesterol and cholesterol esters account for the majority of the neutral lipids; their precise role is not yet determined, but they may aid in stabilizing the lipid structure.

Four important specific surfactant proteins (SPs) constitute a small part (2%–5%) of the weight of surfactant. SP-A, which is expressed in alveolar type II epithelial cells and in Clara cells in the lung, is the most studied surfactant protein. SP-A regulates surfactant turnover and is involved in the immune regulation within the lung and in the formation of tubular myelin. Tubular myelin is a precursor stage of surfactant as it is initially secreted from the type II cell but has not yet spread (see Fig. 1.7C).

SP-B and SP-C are two hydrophobic surfactant-specific proteins. SP-B may be involved in the formation of tubular myelin. SP-B is involved in the surface activity of surfactant and may increase the intermolecular and intramolecular order of the phospholipid bilayer and the lateral stability of the phospholipid layer. The 25 amino-terminal peptides of SP-B may further stabilize the phospholipid layer by increasing the collapse pressure of surfactant phospholipids. This action may prevent the squeezing out of the phospholipids from the monolayers at the alveolar air-liquid interface. A specific charge interaction between the cationic peptide and an anionic lipid, such as PG, may be responsible for this stabilization.

SP-C may be involved in the spreading ability and in the surface activity of surfactant. Another recently discovered surfactant-specific protein, SP-D, is a glycoprotein with an apparent molecular weight of 43 kDa. This substance contains an N-terminal collagenous domain and a carboxy-terminal, glycosylated domain similar to SP-A. The function of SP-D is unknown.

Pulmonary surfactant, synthesized in the alveolar type II epithelial cell, is stored as preformed units in lamellar bodies in the cytoplasm. These preformed lamellar bodies have distinctive swirling patterns that are readily observed by electron microscopy, and they are uniquely characteristic of type II epithelial cells (see Fig. 1.7). Secretion of surfactant into the airway occurs via exocytosis of the lamellar body by both constitutive and regulated mechanisms. Numerous agents, including β-adrenergic agonists, activators of protein kinase C, leukotrienes, and purinergic agonists, have been shown to stimulate the secretion of surfactant.

Pulmonary surfactant is cleared from the alveolus primarily through reuptake by type II cells, with minor contributions through absorption into lymphatics and clearance by alveolar macrophages. After being taken up by the type II cell, the phospholipids either are recycled for future secretion or are degraded and subsequently reutilized in the synthesis of new phospholipids. These processes are regulated developmentally in the fetal lung.

In summary, pulmonary surfactant reduces the work of breathing by reducing surface tension forces, prevents collapse and sticking of alveoli upon exhalation with antistick properties, and stabilizes alveoli, especially those that tend to deflate at low surface tension.

CLINICAL BOX

In 1959 Avery and Mead discovered that the lungs of premature infants who died of hyaline membrane disease (HMD) were deficient in surfactant. HMD, currently known as respiratory distress syndrome (RDS), is characterized by increased work of breathing, progressive atelectasis (lung unit collapse), and respiratory failure in premature infants. It is a major cause of morbidity and mortality in the neonatal period. The major surfactant deficiency in premature infants is the lack of PG. In general, as the level of PG increases in amniotic fluid, the mortality rate decreases. This work culminated in successful attempts to treat HMD in premature infants with surfactant replacement therapy. Today surfactant replacement therapy is the standard care for premature infants.

ALVEOLAR INTERDEPENDENCE

In addition to surfactant, another mechanism, namely interdependence, contributes to the stability of the alveoli (Fig. 2.11). Except for alveoli on the pleural surface, all alveoli are surrounded by other alveoli. The collapse of one alveolus is opposed by the traction exerted by the surrounding alveoli. Thus the collapse of a single alveolus stretches and distorts the surrounding alveoli, which in turn are connected to other alveoli. The pores of Kohn and the canals of Lambert provide collateral ventilation and also prevent alveolar collapse (atelectasis).

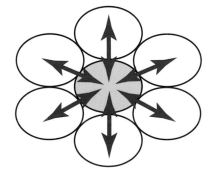

Fig. 2.11 Interdependence. The tendency of one alveolus to collapse (shaded area) is countered by opposing traction from the surrounding alveoli. (From Koeppen BM, Stanton BA (eds): *Berne and Levy's Physiology*, 7th ed. Philadelphia, Elsevier; 2018.)

SUMMARY

1. Lung volumes are determined by the balance between the lung's elastic recoil properties and the properties of the muscles of the chest wall.
2. The vital capacity (VC) is the maximum amount of air that an individual can either inspire or exhale.
3. The functional residual capacity (FRC) is the resting volume of the lung. It is determined by the balance between the lung elastic recoil pressure operating to decrease lung volume and the pressure generated by the chest wall to become larger. At FRC, the pressure across the respiratory system is zero.
4. Limits to respiratory muscle lengthening and shortening are important determinants of TLC and RV, respectively, in young individuals.
5. Lung compliance is a measure of the elastic properties of the lung. A loss of elastic recoil is seen in patients with emphysema and is associated with an increase in lung compliance. In contrast, in diseases associated with pulmonary fibrosis, lung compliance is decreased.
6. The pressure across the lung (transpulmonary pressure [P_L]) is the difference between alveolar pressure and pleural pressure ($P_L = P_A - P_{PL}$). The pressure across the chest wall (P_W) is the difference between pleural and barometric pressure ($P_W = P_{PL} - P_B$). The pressure across the respiratory system is the sum of the recoil pressures of the lung and the chest wall ($P_{RS} = P_L + P_W$).
7. A positive transpulmonary pressure is needed to increase lung volume. The pressure across the respiratory system is zero at points of no airflow (end inspiration and end exhalation).
8. Surfactant in the alveolus changes the surface tension of the air–liquid interface as lung volume changes. Surfactant lowers overall lung compliance. In addition, in the presence of surfactant, the transmural pressure required to keep an alveolus inflated increases as lung volume (and transpulmonary pressure) increases and decreases as lung volume decreases.
9. Alveolar interdependence, the pores of Kohn, and the canals of Lambert help to prevent alveolar collapse (atelectasis).

KEY WORDS AND CONCEPTS

Alveolar interdependence
Atelectasis
Chest wall
Chest wall mechanics
Dipalmitoyl phosphatidylcholine (DPPC)
Dynamic lung mechanics
Emphysema
Functional residual capacity (FRC)
Hysteresis
Lamellar bodies
Laplace's law
Lung compliance
Lung elastic recoil
Obstructive pulmonary disease (OPD)
Phosphatidylcholine (PC)
Pleural effusion
Pressure volume curve

Pulmonary edema
Pulmonary fibrosis
Residual volume (RV)
Respiratory distress syndrome (RDS)
Respiratory system
Restrictive lung disease (RLD)
Static lung mechanics
Surface tension
Surfactant
Surfactant B (SP-B)
Tidal volume (TV or V_T)
Total lung capacity (TLC)
Transmural pressure
Transpulmonary pressure (P_L)
Type I cell
Type II cell
Vital capacity (VC)

SELF-STUDY PROBLEMS

1. What factors determine total lung capacity?
2. What factors determine residual volume?
3. Describe the lung volume changes in an individual with acute hypersensitivity pneumonitis (a condition associated with interstitial pneumonia and the presence of proteinaceous fluid with increased numbers of alveolar macrophages in the alveoli).
4. What are the two major properties of surfactant that decrease the work of breathing?

ADDITIONAL READINGS

1. Brown RH, Mitzner W. Effects of lung inflation and airway muscle tone on airway diameter in vivo. *J Appl Physiol.* 1996;80:1581–1588.

2. Cheung D, Schot R, Zwindermann AH, et al. Relationship between loss in parenchymal recoil pressure and maximal airway narrowing in subjects with alpha-1-antitrypsin deficiency. *Am J Respir Crit Care Med.* 1997;155:135–140.

3. D'Angelo E, Robatto FM, Calderini E, et al. Pulmonary and chest wall mechanics in anesthetized paralyzed humans. *J Appl Physiol.* 1991;70:2602–2610.

4. George RB, Light RW, Matthay MA, Matthay RA, eds. *Chest Medicine: Essentials of Pulmonary and Critical Care Medicine.* 5th ed. Philadelphia: Lippincott-Williams and Wilkins; 2005.

5. Hlastala MP, Berger AJ. *Physiology of Respiration.* 2nd ed. New York: Oxford University Press; 2001.

6. Lai-Fook SJ, Rodarte JR. Pleural pressure distribution and its relationship to lung volume and interstitial pressure. *J Appl Physiol.* 1991;70:967–978.

7. Lumb AB. *Nunn's Applied Respiratory Physiology.* 8th ed. Philadelphia: Elsevier; 2017.

8. Zapletal A, Desmond KJ, Demizio D, et al. Lung recoil and the determination of airflow limitation in cystic fibrosis and asthma. *Pediatr Pulmonol.* 1993;15:13–18.

Dynamic Lung Mechanics

OBJECTIVES

1. Describe how a pressure gradient is created.
2. Define airway resistance and its measurement.
3. Discuss three factors that contribute to or regulate airway resistance in health and disease.

4. Describe the concepts of flow limitation, the equal pressure point, and dynamic airway compression.
5. Define work of breathing and the factors that contribute to work of breathing.

Dynamic lung mechanics studies the lung in motion. To cause air to move from the outside of the body into the distal airways, three opposing forces must be overcome: (1) the elastic recoil of the lungs and chest wall, (2) the frictional resistances of the airways and of the tissues of the lung and chest wall, and (3) the inertance or impedance of acceleration of the respiratory system. The elastic forces of the lung and chest wall (Chapter 2) depend on lung volume and are not affected by motion. Inertance depends on the rate of airflow but is negligible during quiet breathing. Thus the major force that must be overcome to achieve airflow is frictional resistance. Frictional resistance is determined by flow and not by a change in lung volume.

HOW A PRESSURE GRADIENT IS GENERATED

Gases move from regions of higher pressure to regions of lower pressure. The movement of air in and out of the lungs requires the creation of a pressure gradient from the inside of the alveoli to the outside world. Pressure changes within the airways are, by convention, referenced to barometric pressure and are either greater than or less than barometric pressure. Because the absolute barometric pressure is different at different altitudes, again by convention, the pressure surrounding the chest wall (the barometric pressure) is referenced to zero when pressure gradients are being measured. Inspiration occurs when negative pressure is generated inside the alveoli—that is to say, when alveolar pressure is lower than atmospheric pressure.

Alveoli are not capable of expanding on their own. They will expand only when there is an increase in the distending pressure across their walls. The distending pressure across the alveolar wall is called the **transmural** (mural, meaning any wall) or **transpulmonary** (across the lung; that is, from the alveolus to the pleura) pressure gradient and it is generated by the muscles of inspiration. Before airflow begins, the pressure inside the alveoli is the same as atmospheric pressure, which by convention is equal to 0 cm H_2O. An important principle of respiration is that pressures at the pleural surface generated by the muscles of respiration are transmitted through the alveolar walls to the more centrally located alveoli and small airways. Thus alveolar units are structurally interdependent.

During inspiration, as the muscles of inspiration contract, the pressure inside the airways decreases relative to barometric pressure (that is, it becomes less than atmospheric pressure or "negative" relative to the "zero" atmospheric pressure) according to **Boyle's law** (see Appendix C). Thus if the pressure in the alveoli decreases, the volume in the alveoli must increase. For example, during inspiration the pressure inside the airways is −5 cm H_2O. That is, it is 5 cm H_2O less than atmospheric pressure (zero), but the actual pressure, assuming that you are at sea level, would be 760 mm Hg − 5 cm H_2O (note the different units) or 760 mm Hg − ~4 mm Hg. During exhalation, the process is reversed, and the pressure inside the airways becomes greater than atmospheric pressure. The important principle to remember is that gases always flow from an area of higher pressure to an area of lower pressure.

RESISTANCE

The pressure flow characteristics of laminar flow (Appendix C) were first described by the French physician Poiseuille.

In straight circular tubes, the flow rate ($\dot{V}$; the dot above the letter V signifies a change in volume with respect to time—that is, a flow rate) is given by:

$$\dot{V} = \frac{P\pi r^4}{8nl}$$

where P is the driving pressure, r is the radius, n is the viscosity, and l is the length. Thus it can be seen that the driving pressure (P) is proportional to the flow rate ($\dot{V}$)—that is, $P = k \times \dot{V}$. The flow resistance, R, across a set of tubes is defined as the change in driving pressure (ΔP) divided by the flow rate, or

$$R = \frac{\Delta P}{\dot{V}} = \frac{8nl}{\pi r^4}$$

The units of resistance are cm $H_2O/L \cdot$ sec. A number of important observations can be made based on this equation, including the role of the radius in determining resistance. If the radius of the tube is reduced in half, the resistance will increase 16-fold. If, however, the length is increased twofold, the resistance will only increase twofold. Thus the radius of the tube primarily determines resistance. Stated another way, resistance is inversely proportional to the fourth power of the radius and directly proportional to the length of the tube and the gas viscosity. The radius is thus the main factor that affects resistance. The smaller the airway, the greater the resistance of that airway.

Resistance to airflow in the respiratory system is composed of three individual resistances; airway resistance, pulmonary (parenchyma or lung tissue) resistance, and chest wall resistance. Airway resistance is defined as the frictional resistance of the entire system of airways from the tip of the nose (for nasal breathing) or mouth (for mouth breathing) to the alveoli. Pulmonary resistance (or lung resistance) is defined as the frictional resistance afforded by the lungs and the airways combined. Chest wall resistance is the frictional resistance of the chest wall and abdominal structures. In turn, airway resistance is composed of the resistance of the upper airway (from nose to glottis) and the resistance of the lower airways (from glottis to alveoli).

Approximately 25% to 40% of the total resistance to airflow is located in the upper airways—namely the nose, nasal turbinates, oropharynx, nasopharynx, and larynx (Fig. 3.1). Respiratory system resistance is thus higher when breathing through the nose than when breathing through the mouth. During V_T breathing, the vocal cords open slightly during inspiration and close slightly during exhalation. During inspiration, airways inside the chest are surrounded by a negative intrathoracic (pleural) pressure, and airways outside the chest (extrathoracic airways) are surrounded by atmospheric pressure. As a result, the pressure

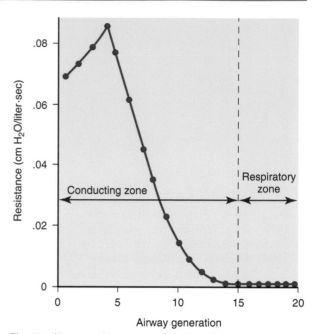

Fig. 3.1 Airway resistance as a function of the airway generation. As the airways branch from the trachea to mainstem bronchi to lobar bronchi, and so on, the daughter airways at each branch point are described as belonging to the next generation. In the normal lung, most of the resistance to airflow occurs in the first eight generations. (Koeppen BM, Stanton BA, eds. *Berne and Levy's Physiology*, 7th ed. Philadelphia: Elsevier; 2018.)

surrounding the extrathoracic airways is greater than the pressure inside the airways, and these extrathoracic airways are pulled inward, resulting in partial or complete airway obstruction, especially during deep inspirations.

This inward pulling of extrathoracic airways during inspiration is most easily demonstrated in the nose. Making a rapid inspiratory effort while breathing through the nose results in collapse of the anterior portion of the nose (a "sniff"). Counteracting the collapse of the extrathoracic airways during inspiration are the muscles of the oropharynx that contract during inspiration. Reflex contraction of these pharyngeal dilator muscles dilates and stabilizes the upper airway. In the anterior nose, active contraction of the alae nasi minimizes the collapse associated with sniffing. Failure of these muscles to contract can occur, especially during sleep, and can result in airway obstruction and obstructive sleep apnea (see Chapter 10).

Airflow resistance in the lower airways (Raw) can be divided between the resistance in the large airways (≥ 4 mm in diameter: first four airway generations), the medium-sized airways (subsegmental bronchi, 1–4 mm in

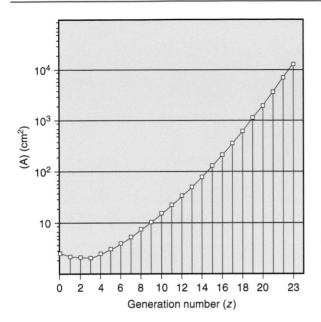

Fig. 3.2 Change in surface area (A) of the airways with increasing airway generation number. Although each individual airway gets smaller with each increase in generation number, (z) the total cross-sectional area of each generation is greater than the total of area of the previous generation. (From Weibel ER. *Morphometry of the Human Lung.* Heidelberg: Springer-Verlag; 1963.)

diameter), and the small airways (bronchioles, <1 mm in diameter). Therefore Raw is equal to the sum of each of these individual resistances; that is,

$$Raw = R_{large} + R_{medium} + R_{small}$$

From Poiseuille's equation you might conclude that the major site of resistance in the airways is in the smallest airways. For many years this was thought to be true. In fact, however, the major site of resistance along the bronchial tree is the large bronchi. The smallest airways contribute little to the overall total resistance of the bronchial tree even though their individual resistance is high. The reason for this is interrelated and twofold. First, for the whole lung, the airways are a complex combination of tubes of different sizes arranged both in parallel and in series. As gas flows into more distal airways, the airway number increases faster than the decrease in individual airway size. As a result, there is a large increase in total airway cross-sectional area and airflow velocity becomes very low as the effective cross-sectional area increases (Fig. 3.2). Second, at the same time that individual airways are becoming smaller with each generation and the resistance from generation to generation is additive (airways in series where $R_{TOT} = Rgen_1 + Rgen_2 + Rgen_3 + ...$), the increase in airway number and airways now in parallel is increasing faster and the resistance within a generation where the airways are in parallel is decreasing (e.g., in generation 10, $1/R_{10} = 1/Rbranch_1 + 1/Rbranch_2 + 1/Rbranch_3 + ...$). Thus the resistance of the airway

generations with small airways is small. As an example, assume that there are three tubes each with a resistance of 3 cm $H_2O/L \cdot sec$ (Fig. 3.3). If the tubes are in series, the total resistance (R_{TOT}) is the sum of the individual resistances:

$$R_{TOT} = R_1 + R_2 + R_3 = 3 + 3 + 3 = 9 \text{ cm } H_2O/L \cdot sec$$

If the tubes are in parallel (as they are in small airways), the total resistance is the sum of the inverse of the individual resistances (see Fig. 3.3).

$$1/R_{TOT} = 1/R_1 + 1/R_2 + 1/R_3 = 1/3 + 1/3 + 1/3$$
$$= 1 \text{ cm } H_2O/L \cdot sec$$

During normal breathing, approximately 80% of the resistance to airflow at functional residual capacity (FRC) occurs in airways with diameters greater than 2 mm. This is in contrast to the pulmonary blood vessels, in which most of the resistance is in the small vessels. Because the small airways contribute so little to total lung resistance, the measurement of airway resistance (see Chapter 4) is a poor test to detect small airway obstruction.

The partitioning of Raw between large and small airways can be further illustrated by the following example. If the resistance of the respiratory system (Raw) equals 2 cm $H_2O/L \cdot sec$, and if the "large" airways (from the trachea to the segmental bronchi) contribute 80% to the total resistance, the subsegmental "medium-sized" airways (1–4 mm in diameter) contribute 15%, and the "small" airways (<1 mm in diameter) contribute the remainder, then the

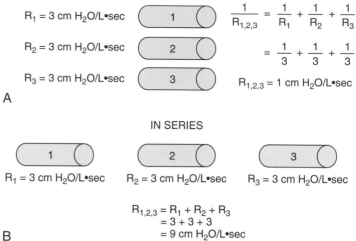

Fig. 3.3 Resistance in airways in parallel and in series. Resistance of airways in parallel **(A)** is always much less than the resistance in airways in series **(B)**. This means that the total resistance of the small airways is less than the total resistance of the large airways even though the individual resistances of the small airways are much greater than the individual resistances of the large airways.

individual resistances of the small, medium, and large airways can be determined as follows:

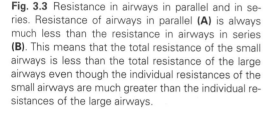

$$\text{Large airways} = 0.80 \times 2 \text{ mm } H_2O/L \cdot \text{sec}$$
$$= 1.6 \text{ cm } H_2O/L \cdot \text{sec}$$

$$\text{Medium airways} = 0.15 \times 2 \text{ mm } H_2O/L \cdot \text{sec}$$
$$= 0.30 \text{ cm } H_2O/L \cdot \text{sec}$$

$$\text{Small airways} = 0.05 \times 2 \text{ mm } H_2O/L \cdot \text{sec}$$
$$= 0.10 \text{ cm } H_2O/L \cdot \text{sec}$$

In this example, tripling of the resistance in the small airways due to obstruction would only increase Raw to 2.2 cm $H_2O/L \cdot$ sec, a 20% change. Thus significant small airway disease can exist without a large change in Raw. This is another reason why small airway disease is "silent" and difficult to detect.

There is also a difference between inspiratory and expiratory resistance. During quiet inspiration, the difference in pressure between the open mouth and the alveoli is 0.5 cm H_2O and the average airflow rate is 0.25 L/sec. Thus Raw = 0.5/0.25 = 2.0 cm $H_2O/L \cdot$ sec during inspiration. During exhalation, there is the same pressure difference, but the airflow rate is slightly slower at 0.2 L/sec. Thus expiratory Raw (0.5/0.2 = 2.5 cm $H_2O/L \cdot$ sec) is slightly greater than inspiratory Raw.

FACTORS CONTRIBUTING TO RESISTANCE

Airway resistance is determined by a number of factors, including the number, length, and cross-sectional area of the conducting airways. The number of airways is established by the 16th week of gestation and is determined by the pattern of branching. Airway length varies from person to person and is dependent on age and body size and the phase of the respiratory cycle. Airways lengthen during inspiration as lung volume increases and shorten during exhalation. Of all the factors contributing to airway resistance, the cross-sectional area of the conducting airways is the most important because Raw varies inversely with the fourth power of the radius of the airway.

LUNG RESISTANCE

In healthy individuals, lung resistance is approximately 1 cm $H_2O/L \cdot$ sec. Lung resistance includes airway resistance and the resistance of the lung parenchyma to changing lung volume. Refer to the pleural pressure diagram shown in Fig. 2.7. In this illustration, when the lung is inflated very slowly (known as a quasi-steady state), the dashed pleural pressure curve is generated. In contrast, during tidal volume breathing, the solid pleural pressure curve is generated. The difference between the two curves represents the additional pressure that is required to overcome the resistance encountered during changing lung volume. It is composed of the resistance due to the acceleration of gas as it moves toward (or away from) the lung periphery as a result of the changing cross-sectional area and the viscous impedance encountered in changing lung volume.

The cross-sectional area of a conducting airway is determined by the balance of two opposing forces (Fig. 3.4). The elastic forces in the airways and the tension

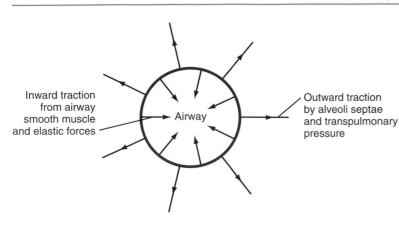

Fig. 3.4 Factors responsible for airway size. Airway smooth muscle and elastic forces in the airways tend to constrict the airways and decrease cross-sectional area. This tendency to constriction is opposed by the outward traction on the airways due to the interdependence of alveoli and terminal bronchioles or because of a positive transpulmonary pressure.

of airway smooth muscle surrounding the airways tend to contract the walls and decrease the cross-sectional area. Increasing the cross-sectional area is the outward traction either from a positive transpulmonary pressure or from the interdependence of alveoli and terminal bronchioles. The strength of these two opposing forces is largely determined by lung volume, elastic recoil, and the effect of neural and humoral agents on smooth muscle tone.

LUNG VOLUME AND AIRWAY RESISTANCE

Lung volume is one of the most important factors affecting airway resistance, because the length and diameter of the airways increase with increasing lung volume and decrease with decreasing lung volume. As a result, resistance to airflow decreases with increasing lung volume and increases with decreasing lung volume. The relationship between Raw and lung volume is, however, curvilinear (Fig. 3.5). Specifically, Raw does not change significantly with changes in lung volume greater than FRC. Between FRC and residual volume (RV), however, Raw increases rapidly and approaches infinity (no airflow) at RV. The reciprocal of Raw is called the conductance (Gaw = 1/Raw). When conductance is plotted against lung volume, the relationship becomes linear (see Fig. 3.5). As can be seen from the graph in Fig. 3.5, conductance varies with lung volume. It also will vary in children compared with adults as a result of differences in body size. Specific airway conductance (SGaw) is airway conductance (Gaw) divided by the lung volume at which it is measured. SGaw takes into account these variations in body size. From this relationship it can be seen that in the presence of increased airway resistance, breathing at a higher lung volume will reduce airway resistance. Individuals with increased airway resistance frequently breathe at higher than normal lung volumes.

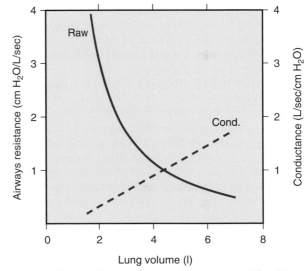

Fig. 3.5 Airway resistance (Raw) and conductance (Cond.) as a function of lung volume. (From Koeppen BM, Stanton BA, eds. *Berne and Levey's Physiology*, 7th ed. Philadelphia: Elsevier; 2018.)

Although this will tend to normalize their Gaw, their SGaw will remain abnormal. Factors known to increase resistance include airway mucus, edema, and contraction of bronchial smooth muscle, all of which decrease the caliber of the airways.

Applying Poiseuille's law, it can be seen that the density and viscosity of the inspired gas also affect resistance. When gas density increases, such as during a dive, airway resistance increases. When an oxygen–helium mixture is breathed instead of oxygen–nitrogen, the decrease in gas density results in a decrease in airway resistance. This decrease has been exploited in the treatment of **status asthmaticus**, a condition associated with airway inflammation and increased airway resistance due to a combination of bronchospasm, edema, and mucus, in which breathing in an oxygen–helium gas admixture results in decreased airway resistance and work of breathing and improved oxygen delivery to the alveoli.

ELASTIC RECOIL AND AIRWAY RESISTANCE

The elastic recoil of the lung also affects airway caliber through direct traction on small intrapulmonary airways and by effects on intrapleural pressure (see Fig. 3.4). Because of its effects on airway size in normal individuals, elastic recoil is the major determinant of intrathoracic airway resistance when individuals are breathing under quiet conditions in which flow is not limited.

As previously mentioned, the airway resistance at FRC in normal adults is 1 to 3 cm $H_2O/L \cdot sec$. Resistance is higher in young children because their airways are smaller. As we shall see later, there is a strong negative correlation between resistance and maximal expiratory flow. A high resistance is associated with decreased expiratory flows.

NEUROHUMORAL REGULATION OF AIRWAY RESISTANCE

Airway resistance is also affected or regulated by neural and humoral agents through their effects on airway smooth muscle (Box 3.1). Airway smooth muscle from the trachea to the alveolar ducts is under the control of efferent fibers of the autonomic nervous system. These submucosal smooth muscle bands encircle the airways and can change the diameter of bronchi and bronchioles independent of lung volume or

---

BOX 3.1 Active Control of the Airways

Constrict
- Parasympathetic stimulation
- Acetylcholine
- Histamine
- Leukotrienes
- Thromboxane A_2
- Serotonin
- Alpha-adrenergic agonists
- Decreased P_{CO_2} in small airways

Dilate
- Sympathetic stimulation β_2 receptors
- Circulating β_2 agonists
- Nitric oxide
- Increased P_{CO_2} in small airways
- Decreased P_{O_2} in small airways

---

pleural pressure. Stimulation of cholinergic, parasympathetic postganglionic fibers, either directly or reflexively, leads to airway constriction (the vagus nerve innervates airway smooth muscle) with an increase in airway resistance and a decrease in anatomic dead space. In contrast, stimulation of the sympathetic nerves and release of the postganglionic neurotransmitter norepinephrine inhibits airway constriction. Airway smooth muscle tone is mediated by β_2-adrenergic receptors that predominate in the airways. In general, parasympathetic tone in bronchial smooth muscle is greater than sympathetic tone, and thus even normal individuals can have a small decrease in airway resistance after inhalation of a bronchodilator.

Reflex stimulation of the vagus nerve due to smoke inhalation, dust, cold air, or other irritants can result in airway constriction and/or cough. Agents such as histamine, acetylcholine, thromboxane A2, prostaglandin F2, and leukotrienes (LTB4, C4, and D4) are released by various resident and recruited airway cells in response to various triggers and act directly on airway smooth muscle, causing constriction and an increase in airway resistance.

O_2 and CO_2 also affect airway caliber. Decreased CO_2 at bifurcations of the airways causes a local constriction of nearby airway smooth muscle, whereas increased CO_2 or decreased O_2 causes dilation. O_2 and CO_2 responsiveness of airway smooth muscle may be an important homeostatic mechanism in balancing ventilation and perfusion when there is a pulmonary embolus.

The responsiveness of airway smooth muscle to humoral agents is used to determine whether an individual has heightened airway sensitivity. Measurement of pulmonary function after inhalation of methacholine, a histamine-like compound, is used in individuals suspected of having asthma to provoke airway constriction. Although all individuals will eventually respond at high concentrations of methacholine, individuals with asthma develop airway obstruction at very low methacholine concentrations.

DYNAMIC COMPLIANCE

Compliance can be described both in terms of static changes (Chapter 2)—that is, compliance at discrete points—and in dynamic changes created by breathing and time. **Dynamic compliance** is defined as the change in the volume of the lungs divided by the distending pressure during the course of a breath.

A dynamic pressure volume curve can be created by having an individual breathe over a normal lung volume range (usually from FRC to FRC + 1 L). The mean dynamic compliance of the lung (dyn CL) is calculated as the slope of the line that joins the end-inspiratory and end-expiratory points of no flow (Fig. 3.6).

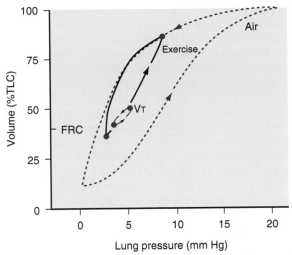

Fig. 3.6 Dynamic pressure–volume loops of the lung: resting tidal volume (VT) *(small loop)* and VT during exercise *(mid-sized loop)*. The maximum air-filled lung pressure–volume loop *(red loop)* from Fig. 2.9 is also shown. The dynamic compliance of the tidal breath (slope of the line connecting end inspiration with end expiration) is less than that of the lung during exercise. FRC, functional residual capacity; TLC, total lung capacity; VT, tidal volume. (Modified from Berne RM, Levy ML, eds. *Principles of Physiology*, 3rd ed. St. Louis: Mosby; 1999.)

Dynamic and static compliance are closely related in normal individuals. At a respiratory frequency of 15 breaths per minute or lower, dynamic compliance is slightly less than static compliance. This is because during tidal volume breathing there is a small change in alveolar surface area that is insufficient to bring additional surfactant molecules to the surface, and so the lung is less compliant. At higher respiratory frequencies, such as during exercise, dynamic compliance is slightly greater than static compliance. This is because during exercise there are large changes in tidal volume and more surfactant is incorporated into the air–liquid interface; thus the lung is more compliant. In individuals with increased airway resistance, the ratio of dynamic compliance to static compliance decreases significantly as respiratory rate increases. Thus dynamic compliance is affected not only by changes in lung compliance but also by changes in airway resistance.

Airway resistance contributes to the difference between static and dynamic compliance in individuals with obstructive pulmonary disease. Consider two alveoli supplied by the same airway (Fig. 3.7). If the resistance and compliance of the two units were equal, the two units would fill and empty with identical time courses. If, however, the resistance of the airways supplying each of the units were equal but the compliance of one of the units were decreased by half, the two units would fill with the same time course,

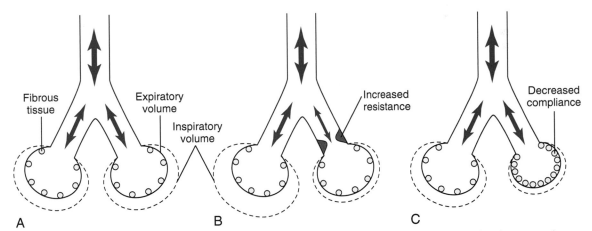

Fig. 3.7 Relationship between compliance and resistance. **A,** Two respiratory units with equal resistance and compliance will fill and empty with identical time courses. **B,** If the resistance of one airway is increased, the unit with the higher resistance will fill more slowly (note smaller arrow), and more of the ventilation will be distributed to the other unit (note larger inspiratory volume). **C,** If the compliance of one unit is decreased, the two units will fill with the same time course, but the volume of the unit with the decreased compliance will be less than the volume of the other unit. (Modified from Berne RM, Levy ML, eds. *Principles of Physiology*, 3rd ed. St. Louis: Mosby; 1999.)

but the unit with the lower compliance would receive only half of the volume of air of the other unit. Conversely, if the compliance of the two lung units were the same but the resistance of one unit were twice the resistance of the other unit, the unit with the higher resistance would fill more slowly than the other lung unit, although, given sufficient time, both units would fill to the same volume.

As respiratory rate increases, the unit with the lower resistance will accommodate a larger volume of air per breath. In addition, there will be a redistribution of air at the end of inspiration, because one alveolus will have more air than the other. As a result, because the compliance characteristics are the same, the more distended alveolus will have a higher elastic recoil pressure, and air will follow the pressure gradient and move to the other alveolus.

Alveoli supplied by airways with increased resistance (e.g., airway obstruction/disease) are referred to as having long time constants. The **time constant** (τ, or tau) of the lung is defined as the time (in seconds) necessary to inflate a particular lung region to 60% of its potential filling capacity. It is the product of airway resistance and lung compliance, and it is increased in diseases associated with either an increase in resistance or an increase in compliance (e.g., emphysema). For example, as respiratory frequency increases in individuals with small airway obstruction, alveoli with long time constants will have insufficient time to fill and will not contribute to the dynamic compliance. Dynamic compliance will decrease as the respiratory rate increases, and more and more of these alveoli with long time constants will drop out.

Sighing and yawning increase dynamic compliance by increasing tidal volume via restoring the normal surfactant layer. Both of these activities are important to maintaining normal compliance. In contrast to the lung, the dynamic compliance of the chest wall is not significantly different from its static compliance.

DYNAMIC AIRWAY COMPRESSION AND FLOW LIMITATION

Take a deep breath in and blow the air out while feeling the force of air movement against your hand. Note that as lung volume decreases, the flow rate felt by your hand decreases. Try now to increase that flow rate at low lung volumes by exerting greater expiratory effort. No matter how hard you try, expiratory flow rates decrease as lung volume decreases, and the maximum expiratory flow rate occurs at a relatively modest level of effort. This is called **expiratory flow limitation**. Expiratory flow limitation occurs when the airways, which are intrinsically floppy, distensible tubes, become compressed (**dynamic airway compression**). Airways become compressed when the pressure outside the airway is greater than the pressure inside the airway.

Consider the events that occur during expiratory flow at two different lung volumes (Fig. 3.8). The collective airways and alveoli are shown surrounded by the pleural space and the chest wall. In Fig. 3.8, the airways are shown as tapered tubes because the total or collective airway cross-sectional area decreases from the alveoli to the trachea. At the start of exhalation, but before any gas flow occurs, the alveolar pressure (P_A) is zero (no airflow), and the pleural pressure (P_{PL}), in this example, is -30 cm H_2O. The transpulmonary pressure (P_L) is thus $+30$ cm H_2O ($P_L = P_A - P_{PL}$). Because there is no flow, the pressure inside the airways is zero, and the pressure across the airways (P_{TA}, transairway pressure) is $+30$ cm H_2O ($P_{TA} = P_{airway} - P_{PL} = 0 - [-30$ cm $H_2O]$). This positive transpulmonary and transairway pressure holds the alveoli and the airways open.

When exhalation begins, the diaphragm relaxes and the pleural pressure rises to $+60$ cm H_2O. Alveolar pressure also rises; in part, this is due to the increase in pleural pressure (60 cm H_2O) (recall that at zero flow, pleural pressure and alveolar pressure are equal), and in part this is due to the elastic recoil pressure (P_{EL}) of the lung at that lung volume. The alveolar pressure is thus the sum of the pleural pressure and the elastic recoil pressure (which in this case is $+30$ cm H_2O). This is the driving pressure for expiratory gas flow. Because alveolar pressure ($P_A = P_{EL} + P_{PL} = 30$ cm $H_2O + 60$ cm $H_2O = 90$ cm H_2O in this example) is greater than atmospheric pressure, gas begins to flow from the alveolus to the mouth when the glottis opens. As gas flows out of the alveoli, the transmural pressure across the airways decreases (i.e., the pressure head for expiratory gas flow dissipates). This occurs for two reasons: first, there is a resistive pressure drop caused by the frictional pressure loss associated with flow (expiratory airflow resistance). The second reason is that as the cross-sectional area of the airways decreases toward the trachea, the gas velocity increases. This acceleration of gas flow further decreases the pressure due to the **Bernoulli principle** effect (Fig. 3.9).

Thus as air moves out of the lung, the driving pressure for expiratory gas flow decreases. In addition, the mechanical tethering (traction) that helps hold the airways open at high lung volumes decreases as lung volume decreases. There is a point between the alveoli and the mouth at which the pressure inside the airways is equal to the pressure surrounding the airways. This point is called the **equal pressure point**. Airways toward the mouth become compressed because the pressure outside is greater than the pressure inside (**dynamic airway compression**). As a consequence, the transairway pressure now becomes negative ($P_{TA} = P_{airway} - P_{PL} = 58 - [+60] = -2$ cm H_2O just beyond the

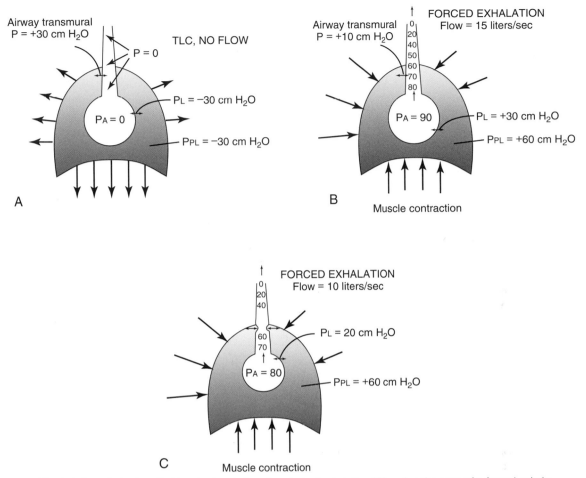

Fig. 3.8 Flow limitation. End inspiration, before the start of exhalation **(A)** and at the start of a forced exhalation **(B)**. **C,** Expiratory flow limitation later, in a forced exhalation. Expiratory flow limitation occurs at locations where airway diameter is narrowed as a result of a negative transmural pressure. See text for further explanation. (From Koeppen BM, Stanton BA, eds. *Berne and Levey's Physiology*, 7th ed. Philadelphia: Elsevier; 2018.)

equal pressure point), and no amount of greater effort will increase the flow further, because the higher pleural pressure will tend to collapse the airway at the equal pressure point just as much as it tends to increase the driving gradient for expiratory gas flow. Under these conditions, airflow is independent of the total driving pressure. This is why effort *independent expiratory flow limitation* occurs. It is also why airway resistance is higher during exhalation than inspiration.

In normal individuals, dynamic airway compression does not occur during a passive exhalation (Fig. 3.10). Consider a lung inflated to the same lung volume as before with the same elastic recoil. In the absence of forceful contraction of the muscles of exhalation, pleural pressure is slightly negative. The driving pressure for expiratory gas flow is the sum of the pleural pressure (-5 cm H_2O in this example) and elastic recoil pressure ($+30$ cm H_2O in this case) or 25 cm H_2O. Gas flows out of the lung when the glottis opens, and the pressure head is dissipated as lung volume decreases secondary to frictional resistance. However, at every point in which there is gas flow (alveolar pressure $-$ atmospheric pressure >0), the transmural pressure across the airway is positive, tending to hold the airway open. Thus during quiet breathing in normal individuals, there is no flow limitation and no dynamic airway compression.

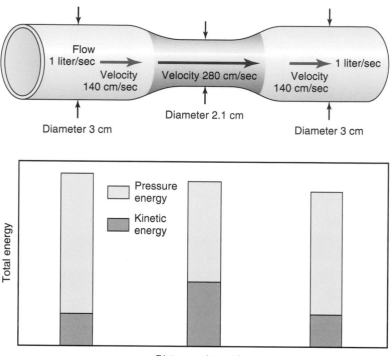

Fig. 3.9 The Bernoulli principle. As fluid moves through a tube at a constant flow rate, the total energy (kinetic plus potential energy) decreases as a result of frictional resistance (converting some of the energy into heat). At points of narrowing, fluid velocity increases, causing an increase in kinetic energy at the expense of potential energy. When the tube then widens, the fluid decelerates, and the kinetic energy is converted into pressure energy. Thus, as air moves from the larger to the smaller airways, rates of airflow decrease. Similarly, during exhalation, as small airways empty into large airways, rates of airflow increase. (Redrawn from Leff A, Schumacker P. *Respiratory Physiology: Basics and Applications.* Philadelphia: W.B. Saunders; 1993.)

In contrast, coughing is the best example of dynamic compression in normal individuals. At the start of a cough, the individual takes a deep breath (usually 1.5 times tidal volume), increasing elastic recoil; the glottis closes and the chest wall muscles contract, increasing pleural pressure. The glottis then opens and gas is forcefully expelled.

During the cough, the posterior membranous portion of the trachea is compressed and the tracheal diameter is narrowed (Fig. 3.11). Airflow at the site of compression is turbulent and makes the sound that we call a cough.

The measurement of expiratory flow rates is discussed in Chapter 4.

In the absence of lung disease, the equal pressure point occurs in airways that contain cartilage and thus resist deformation. The equal pressure point, however, is not static. As lung volume decreases and the elastic recoil pressure decreases, the equal pressure point moves closer to the alveoli. The smallest airways, which have no cartilaginous support and rely on the traction of alveolar septa to help keep them open, may be compressed or even collapse. Whether they actually collapse depends on the transmural pressure gradient across the walls of the smallest airways.

In individuals with lung disease such as airway obstruction secondary to a combination of mucus and airway inflammation, at the start of exhalation, the driving pressure for expiratory gas flow is the same as in a normal individual—that is, it is the sum of the elastic recoil pressure and the pleural pressure. As exhalation proceeds, however, there is a greater resistive drop in the pressure head due to the decrease in airway radius secondary to mucus and inflammation. As a result, the point at which the pressure inside the airway is equal to the pressure outside now occurs in smaller airways without cartilage. These airways become compressed and readily collapse as the equal pressure point moves even closer to the alveolus. **Premature airway closure** occurs, resulting in air trapping and an increase in lung volume. The increase in lung volume initially helps offset the increase in airway resistance due to the mucus and inflammation by increasing airway caliber and increasing elastic recoil. As inflammation progresses or mucus increases, flow

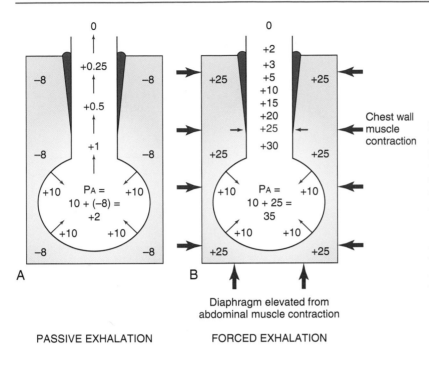

A   PASSIVE EXHALATION

B   FORCED EXHALATION

Diaphragm elevated from
abdominal muscle contraction

Fig. 3.10 Dynamic airway compression. **A,** During passive exhalation, intraairway pressure remains positive and greater than pleural pressure; no dynamic compression occurs. **B,** With a forced exhalation, the driving pressure for expiratory gas flow is still the sum of the elastic recoil pressure (+10 cm H_2O) and the pleural pressure (+25 H_2O). As gas moves out of the alveoli, the pressure head is dissipated due to frictional resistance. At some point in the airways, the intraairway pressure is equal to the pleural pressure (equal pressure point; red arrows). Beyond this point, the pleural (outside) pressure is greater than airway (inside) pressure and airways are compressed. P_A, alveolar pressure.

limitation occurs, and maximal expiratory flow rates decrease. Premature airway closure is the mechanism responsible for the appearance of crackles on auscultation in individuals with lung disease. It can be due to mucus, airway inflammation, fluid in the airways, or any mechanism responsible for airway narrowing or compression and can also be due to loss of elastic recoil (emphysema). In fact, acute and chronic lung diseases can alter the expiratory flow volume relationship as a result of any of the following:

- Changes in static lung recoil pressures
- Changes in airway resistance and the distribution of resistance along the airways
- Loss of mechanical tethering of intraparenchymal airways
- Changes in stiffness or mechanical properties of the airways
- Differences in the severity of the previous changes among lung regions

Airway closure can be demonstrated only at especially low lung volumes in healthy individuals, but the lung volume at which airway closure occurs (the closing volume) in individuals with obstructive pulmonary diseases is much higher. The measurement of this closing volume is discussed in Chapter 4.

THE WORK OF BREATHING

Breathing requires the use of respiratory muscles (e.g., diaphragm, intercostals) that expend energy; thus work is involved in inspiration and (to a lesser extent) in exhalation. Work is required to overcome the inherent mechanical properties of the lung (i.e., elastic and flow resistive forces) to move both the lungs and the chest wall. In the respiratory system, the work of breathing is the change in volume multiplied by the pressure exerted across the respiratory system. The pressure change is the change in transpulmonary pressure that is required to overcome the elastic work of breathing and the resistance work of breathing. The volume change is the volume of air that is moving in and out of the lung (e.g., the tidal volume at rest); that is,

$$\text{Work of breathing (W)} = \text{pressure (P)} \times \text{change in volume } (\Delta V)$$

The elastic component of the work of breathing is composed of the work associated with overcoming the elastic recoil of the chest wall and lung parenchyma and the work associated with overcoming the surface tension of the

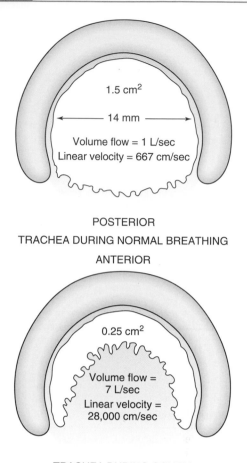

TRACHEA DURING COUGH

Fig. 3.11 Tracheal dimensions and air velocity during cough. With coughing, the noncartilaginous posterior membrane of the trachea is inverted, decreasing the size of the tracheal lumen to one-sixth of normal. With an increase in flow rate of 7-fold during a cough, the linear velocity of air increases 42-fold. (Redrawn from Comroe JH. *Physiology of Respiration.* Chicago: Year Book Medical Publishers; 1965.)

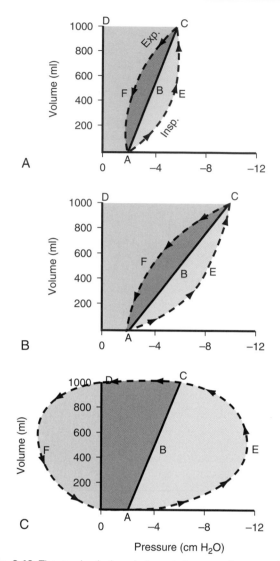

Fig. 3.12 The mechanical work done during a respiratory cycle in a normal lung **(A)**, a lung with reduced compliance **(B)**, and a lung with increased airway resistance **(C)**. Exp., expiratory; F, flow; Insp., inspiratory. (From Koeppen BM, Stanton BA, eds. *Berne and Levey's Physiology*, 7th ed. Philadelphia: Elsevier; 2018.)

alveoli. The resistive component of the work of breathing is the work associated with overcoming the tissue (lung) and airway resistance.

Although methods are not available to measure the total amount of work involved in breathing, one can estimate the mechanical work necessary by measuring volume and pressure changes during a respiratory cycle. Work of breathing can be illustrated by analysis of the pressure–volume curves shown in Fig. 3.12. Panel A is representative of a respiratory cycle of a normal lung. The static inflation–deflation curve is represented by line ABC. The total mechanical workload is represented by the trapezoidal area 0AECD. A breakdown of the trapezoidal areas in Panel A enables one to appreciate individual aspects of the mechanical work load, which includes the following areas:

0ABCD—work necessary to overcome elastic resistance

AECF—work necessary to overcome nonelastic resistance

AECB—work necessary to overcome nonelastic resistance during inspiration

ABCF—work necessary to overcome nonelastic resistance during exhalation (represents stored elastic energy from inspiration)

In restrictive lung diseases such as pulmonary fibrosis in which lung compliance is decreased or in obese individuals who have increased inward chest elastic recoil pressure, the elastic work of breathing is increased, the pressure–volume curve is shifted to the right, and thus the work of breathing is increased significantly (see Panel B in Fig. 3.12), as seen by the increase in the trapezoidal area 0AECD. In obstructive lung diseases such as asthma and chronic bronchitis, in which airway resistance is elevated, or in diseases associated with increased tissue resistance such as sarcoidosis, greater negative pleural pressures are needed to maintain proper inspiratory flow rates. In addition to the increase in total inspiratory work (area 0AECD), individuals with such conditions have an increase in positive pleural pressure during exhalation due to the increase in resistance and also an increased expiratory workload visualized as area DF0. This is because the stored elastic energy in area ABCF in Panel A is not sufficient, and additional energy is needed for exhalation. For these individuals, the resistive work of breathing can be extremely high during a forced exhalation associated with dynamic compression. Respiratory muscles are capable of performing increased work over long periods of time, but like other skeletal muscles, they can fatigue. **Respiratory muscle fatigue** is a major problem in individuals with lung disease and can result in respiratory failure.

In addition to the diseases just mentioned, work of breathing is influenced by breathing patterns. Work of breathing is increased when deeper breaths are taken (increase in tidal volume requires more elastic work to overcome) or when there is an increase in the respiratory rate (increase in minute ventilation requires more flow-resistance forces to overcome) (Fig. 3.13). As would be anticipated, individuals with normal lungs and individuals with lung disease adopt the respiratory patterns at which the work of breathing is the lowest. Individuals with pulmonary fibrosis (high elastic work) breathe more shallowly and rapidly, whereas individuals with obstructive lung disease (nonelastic work, high resistive work) breathe more slowly and deeply.

In normal individuals, the oxygen cost of quiet breathing is less than 5% of the total body oxygen uptake. This oxygen cost can increase to 30% during maximal exercise. In individuals with obstructive pulmonary disease, the work of breathing is high and can become the limiting factor in exercise.

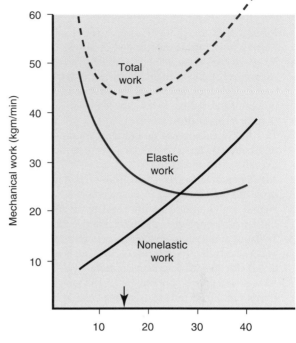

Fig. 3.13 The effect of respiratory rate on the elastic, nonelastic, and total mechanical work of breathing at a given level of alveolar ventilation. Subjects tend to adopt the respiratory rate at which the total of work of breathing (the sum of the elastic work and the nonelastic work) is minimal *(arrow)*. (From Koeppen BM, Stanton BA, eds. *Berne and Levey's Physiology*, 7th ed. Philadelphia: Elsevier; 2018.)

CLINICAL BOX

Cystic fibrosis is an inherited disease associated with the production of thick, sticky mucus that is difficult to remove. One of the earliest changes in pulmonary physiology associated with the disease is obstruction of the small, peripheral airways. Although these changes result in airway obstruction, the earliest abnormality that is detected in the disease is not an increase in airway resistance but an increase in residual volume secondary to air trapping. This increase in residual volume alters the position of the equal pressure point (moving it from the peripheral, small airways to the larger airways secondary to an increase in alveolar volume and thus an increase in elastic recoil pressure). As a result, there are no crackles (or rales) and no symptoms may be present. Only with further mucus retention and an inability to compensate for further air trapping are both symptoms of cough and crackles on physical examination apparent. It is important in a progressive disease such as cystic fibrosis to detect these abnormalities early and institute appropriate preventive therapy and treatment.

SUMMARY

1. Resistance is the change in pressure per unit of flow. Airway resistance is determined by airway caliber and length as well as gas velocity and density.
2. Airway resistance is highly sensitive to changes in airway radius and varies with the inverse of the fourth power of the radius. Resistance is higher in turbulent than in laminar flow.
3. The first eight airway generations are the major site of airway resistance. Small airways contribute little to overall airway resistance.
4. Airway resistance decreases with increases in lung volume and with increases in elastic recoil.
5. Neural and humoral agents regulate or affect airway resistance through their effects on airway smooth muscle.
6. Dynamic and static compliance are closely related in normal individuals, but dynamic compliance is much lower in individuals with obstructive pulmonary disease.
7. Airway resistance contributes to the long time constants present in individuals with obstructive pulmonary disease.
8. Flow limitation occurs when dynamic airway compression is present.
9. The equal pressure point is the point at which the pressure inside and the pressure surrounding the airway are the same. As lung volume and elastic recoil decrease during exhalation, the equal pressure point moves toward the alveolus in normal individuals, resulting in dynamic compression and expiratory flow limitation. In individuals with chronic obstructive pulmonary disease (COPD), at any lung volume the equal pressure point is closer to the alveolus, resulting in greater expiratory flow limitation and decreased expiratory flow rates.
10. Work of breathing is the change in volume times the pressure exerted across the respiratory system and is composed of elastic and nonelastic (resistive) components. Work of breathing is elevated in individuals with obstructive pulmonary diseases. All individuals breathe at a respiratory frequency that minimizes the work of breathing.

KEYWORDS AND CONCEPTS

Airway resistance (Raw)
Alveolar interdependence
Bernoulli principle
Dynamic airway compression
Dynamic compliance
Equal pressure point
Expiratory flow limitation
Flow limitation

Frictional resistance
Poiseuille's law
Premature airway closure
Respiratory muscle fatigue
Status asthmaticus
Time constant
Velocity profile
Work of breathing

SELF-STUDY PROBLEMS

1. What is the effect of lung volume on airway resistance?
2. What are the factors that control the cross-sectional area of an airway?
3. What is the effect of a reduction in elastic recoil pressure on the location of the equal pressure point?
4. Why are large airways the major contributors to the resistance of the respiratory system compared with small airways?

ADDITIONAL READINGS

Brown RH, Mitzner W. Effects of lung inflation and airway muscle tone on airway diameter in vivo. *J Appl Physiol.* 1996;(80):1581–1588.

Cheung D, Schot R, Zwindermann AH, et al. Relationship between loss in parenchymal recoil pressure and maximal airway narrowing in subjects with alpha-1-antitrypsin deficiency. *Am J Respir Crit Care Med.* 1997;155:135–140.

D'Angelo E, Robatto FM, Calderini E, et al. Pulmonary and chest wall mechanics in anesthetized paralyzed humans. *J Appl Physiol.* 1991;70:2602–2610.

George RB, Light RW, Matthay MA, Matthay RA, eds. *Chest Medicine: Essentials of Pulmonary and Critical Care Medicine.* 5th ed. Philadelphia: Lippincott-Williams and Wilkins; 2005.

Lai-Fook SJ, Rodarte JR. Pleural pressure distribution and its relationship to lung volume and interstitial pressure. *J Appl Physiol.* 1991;70:967–978.

Zapletal A, Desmond KJ, Demizio D, et al. Lung recoil and the determination of airflow limitation in cystic fibrosis and asthma. *Pediatr Pulmonol.* 1993;15:13–18.

4

Tests of Lung Function

OBJECTIVES

1. Describe lung volumes and their measurement using three methods.
2. Discuss the uses of spirometry in clinical practice.
3. Define the effort-dependent and effort-independent portions of the flow volume curve.
4. Outline an approach to the interpretation of lung volumes, spirometry, and flow volume curves.
5. Describe the physiology behind the diffusion capacity for carbon monoxide and list three diseases associated with abnormal results.
6. Briefly outline the measurement of resistance and compliance.

Pulmonary function tests are designed to identify and quantify abnormalities in lung function. With the exception of exercise-induced asthma, pulmonary function tests do not diagnose disease. Rather, they describe pathophysiologic processes and help distinguish between cardiac and pulmonary disease. The two major groups of pathophysiologic processes that can be distinguished using pulmonary function tests are obstructive pulmonary disease (OPD) and restrictive pulmonary disease (RLD). Pulmonary function test results are a major contributing element of the history, physical examination, and laboratory data that aid clinicians in making a diagnosis and in assessing response to therapy and disease progression.

LUNG VOLUME MEASUREMENT

As a general rule, all lung volumes are measured in liters. The most important lung volume measurement is the vital capacity (VC) or the total volume of air that an individual is able to exhale from a full and maximal inspiration to a maximal exhalation (see Chapter 2). When measured as a rapid exhalation, it is called the **forced vital capacity** (FVC). The FVC varies with age, height, sex, and ethnicity but is approximately 4 L in a healthy adult male.

The VC can also be measured as a slow exhalation (called the **slow vital capacity** [SVC]). In individuals with normal lung function, the FVC and the SVC are the same. In the presence of premature airway closure, however, the SVC is greater than the FVC because air trapping occurs during a forced maneuver secondary to dynamic airway closure (see Chapter 3). The difference between the SVC and the FVC is thus a measure of dynamic airway closure and is used more often by physiologists than clinicians.

Many lung volumes are altered in the presence of disease (Table 4.1). The vital capacity is decreased in both obstructive and restrictive lung diseases. In the presence of chest wall muscle weakness, the chest wall outward recoil pressure is decreased, the lung recoil pressure is less opposed, and the functional residual capacity (FRC) decreases. In contrast, in the presence of air trapping, the FRC increases.

The relationship between residual volume (RV) and total lung capacity (TLC) is called the **RV/TLC** ratio and is often used to help distinguish between restrictive pulmonary disease and OPD. In normal individuals, the RV/TLC ratio is less than 25%. An elevated RV/TLC ratio due to an increase in RV out of proportion to any change in TLC is caused by air trapping secondary to airway obstruction. An elevated RV/TLC ratio due to a decrease in TLC out of proportion to any change in RV is seen in individuals with restrictive lung disease.

MEASUREMENT OF LUNG VOLUMES

There are three commonly used methods to measure lung volumes: inert gas dilution, plethysmography, and nitrogen washout.

Inert Gas Dilution Technique

In the inert gas dilution technique (Fig. 4.1), a known concentration of an inert gas such as helium, argon, or neon (this example uses helium) is added to a spirometer system that has a known volume. At FRC, the subject is connected to the system and breathes in the closed system until the helium concentration reaches a plateau, indicating equal concentrations of helium in the spirometer system and in the subject's lung. Because helium is inert, the new helium concentration after equilibrium in the subject's lung has occurred can be used to determine the subject's FRC by solving for V_2 using the mass balance equation:

$$C_1 V_1 = C_2 (V_1 + V_2)$$

where C_1 is the initial concentration of helium in the spirometer system, V_1 is the volume of the spirometer system, C_2 is the new concentration of helium at equilibrium in the subject's lung and spirometer, and V_2 is the subject's FRC. By measuring the FRC, other lung volumes such as RV and TLC can be determined by subtracting the ERV from the FRC to get RV and by adding the RV to the FVC to get TLC.

Plethysmography

Plethysmography can also measure lung volumes and is the preferred method. The principle of plethysmography is based on Boyle's law ($P_1 V_1 = P_2 V_2$ at a constant [isothermal] temperature [Appendix C]). The gas in the lungs is isothermal because of its intimate contact with capillary blood.

TABLE 4.1 Lung Volume Abnormalities in Obstructive and Restrictive Pulmonary Diseases

	Obstructive Lung Disease	Restrictive Lung Disease
TLC	N→↑	↓
RV	↑	↓→N
FRC	↑	↓
RV/TLC (%)	↑	N→↑

FRC, functional residual capacity; RV, residual volume; TLC, total lung capacity; N, normal; ↑, increased; ↓, decreased.

A plethysmograph (also known as a body box) is an airtight box with pressure transducers for measuring the pressure inside the box and at the mouth (Fig. 4.2). The mouth pressure measured with an open glottis and no airflow reflects alveolar pressure. The change in pressure inside the box is related to volume by introducing a small volume of gas into the box and measuring the change in pressure. The subject sits inside the airtight box and breathes through a mouthpiece connected to the outside. With temperature constant, the shutter on the mouthpiece closes and the individual gently and slowly pants against the closed mouthpiece (Fig. 4.3). The change in pressure in the mouthpiece reflects alveolar pressure (there is essentially no airflow). Pressure changes inside the box reflect changes in pulmonary gas volume as gas within the chest is alternately compressed and decompressed by the action of the respiratory muscles. If the valve at the mouth closes while the subject is making an expiratory effort, alveolar pressure increases by an amount that is measured by the mouth pressure sensor, lung volume decreases as a result of gas compression, and, with no airflow, the pressure inside the plethysmograph decreases. This pressure change is related back to a change in volume, and all the elements of Boyle's law are now present to solve for lung volume at FRC.

In individuals with normal lungs, FRC measured by helium dilution and by plethysmography are the same. The inert gas technique, however, can markedly underestimate FRC in individuals with OPD, because equilibration of the helium in markedly obstructed airways may not have occurred during the test (these areas have very long time constants). In contrast, plethysmography measures all gas in the lung at FRC, including trapped gas. Because of this, the difference in FRC measured by plethysmography and FRC measured by helium dilution has been used (primarily by physiologists) as a measure of trapped gas.

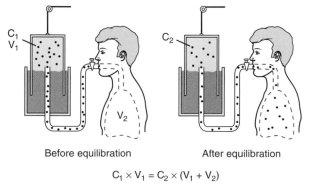

Before equilibration   After equilibration

$$C_1 \times V_1 = C_2 \times (V_1 + V_2)$$

Fig. 4.1 Measurement of lung volume by helium dilution. C, concentration of helium; V, volume. (From Koeppen BM, Stanton BA, eds. *Berne and Levy Physiology*, 7th ed. Philadelphia: Elsevier; 2018.)

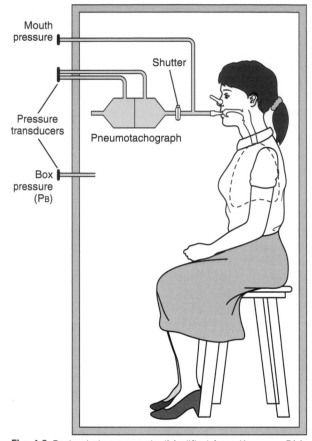

Mouth
pressure

Shutter

Pressure
transducers

Pneumotachograph

Box
pressure
(PB)

Fig. 4.2 Body plethysmograph. (Modified from Koeppen BM, Stanton BA, eds. *Berne and Levy's Physiology*, 7th ed. Philadelphia: Elsevier; 2018.)

Nitrogen Washout Technique

The nitrogen washout technique is similar in many ways to the inert gas technique. The subject is connected to the system at end exhalation and breathes nitrogen-free air (Fig. 4.4). At the start of the test, the lung contains 80% nitrogen that is evenly distributed. The volume of exhaled gas is collected into a bag and the nitrogen concentration is measured. Using the simple mass balance equation ($C_1V_1 = C_2V_2$), the concentration of nitrogen at the start (C_1) (i.e., in the lung) and at the end (C_2) (i.e., in the bag) is known, and the volume in the bag is known (V_2). The equation is then solved for the volume in the lung (V_1). The nitrogen washout technique is used infrequently because, like the inert gas technique, it underestimates FRC in individuals with airway obstruction; it can also be uncomfortable for subjects, and it requires a nitrogen analyzer and bags to collect expiratory gas.

SPIROMETRY

The rapidity with which air flows out of the lung (known as the expiratory flow rate) can be measured using spirometry. Spirometry measures the rate at which the lung changes volume during a forced breathing maneuver (Fig. 4.5). When performed from TLC, spirometry measures the FVC. In the "FVC maneuver," the subject breathes in and out of a mouthpiece that is connected to a spirometry machine. The subject is then instructed to inhale maximally and then exhale as rapidly, as forcibly, and as completely as possible until he or she is unable to exhale further.

The FVC maneuver can be displayed in two ways: as a spirogram (volume/time curve) and as a flow volume loop.

Spirogram Display

In a spirogram, the volume of gas exhaled is plotted against time (Fig. 4.6A). The spirogram reports four major test results:

1. The forced vital capacity (FVC)
2. The forced expiratory volume in 1 second (FEV_1)
3. The ratio of the FEV_1 to the FVC (FEV_1/FVC)
4. The average midmaximal expiratory flow (MMEF), also known as the forced expiratory flow between 25% and 75% of the VC (FEF_{25-75}).

The FVC is measured directly from the spirogram tracing and is the total volume of air that is exhaled during a forced exhalation; it is reported in liters. The volume of air that is exhaled in the first second during the maneuver is called the FEV_1, and it is also measured directly from the spirogram tracing and is reported in liters. The FEV_1/FVC ratio varies with age. It is 85% in children and decreases with age, but even in the elderly it is greater than 70%. An FEV_1/FVC ratio less than 70% suggests obstruction to expiratory gas flow and is a hallmark of OPD. The fourth test that can be measured from the spirogram is the average flow rate over the middle section of the VC. This test has several names, including MMEF (midmaximal expiratory flow) and FEF_{25-75}. It can be calculated from the spirogram tracing by dividing the VC into quarters, dropping a line from the first (25%) and third (75%) quartiles, and then connecting the lines and measuring the slope (see Fig. 4.6A). Volume/time is a flow rate and thus the slope of this line is an expiratory flow rate, the only flow rate that can easily be obtained from the spirogram. Although the maximum or peak expiratory flow rate (PEFR) can also be obtained from the spirogram by measuring the maximum slope, this is rarely done because there are easier and more accurate ways of making this measurement. Occasionally, other measures are obtained using the

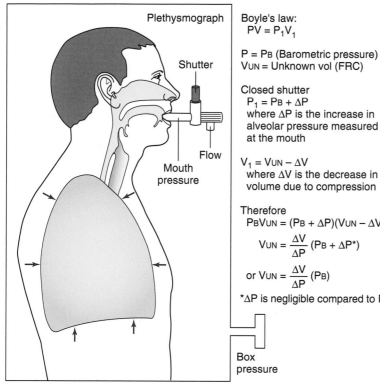

Plethysmograph

Shutter

Flow

Mouth
pressure

Box
pressure

Boyle's law:
$$PV = P_1V_1$$

$P = P_B$ (Barometric pressure)
V_{UN} = Unknown vol (FRC)

Closed shutter
$$P_1 = P_B + \Delta P$$
where ΔP is the increase in
alveolar pressure measured
at the mouth

$$V_1 = V_{UN} - \Delta V$$
where ΔV is the decrease in
volume due to compression

Therefore
$$P_B V_{UN} = (P_B + \Delta P)(V_{UN} - \Delta V)$$

$$V_{UN} = \frac{\Delta V}{\Delta P}(P_B + \Delta P^*)$$

or $$V_{UN} = \frac{\Delta V}{\Delta P}(P_B)$$

*ΔP is negligible compared to P_B.

Fig. 4.3 Measurement of functional residual capacity by body plethysmography. See text for details. (Modified from Hyatt RE, Scanlon PD, Nakamura M. *Interpretation of Pulmonary Function Tests: A Practical Guide*, 4th ed. Rochester, MN: Scientific Publications; 2014.)

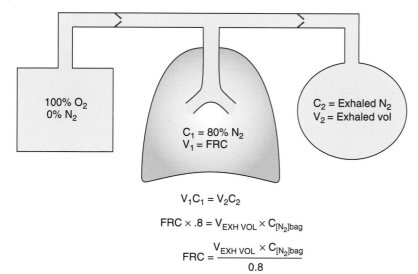

100% O_2
0% N_2

C_1 = 80% N_2
V_1 = FRC

C_2 = Exhaled N_2
V_2 = Exhaled vol

$$V_1C_1 = V_2C_2$$

$$FRC \times .8 = V_{EXH\ VOL} \times C_{[N_2]bag}$$

$$FRC = \frac{V_{EXH\ VOL} \times C_{[N_2]bag}}{0.8}$$

Fig. 4.4 Measurement of functional residual capacity (FRC) by the nitrogen washout method. See text for details. $V_{EXH\ VOL}$, Volume of the bag in which the exhaled gas is collected, or the exhaled volume of gas. (Modified from Hyatt RE, Scanlon PD, Nakamura M. *Interpretation of Pulmonary Function Tests: A Practical Guide*, 4th ed. Rochester, MN: Scientific Publications; 2014.)

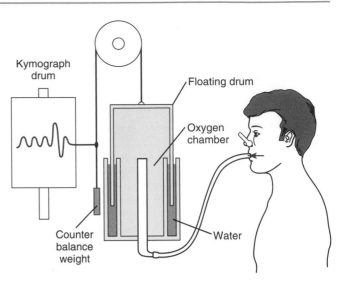

Fig. 4.5 Simple water-seal spirometer. (From Koeppen BM, Stanton BA, eds. *Physiology,* 7th ed. Philadelphia: Elsevier; 2018.)

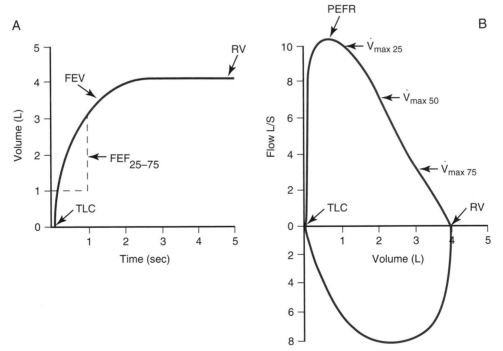

Fig. 4.6 The clinical spirogram **(A)** and expiratory flow volume curve **(B)**. The subject takes a maximal inspiration and then exhales as rapidly, forcefully, and maximally as possible. The volume exhaled is plotted as a function of time. In the spirogram that is reported in clinical settings, exhaled volume increases from the bottom of the trace to the top **(A)**. This is in contrast to the physiologist's view of the same maneuver (see Fig. 2.1) in which the exhaled volume increases from the top to the bottom of the trace. Note the locations of TLC and RV on both tracings. FEF, forced expiratory flow; FEV, forced expiratory volume; PEFR, peak expiratory flow rate; RV, residual volume; TLC, total lung capacity; $\dot{V}_{max}$, maximal expiratory flow rate. (From Koeppen BM, Stanton BA, eds. *Physiology,* 7th ed. Philadelphia: Elsevier; 2018.)

spirogram, including FEV_3 and FEV_6, forced expiratory volume exhaled at 3 seconds and 6 seconds, respectively. The value of these additional measurements compared with FEV_1 and FVC is not clear except in individuals with severe obstruction.

Flow Volume Loop Display

The FVC maneuver can also be displayed as a flow volume loop in which the instantaneous inspiratory and expiratory flow rates are plotted against volume (see Fig. 4.6B). It is created in the same way as the spirogram. The subject puts his mouth around a mouthpiece and breathes normally (tidal volume [V_T]). The subject is then asked to take a maximal inspiration to TLC and to breathe out as fast, forcefully, and rapidly as he can until he can exhale no further (a maximal exhalation to RV), at which time he takes a rapid and maximal inspiration back to TLC. Flow rates above the horizontal line are expiratory, whereas flow rates below the horizontal line are inspiratory. The point on the flow volume loop at which maximal inspiration has occurred is the TLC, and the point at which maximal exhalation has occurred is the RV.

Expiratory Flow Volume Curve

The expiratory flow volume curve gives results for four main pulmonary function tests. Again, the total amount of air that can be exhaled is the FVC. The greatest flow rate achieved during the maneuver is the PEFR. The expiratory flow volume curve can also be divided into quarters. The instantaneous flow rate at which 50% of the VC remains to be exhaled is called the FEF_{50} (also known as the $\dot{V}_{max50}$). The flow rate at which 75% of the VC has been exhaled is called the $\dot{V}_{max75}$, and the flow rate at which 25% of the VC has been exhaled is called the $\dot{V}_{max25}$.*

DETERMINANTS OF MAXIMAL FLOW

In general, the maximum inspiratory flow rate is the same or slightly greater than the maximal expiratory flow rate. Three major factors are responsible for the maximum inspiratory flow rate. The first factor is the force generated by the inspiratory muscles that is greatest at RV and then decreases as lung volume increases above RV; the second factor is the increase of the static

recoil pressure of the lung as the lung volume increases above RV and as lung elastic fibers are stretched. This opposes the force generated by the inspiratory muscles and tends to reduce maximum inspiratory flow rates. The third factor is the airway resistance that decreases with increasing lung volume as airway caliber increases. The combination of the inspiratory muscle force, the static recoil of the lung, and the changes in airway resistance causes maximal inspiratory flow to occur about halfway between TLC and RV.

During exhalation, maximal flow occurs early (in the first 20%) in the maneuver, and flow rates decrease progressively as lung volume decreases. Even with increasing effort, maximal flow will decrease as RV is approached ("expiratory flow limitation"; see Chapter 3). Expiratory flow limitation can be demonstrated by asking an individual to perform three forced expiratory maneuvers with increasing effort. Fig. 4.7 shows the superimposed results of these maneuvers. As effort increases, peak expiratory flow increases. However, the flow rates at lower lung volumes converge, indicating that with modest effort maximal expiratory flow is achieved. No amount of effort will increase these flow rates at lower lung volumes. For this reason, expiratory flow rates at lower lung volumes are said to be **effort-independent** because maximal flow is achieved with modest effort. In this range, the expiratory flow rate is flow-limited by the lung and no amount of additional effort can increase the flow rate beyond this limit. In contrast, events early in the expiratory maneuver are said to be **effort-dependent**. That is, increasing effort generates increasing flow rates. In general, the first 20% of the flow in the expiratory flow volume loop is effort-dependent.

INTERPRETING THE VITAL CAPACITY MANEUVER

Two important principles are useful in interpreting the VC maneuver: (1) events that occur early in the maneuver reflect large airway function, and (2) different patterns of abnormalities are found in obstructive and restrictive lung disease. It is important not only to look at the values reported for the various tests but also to examine carefully the shape of the spirogram or flow volume curve.

In general, OPD is categorized by premature airway closure, which is manifested in pulmonary function tests by decreases in expiratory flow rates secondary to airway obstruction, and by increases in lung volumes due to air trapping. In OPD, the usual sequence of abnormalities in pulmonary function is an increase in RV and in

---

*In the pediatric literature, the flow rate at which 75% of the FVC has been exhaled is called the $\dot{V}_{max25}$ (25% of the FVC remained to be exhaled), and the flow rate at which 25% of the VC has been exhaled is called the $\dot{V}_{max75}$ (75% of the FVC remained to be exhaled). To distinguish which nomenclature system is being used, look at the lowest of th $\dot{V}_{e_{max}}$ flow rates. This is the flow rate closest to residual volume.

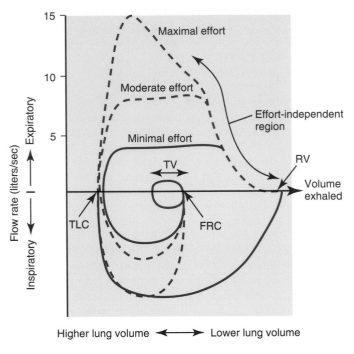

Fig. 4.7 Isovolume curves. Three superimposed expiratory flow maneuvers are made with increasing effort. Note that peak inspiratory and expiratory flow rates are effort-dependent, whereas expiratory flow rates later in expiration are effort-independent. FRC, functional residual capacity; RV, residual volume; TLC, total lung capacity; TV, tidal volume. (From Koeppen BM, Stanton BA, eds. *Physiology,* 7th ed. Philadelphia: Elsevier; 2018.)

the RV/TLC ratio, followed by a decrease in expiratory flow rates, then by a decrease in FEV_1, and finally by a decrease in FVC; that is, air trapping and decreases in expiratory flow rates are seen with early airway obstruction or mild disease. Decreases in FEV_1 (in addition to greater decreases in expiratory flow rates) occur with moderate airway obstruction and decreases in FVC (in conjunction with a marked decrease in FEV_1 and in expiratory flow rates) occur with more advanced airway obstructive disease.

In OPD, the FEV_1 is decreased out of proportion to any change in FVC. Thus the hallmark of OPD is a decrease in the FEV_1/FVC ratio due to a decrease in FEV_1 out of proportion to any change in FVC. This latter distinction is important because the FEV_1 is also decreased in restrictive pulmonary disease (Table 4.2).

Early events, such as the PEFR, reflect large airway function, whereas events that occur late (the last 80%) reflect small airway obstruction. For example, in someone with small airway obstruction, the only abnormality on spirometry might be a decrease in the $\dot{V}_{max75}$. In contrast, in someone with large airway obstruction such as paralysis of a vocal cord, the only abnormality might be a decrease in PEFR.

TABLE 4.2   Patterns of Abnormalities in Pulmonary Function Tests

Pulmonary Function Measurement	OPD	RLD
FVC (L)	↓	↓
FEV_1 (L)	↓	↓
FEV_1/FVC	↓	N
FEF_{25-75} (L/sec)	↓	N
PEFR (L/sec)	↓	N
FEF_{50} (L/sec)	↓	N
FEF_{75} (L/sec)	↓	N
Slope of FVC curve	↓	N to ↑

OPD, obstructive pulmonary disease; FEV, forced expiratory volume; FVC, forced vital capacity; FEF, forced expiratory flow; PEFR, peak expiratory flow rate; RLD, restrictive lung disease; N, normal; ↑, increased; ↓, decreased.

The shapes of the spirogram and flow volume curve can also help in determining the presence of airway obstruction. In OPD, the slope of the rise in volume with time is reduced; these changes are reflected both in the FEF_{25-75} and in the FEV_1. On the flow volume

---

> **BOX 4.1   Causes of Abnormal Vital Capacity**
>
> **Pulmonary Lesions**
> - Loss of distensible lung tissue
> - Pulmonary edema
> - Pneumonia
> - Atelectasis
> - Surgical resection
> - Bronchogenic carcinoma
>
> **Nonpulmonary Lesions**
> - Neuromuscular disease
> - Thoracic space reduction (pleural effusion, pneumothorax, cardiac enlargement)
> - Diaphragm movement limitation (pregnancy, ascites)
> - Chest wall movement limitation (scleroderma, kyphoscoliosis, pain)

curve, the shape of the downward slope changes and becomes concave or sags. As disease progresses, these changes become more severe. A flattening of the expiratory or inspiratory limbs of the flow volume curve also has significance and is indicative of extrathoracic airway obstruction.

In restrictive lung diseases, volumes are decreased whereas flow rates are maintained until late in the disease process. In individuals with restrictive lung diseases, VC and FEV_1 are reduced; however, in contrast to OPD, the decreases are proportional; that is, the FEV_1/FVC ratio is normal (Table 4.2). The shape of the flow volume curve and the spirogram appear normal but are reduced in size, reflecting the reductions in FVC with normal (or even supranormal) expiratory flow rates.

APPROACH TO INTERPRETING LUNG VOLUMES, SPIROGRAMS, AND FLOW VOLUME CURVES

The first step to interpreting pulmonary function tests is to examine the quality and reproducibility of the test (Fig. 4.8). This is especially important in regard to the spirogram and flow volume curve because patient cooperation and maximal effort are required. The test is reproducible if the FVC and FEV_1 on three maneuvers are within 5% to 10% of each other. On inspection, a good test is associated with a rapid rise in expiratory flow with a smooth decline as the RV is approached.

On the spirogram, there should be a clear plateau with a change of less than 200 mL in exhaled volume over the last 2 seconds of the maneuver and a total expiratory time of 6 seconds or greater in adults (2 seconds or greater in children).

If the spirogram and flow volume curve are reproducible and of high quality, the results can be interpreted. Next, examine the shape of the flow volume curve and its relationship to normal (Fig. 4.9). The greater the discrepancy between the subject's curve and the normal curve, the greater the ventilatory abnormality. A concave shape with a decreased slope is indicative of an obstructive process. In contrast, a steep slope with a reduced FVC is consistent with restrictive lung disease.

Next, examine the test values. A reduced FEV_1 out of proportion to a change in FVC with low expiratory flow rates and elevated lung volumes with an increase in the RV/TLC ratio due to an increase in RV out of proportion to any change in TLC are indicative of OPD. A reduced FEV_1 with a reduced FVC and a normal FEV_1/FVC ratio in conjunction with preserved expiratory flow rates (except in severe disease) with reduced lung volumes and an elevated RV/TLC ratio secondary to a reduction in TLC out of proportion to a change in RV are hallmarks of restrictive pulmonary disease. The degree of ventilatory limitation can be defined by the loss of area under the normal curve. An area loss of 25% is defined as mild, 50% as moderate, and 75% as severe ventilatory limitation.

PEAK EXPIRATORY FLOW RATE

The peak expiratory flow rate (PEFR) can be read directly from the expiratory flow volume curve and can be measured using a peak flow meter. Peak flow meters are portable, inexpensive, and easy to use. As a result, they are often used at home, especially by individuals with asthma, to monitor airway caliber and disease status. More than other measures, peak expiratory flow is very dependent on patient effort. The individual must exhale as forcefully as possible to obtain reproducible results. Another limitation is that peak expiratory flow measures large airway function; thus the PEFR can both underestimate and overestimate the overall degree of airway obstruction.

OTHER USEFUL TESTS OF LUNG FUNCTION

Although the VC maneuver is the single most important pulmonary function test, other tests are useful in helping

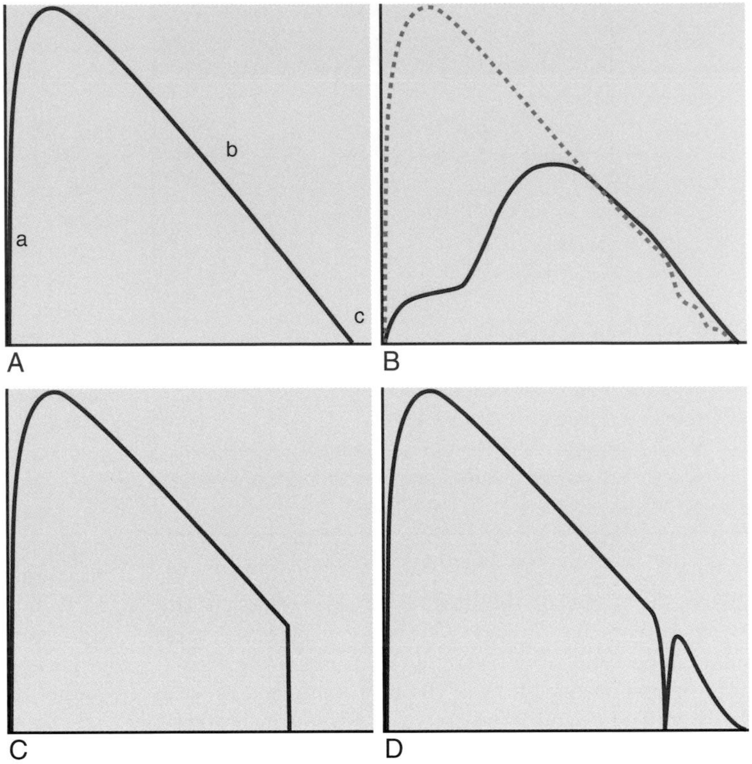

Fig. 4.8 Interpreting the quality of the expiratory flow volume curve. **A,** Excellent effort and test quality. Important elements of an excellent test are a rapid rise (a), a smooth decrease in expiratory flow (b), and a decrease in flow to the baseline (c). **B,** A hesitant start; compare with normal curve as shown by dotted line. This curve is unacceptable. **C,** Good effort at the start, but the individual abruptly stopped exhalation before reaching residual volume; this curve is unacceptable. **D,** Good effort at the start, but the individual stopped exhaling momentarily, closed the glottis, and then continued the effort; test should be repeated.

diagnose underlying lung disease. Some of these clinically important tests are described here.

The **diffusion capacity for carbon monoxide (Dlco)** is a measure of the surface available for gas diffusion. An abnormal test is indicative of a loss of surface area usually because of destruction of the capillary bed. Carbon monoxide (CO) is used as the test gas in part because it is easier to measure than O_2 and in part because there is no limitation to the diffusion of CO. There are two ways that the test can be done: either as a single breath or in a steady state. The single breath test is easiest and quickest. In this test the subject exhales to residual volume and then inhales a gas mixture containing a very low concentration of carbon monoxide and an inert gas (usually helium) to TLC. At TLC, the subject holds his/her breath for 10 seconds and then exhales; the exhaled gas is measured for carbon monoxide and helium. The helium is used to measure TLC, and the difference between the inhaled and the exhaled CO is used to calculate the surface area for diffusion.

The normal value for Dlco is 20 to 30 mL. Because the surface area for diffusion will vary with lung size, dividing Dlco by the total alveolar volume (Va) estimated from the helium concentration normalizes the value for differences in size. The Dlco/Va is called the **Krogh constant**.

Of the numerous conditions in which the Dlco may be elevated, the most important causes of an abnormal Dlco are those that result in a decrease (Box 4.2). Any process that alters or decreases the surface area for gas diffusion will result in a decrease in the Dlco. Some of these conditions deserve further discussion.

Emphysema

Emphysema produces a contradiction of sorts. Lung volumes in patients with emphysema are increased, but alveolar walls and capillaries are destroyed. Thus the surface area for gas exchange is reduced. A reduction in the Dlco is the single best test to distinguish between emphysema and chronic bronchitis in an individual with COPD.

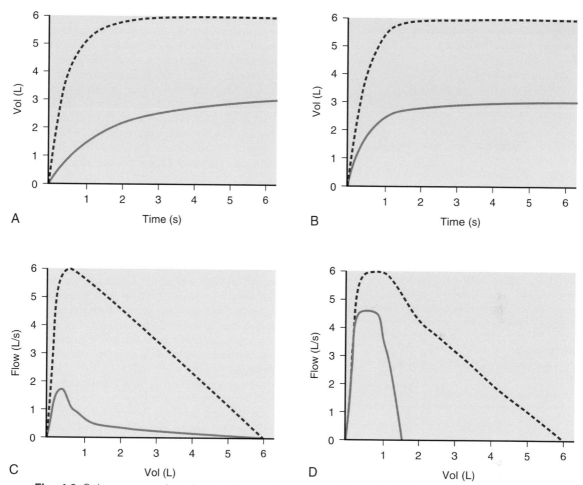

Fig. 4.9 Spirograms and expiratory flow volume curves for an individual with obstructive pulmonary disease (OPD) (**A** and **C**) and with restrictive pulmonary disease (**B** and **D**). *Dashed lines* represent normal values. For the individual with OPD, note the prolonged time to reach the vital capacity (**A**) and the marked decrease in expiratory flow rates (**C**). For the individual with restrictive pulmonary disease, note the reasonably normal shape of the spirogram (**B**) and the flow volume curve (**D**). Volumes, however, are reduced.

Lung Resection

If a significant amount of lung has been removed, the D_{LCO} will be decreased. However, the D_{LCO}/V_A, which corrects for lung volume, will be normal.

Bronchial Obstruction

If there is a tumor obstructing a large airway, the D_{LCO} will be reduced, but the D_{LCO} corrected for lung volume will be normal.

Multiple Pulmonary Emboli

Emboli in the pulmonary circulation decrease perfusion to alveoli and effectively decrease the surface area for diffusion. Also, pulmonary hypertension causes a decrease in capillary area for diffusion.

Anemia

Any condition that lowers capillary blood volume, including conditions that lower the hemoglobin (Hgb)

BOX 4.2 Causes of Abnormal DLCO

Decreased Area for Diffusion
- Emphysema
- Lung/lobe resection
- Bronchial obstruction, as by tumor
- Multiple pulmonary emboli
- Anemia

Increased Thickness of the Alveolar–Capillary Membrane
- Idiopathic pulmonary fibrosis
- Sarcoidosis involving parenchyma
- Asbestosis
- Alveolar proteinosis
- Hypersensitivity pneumonitis, including farmer's lung
- Histiocytosis X (eosinophilic granuloma)
- Congestive heart failure
- Collagen vascular disease (scleroderma, lupus erythematosus)
- Alveolitis or fibrosis—drug-induced (bleomycin, nitrofurantoin, amiodarone, methotrexate)

Miscellaneous
- High carbon monoxide from smoking
- Pregnancy
- Ventilation/perfusion mismatch

DLCO, diffusion capacity for carbon monoxide

in the capillaries, effectively reduce the area for diffusion. Anemia can be corrected using the following equation:

$$DLCO\,(corr) = DLCO\,(uncorr) \times \frac{[10.22 + Hgb]}{[1.7 \times Hgb]}$$

This is particularly important in individuals who have cancer and are receiving chemotherapeutic drugs that can induce pulmonary toxicity and reduce DLCO. Many of these same individuals are also anemic as a result of chemotherapy-induced bone marrow suppression.

USES OF THE MEASUREMENT OF THE DLCO

The DLCO can distinguish between chronic bronchitis and emphysema in individuals with chronic obstructive pulmonary disease (COPD). In chronic bronchitis the DLCO is normal, whereas in emphysema it is reduced. The DLCO is also useful to follow the course of disease progression in patients with pulmonary fibrosis or the extent of intraalveolar hemorrhage in diseases

such as Goodpasture's. In individuals with **interstitial pulmonary fibrosis**, there is an initial alveolar inflammatory response, with subsequent scar formation (connective tissue deposition—collagen) within the interstitial space. The inflammation and scar tissue thicken the interstitial space, making it more difficult for gas diffusion, resulting in a decreased DLCO. This is a classic characteristic of a restrictive lung disease process; gas readily enters the alveolus but is restricted in its ability to diffuse into the blood. DLCO can also determine the presence of pulmonary toxicity in patients without respiratory symptoms who are undergoing chemotherapy.

AIRWAY RESISTANCE AND LUNG COMPLIANCE

Airway resistance (Raw) measurements are routinely performed in fully equipped pulmonary function laboratories, whereas measurements of lung compliance (CL) are performed in fully equipped research pulmonary function laboratories at academic institutions. The latter add little to what has already been learned using spirometry and lung volumes coupled with an appropriately taken arterial blood gas.

Raw can be measured in two ways: using a flow meter and by body plethysmography.

In the first method, flow at the mouth is measured with the flow meter (Fig. 4.10). A small balloon is passed into the midportion of the esophagus and is connected to a pressure transducer. The pressure in the esophagus, which is a reflection of the pressure in the pleura, is then measured. The difference between the pressure in the pleura (**esophageal pressure**) and the pressure at the mouth is the driving force for gas flow. This difference is divided by the expiratory flow to give pulmonary resistance (RPULM).

In body plethysmography, alveolar pressure relative to mouth pressure is measured. For this measurement of resistance, flow is measured with a pneumotachometer. The subject sits in the airtight box and pants through a mouthpiece with the shutter open. Flow is plotted again box pressure. The shutter is briefly closed, usually at end exhalation, and alveolar pressure is recorded. The difference between alveolar pressure and mouth pressure divided by the flow is the Raw. The esophageal balloon method actually measures pulmonary resistance (RPULM), whereas the body box method measures airway resistance (Raw). Because RPULM is composed of both Raw and lung tissue resistance, Raw is always slightly lower than RPULM.

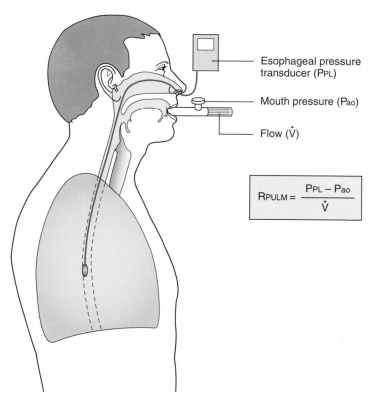

Esophageal pressure
transducer (PPL)

Mouth pressure (Pao)

Flow (V̇)

$$R_{PULM} = \frac{P_{PL} - P_{ao}}{\dot{V}}$$

Fig. 4.10 Measurement of pulmonary resistance (Rpulm) using an esophageal balloon. The esophageal balloon measures pleural pressure (Ppl). The difference between the pressure at the mouth (Pao) and the Ppl divided by the flow rate (V̇) equals Rpulm.

Normal Raw is 1 to 3 cm $H_2O/L \cdot$ sec. Raw varies with lung size. In young infants with smaller airways, Raw is higher than in adults. Raw also varies with lung volume—the greater the lung volume, the lower the resistance, because airway size varies with lung volume. Raw is usually measured at FRC to control for this effect of lung volume. Raw is also increased when the airways are narrowed because of bronchospasm, edema, or infection. Because these processes alter airway caliber, there is a strong negative correlation between Raw and maximal expiratory flow.

MEASUREMENT OF LUNG COMPLIANCE

Clinically, C_L can be measured using an esophageal balloon connected to a pressure transducer and a spirometer. Esophageal balloon pressure is a measure of pleural pressure (P_{PL}). When the lung is not moving (that is, when airflow is zero), P_{PL} is subatmospheric or negative. This is because the lungs are elastic and are always tending to

collapse. Because this tendency of the lung to collapse is resisted by the chest wall, the P_{PL}, when volume is not changing, reflects the elastic pressure or recoil of the lung at that volume. If lung volume is increased by a known amount (ΔV) and volume is then held constant, the new P_{PL} is more negative (lung recoil is greater). The ΔV divided by the change in P_{PL} is the C_L. Because this compliance is measured in the absence of airflow, it is a measure of static compliance ($C_L$stat).

Dynamic lung compliance, or compliance during breathing, also can be measured. At end inspiration and end exhalation, airflow is zero. The difference between P_{PL} at end inspiration and end exhalation divided by the tidal volume is called the dynamic compliance of the lung ($C_L$dyn) (see Fig. 3.6).

In normal individuals, $C_L$stat and $C_L$dyn are nearly the same (0.150–0.250 L/cm H_2O). C_L is lower in smaller lungs and is reduced in individuals with pulmonary fibrosis. $C_L$stat is elevated in individuals with emphysema, reflecting the floppy, inelastic lungs.

In emphysema, CLdyn is reduced and CLstat is increased. The reason for this difference is the nonuniform ventilation in this disease. In patients with emphysema, air flows preferentially into and out of the more normal regions of the lung. Because the elasticity of these regions is not as severely impaired, CLdyn is nearer normal volumes. The difference between CLstat and CLdyn is referred to as **frequency dependence of compliance**. A low CLdyn in patients with emphysema does not mean that the lung is stiff or fibrotic.

USES OF SPIROMETRY AND BODY PLETHYSMOGRAPHY

As previously mentioned, pulmonary function tests are most useful to follow the course of a disease, especially the progression of OPD, and the response to therapy. They quantify defects in function and can sometimes suggest appropriate therapy (bronchodilators). They are least useful to diagnose clinical disease and as a single, isolated test. The reason for this is that pulmonary function tests have greater intersubject variability than intrasubject variability. Different pulmonary function tests have different levels of variability.

Thus pulmonary function tests have a wide range of normal values. For example, a patient may have an FVC of 90% of predicted or expected, which is well within the normal range. It is not known if this individual had an FVC of 120% of predicted values 3 months earlier (in which case the patient has experienced a significant decline in function) or if the FVC has always been 90% of predicted values. This is why longitudinal pulmonary function tests are the most useful to follow the course of a disease.

Pulmonary function tests are also helpful in determining surgical risk and can aid in detecting nonsymptomatic disease in patients at risk for pulmonary function abnormality. For example, pulmonary function tests can be helpful in diagnosing early COPD in a smoker before the individual becomes symptomatic. In individuals with cystic fibrosis, the development of pulmonary function abnormalities in the absence of symptoms is quite common (see Chapter 3, Clinical box). When these abnormalities are identified, changes in therapy that may reverse the early abnormalities and delay disease progression can be tried.

Spirometry and lung volume measurements thus can provide important clinical information. Individual results are compared with predicted values derived from tests performed in large numbers of normal individuals. Predicted values vary by age, sex, ethnicity, height,

TABLE 4.3 Normal Values for Lung Volumes and Pulmonary Function Mechanics	
Lung Volumes	
Functional residual capacity (FRC)	2.4 L
Total lung capacity	6 L
Tidal volume	0.5 L
Breathing frequency	12/min
Pulmonary Function Mechanics	
Pleural pressure (mean)	-5 cm H_2O
Chest wall compliance (at FRC)	0.2 L/cm H_2O
Lung compliance (at FRC)	0.2 L/cm H_2O
Airway resistance	2.0 cm H_2O/ L · sec

and to a lesser extent weight. Normal ranges vary by test but in general are larger for flow rates than for volumes (Table 4.3). Abnormalities in values are indicative of abnormal pulmonary function and can be used to predict eventual abnormalities in gas exchange. They can detect the presence of abnormal lung function long before the development of respiratory symptoms, determine disease severity, and demonstrate response to therapy. An improved response of >12% in FEV_1 after administration of a bronchodilator, for example, is considered clinically significant and suggests that bronchodilator administration may be beneficial.

WHEN SHOULD PULMONARY FUNCTION TESTS BE USED?

Because almost all pulmonary function tests require the cooperation of the subject and a trained technician, pulmonary function tests are not useful in all cases. The subject must be instructed in how to perform pulmonary function testing. In general, the subject must have a natural airway (e.g., no tracheostomy), although some experienced laboratories can test individuals who have a tracheostomy or an endotracheal tube. Pulmonary function tests cannot be successfully performed in a person who cannot follow instructions for whatever reason (mental incapacity, age, etc.).

Pulmonary function tests are underused by clinicians. The following groups of individuals should be considered for regular pulmonary function testing: any patient who smokes, any individual with respiratory symptoms, any individual with asthma, and anyone at risk for lung disease because of environmental exposures on the job or at home.

CLINICAL BOX

Vocal cord dysfunction (VCD) is associated with inappropriate adduction of the vocal cords during inspiration. It presents with symptoms of shortness of breath, wheezing, and occasionally stridor that most often occurs during exercise. VCD is frequently mistaken for exercise-induced asthma and occurs in both adults and adolescents, particularly women. Most individuals are initially treated for asthma, and, often after many years of treatment, they are diagnosed with refractory disease. Pulmonary function tests can be helpful in suggesting a diagnosis. The inspiratory and expiratory flow volumes are normal at rest but when symptomatic, demonstrate a flattened inspiratory loop consistent with a variable extrathoracic airway obstruction. Laryngoscopy during exercise reveals the paradoxical vocal cord adduction during inspiration and the obstruction. Speech therapy using various breathing techniques is effective in treating most patients.

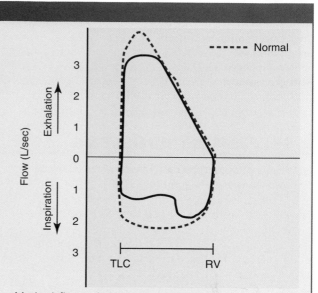

Maximal flow volume curve in an individual with variable extrathoracic airway obstruction. Note the flattening of the inspiratory loop. RV, residual volume; TLC, total lung capacity.

SUMMARY

1. Vital capacity (VC) is the single most important pulmonary function measurement and is the maximal amount of air that an individual can either inspire or exhale.

2. Pulmonary function tests (spirometry, flow volume loop, body plethysmography) can detect abnormalities in lung function before diseases become symptomatic.

3. Obstructive pulmonary disease (OPD) is characterized by increases in lung volumes and airway resistance and decreases in expiratory flow rates. Emphysema, a specific type of COPD, is further characterized by increased lung compliance and decreased diffusion capacity for carbon monoxide (DLco).

4. In OPD, the FEV_1 is decreased out of proportion to any change in the FVC, and as a result the FEV_1/FVC ratio is decreased. In restrictive lung disease, the FEV_1 and FVC are reduced proportionately, resulting in a normal FEV_1/FVC ratio.

5. Restrictive lung diseases are characterized by decreases in lung volume, normal expiratory flow rates and resistance, and a marked decrease in lung compliance.

6. The RV/TLC ratio can be increased in both OPD and restrictive lung disease, although for different reasons.

7. Events that occur early in the forced vital capacity (FVC) maneuver reflect large airway function and are effort-dependent. Events that occur later in the FVC maneuver reflect small airway function and are effort-independent.

8. Predicted values for lung volumes and expiratory flow rates vary by age, sex, ethnicity, height, and, to a lesser extent, weight.

KEYWORDS AND CONCEPTS

Airway resistance (Raw)
Body plethysmography
Boyle's law
Bronchodilator response
Chronic bronchitis
Diffusion capacity for carbon monoxide (DLco)

Effort-dependent expiratory flow
Effort-independent expiratory flow
Emphysema
Esophageal pressure
Flow volume loop
Forced vital capacity (FVC)

Frequency dependence of compliance
Helium dilution
Interstitial pulmonary fibrosis
Krogh constant
Lung compliance (CL)
Nitrogen washout
Obstructive pulmonary disease (OPD)

Peak expiratory flow rate (PEFR)
Pulmonary function tests
Residual volume/total lung capacity (RV/TLC) ratio
Restrictive pulmonary disease
Slow vital capacity (SVC)
Spirometry
Vocal cord dysfunction

SELF-STUDY PROBLEMS

1. What is your interpretation of each of the following
   flow volume curves (A through D)?

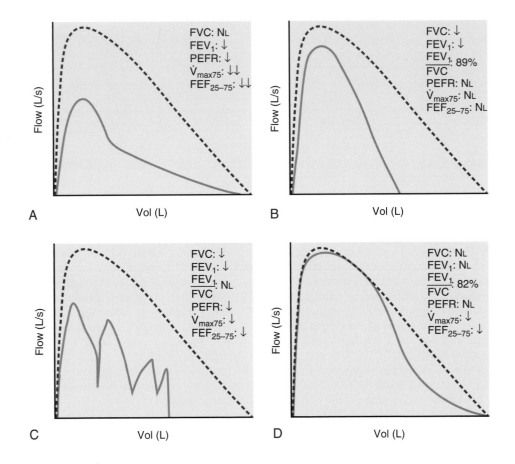

A

FVC: NL
FEV$_1$: ↓
PEFR: ↓
$\dot{V}_{max75}$: ↓↓
FEF$_{25-75}$: ↓↓

B

FVC: ↓
FEV$_1$: ↓
$\dfrac{FEV_1}{FVC}$: 89%
PEFR: NL
$\dot{V}_{max75}$: NL
FEF$_{25-75}$: NL

C

FVC: ↓
FEV$_1$: ↓
$\dfrac{FEV_1}{FVC}$: NL
PEFR: ↓
$\dot{V}_{max75}$: ↓
FEF$_{25-75}$: ↓

D

FVC: NL
FEV$_1$: NL
$\dfrac{FEV_1}{FVC}$: 82%
PEFR: NL
$\dot{V}_{max75}$: ↓
FEF$_{25-75}$: ↓

2. Describe the pulmonary function abnormalities in
   obstructive pulmonary disease. How would you distinguish emphysema from chronic bronchitis?

3. Describe the pulmonary function test abnormalities in
   individuals with restrictive lung disease.
4. List the requirements for a normal DLco.

ADDITIONAL READINGS

1. Altose MD. The physiological basis of pulmonary function testing. *Clin Symp.* 1979;31:1–39.
2. Brand PL, Roorda RJ. Usefulness of monitoring lung function in asthma. *Arch Dis Child.* 2003;88:1021–1025.
3. Chetta A, Marangio E, Olivieri D. Pulmonary function testing in interstitial lung diseases. *Respiration.* 2004;71:209–213.
4. Contreras G, Gutierrez M, Beroiza T, et al. Ventilatory drive and respiratory muscle function in pregnancy. *Am Rev Respir Dis.* 199;144:837–844.
5. Crapo RO, Jensen RL. Standards and interpretive issues in lung function testing. *Respir Care.* 2003;48:764–772.
6. Dunn NM, Katial K, Hoyte FCL. Vocal cord dysfunction: a review. *Asthma Res Pract.* 2015;1:9. 10:1186/s40733-015-0009-z.
7. Evans SE, Scanlon PD. Current practice in pulmonary function testing. *Mayo Clinic Proc.* 2003;78:758–763.
8. Hyatt RE, Scanlon PD, Nakamura M, eds. *Interpretation of Pulmonary Function Tests. A Practical Guide.* 4th ed. Rochester: MN Scientific Publications; 2014.
9. Motram CD. *Ruppel's Manual of Pulmonary Function Testing.* 11th ed. St. Louis: Elsevier; 2018.
10. Wang JS. Pulmonary function tests in preoperative pulmonary evaluation. *Respir Med.* 2004;98:598–605.

5

Alveolar Ventilation

OBJECTIVES

1. Understand the composition of gases from ambient air to the alveoli.
2. Describe the alveolar air equation and its use.
3. Define the alveolar carbon dioxide equation and the relationship between alveolar ventilation and arterial P_{CO_2}.
4. Describe the distribution of ventilation at the apex and at the base in upright individuals.
5. Describe how the nitrogen washout test can be used to examine the distribution of ventilation.
6. Define anatomic and physiologic dead space and their measurement.
7. Outline the effects of aging on lung growth, lung volumes, elastic recoil, expiratory muscle strength, airway closure, and the diffusion capacity for carbon monoxide.

Ventilation is the process by which fresh gas moves in and out of the lung. Alveolar ventilation is the process by which gas moves between the alveoli and the external environment. It includes both the volume of fresh air entering the alveoli and the (similar) volume of alveolar air leaving the body. Minute (or total) ventilation (MV), also referred to as $\dot{V}E$, is the volume of air that enters or leaves the lung per minute and is described by:

$$MV = f \times V_T$$

where f is the frequency or number of breaths per minute, and V_T (also expressed as TV) is the tidal volume or volume of air inspired (or exhaled) per breath. V_T varies with age, sex, body position, and metabolic activity. In an average-sized adult, V_T is 500 mL; in children, V_T is 3 to 5 mL/kg of body weight.

COMPOSITION OF A GAS MIXTURE

The process of respiration brings ambient (or atmospheric) air to the alveoli where oxygen in the ambient air is taken up and carbon dioxide, produced by tissue metabolism, is excreted. Ambient air is a gas mixture composed of nitrogen and oxygen with minute quantities of carbon dioxide, argon, and other inert gases. The composition of a gas mixture can be described either in terms of gas fractions or as the corresponding partial pressures. Because ambient air is a gas, it obeys the gas laws (see Appendix C to review Boyle's law and Dalton's law).

Using the gas laws and applying them to ambient air, two important principles arise (Box 5.1). The first is that when viewed in terms of gas fractions (F), the sum of the individual gas fractions of nitrogen (F_N), oxygen (F_{O_2}), and argon and other gases ($F_{argon\ and\ other\ gases}$) must equal 1; that is, for ambient air,

$$1.0 = F_N + F_{O_2} + F_{argon\ and\ other\ gases}$$

When viewed using Boyle's gas law, the sum of the partial pressures (in mm Hg) or tensions (in torr) of a gas must be equal to the total pressure. (mm Hg also can be expressed as torr, named for Evangelista Torricelli, the inventor of the barometer. The two terms are equal and interchangeable.) Thus at sea level, where the total pressure (also known as the barometric pressure or P_B) is 760 mm Hg, the partial pressure of the individual gases in ambient air is:

$$P_B = P_{O_2} + P_{N_2} + P_{argon\ and\ other\ gases}$$

$$760\ mm\ Hg = P_{O_2} + P_{N_2} + P_{argon\ and\ other\ gases}$$

The second important principle is that the partial pressure of a gas (P_{gas}) is equal to the fraction of gas in the gas mixture (F_{gas}) times the total or ambient (barometric) pressure (an application of Dalton's law).

BOX 5.1 Gas Pressure Units and Their Conversion

Respiratory pressures can be expressed in units of torr, mm Hg, or cm H_2O. Torr is a unit of pressure equal to 1 mm Hg. Pressures used in conjunction with gases in gaseous or liquid phases are usually expressed in units of torr or mm Hg with a vacuum as the reference point. In contrast, pressure gradients, differences in the pressure surrounding a structure with ambient barometric pressure as a reference, are usually expressed in cm H_2O. To convert, 1 mm Hg = 1.35 cm H_2O.

$$P_{gas} = F_{gas} \times P_B$$

Ambient air is composed of approximately 21% oxygen and 79% nitrogen. Therefore the partial pressure of oxygen in ambient air (Po_2) is:

$$\begin{aligned} Po_2 &= Fo_2 \times P_B \\ &= 0.21 \times 760 \text{ mm Hg} \\ &= 159 \text{ mm Hg (or 159 torr)} \end{aligned}$$

This is the oxygen tension (i.e., the partial pressure of oxygen) at the mouth at the start of inspiration. The oxygen tension at the mouth can be altered in one of two ways: by changing the fraction of oxygen or by changing the barometric (atmospheric) pressure. For example, if the fraction of oxygen is increased through the administration of supplemental oxygen, the partial pressure of oxygen will be increased. On the other hand, if the barometric (atmospheric) pressure is decreased—for example, by high altitude—the partial pressure of ambient oxygen will decrease.

At the start of inspiration, ambient gases are brought into the airways, where they become warmed to body temperature and humidified. By the time the inspired gas reaches the larynx, it has become saturated with water vapor; water vapor is a gas that exerts a partial pressure equal to 47 mm Hg at body temperature (see Appendix C for the reason). Because the total pressure remains constant at the barometric pressure, water vapor dilutes the pressure exerted by the other gases. This can be best understood by considering that humidification of a liter of dry gas in a container at 760 torr would increase its total pressure to 807 torr (i.e., 760 torr + 47 torr). In the body, however, barometric pressure remains constant, and therefore the gas simply expands, according to Boyle's law. As a result, the partial pressures of the other gases in the 1 L of gas at 760 torr are diluted by the added water vapor pressure. To calculate the partial pressure of a gas in a humidified mixture, the water vapor partial pressure must be subtracted

from the total barometric pressure. Thus in the conducting airways, the partial pressure of oxygen is:

$$\begin{aligned} P_{trachea}O_2 &= (P_B - P_{H_2O}) \times Fo_2 \\ &= 760 - 47 \text{ mm Hg} \times 0.21 \\ &= 150 \text{ mm Hg} \end{aligned}$$

and the partial pressure of nitrogen is:

$$\begin{aligned} P_{trachea}N_2 &= 760 - 47 \text{ mm Hg} \times 0.79 \\ &= 563 \text{ mm Hg} \end{aligned}$$

Note that the total pressure has remained at 760 mm Hg (150 + 563 + 47 mm Hg). Water vapor pressure, however, has reduced (diluted) the partial pressures of oxygen and nitrogen. The conducting airways do not participate in gas exchange, and therefore the partial pressures of oxygen, nitrogen, and water vapor remain unchanged in the airways until the gas reaches the alveolus.

ALVEOLAR GAS COMPOSITION

At functional residual capacity, the alveoli contain 2.5 to 3 L of gas; an additional 350 mL of gas will enter and leave the alveoli with each breath (Fig. 5.1). Diffusion of O_2 from the alveoli into the pulmonary capillary blood and of CO_2 from the pulmonary capillary blood into the alveoli is a continuous process. Each minute at rest, on average, 300 mL of O_2 are taken up and 250 mL of CO_2 are removed by alveolar ventilation. Thus the partial pressures of O_2 and CO_2 in the alveolar air are determined by alveolar ventilation, by O_2 consumption, and by CO_2 production. The process by which oxygen is taken up and carbon dioxide is removed by the pulmonary capillary blood is described in Chapter 8.

Here we describe only alveolar ventilation. At the end of inspiration with the glottis open, the total pressure in the alveolus is atmospheric; the same gas laws apply, namely the partial pressures of the gases in the alveolus must equal the total pressure, which in this case is atmospheric. The composition of the gas mixture however is changed and can be described as:

$$1.0 = Fo_2 + F_{N_2} + F_{H_2O} + F_{CO_2} + F_{argon \text{ and other gases}}$$

Nitrogen and argon are inert gases, and therefore the fraction of these gases in the alveolus does not change. The fraction of water vapor also does not change because the gas is already fully saturated and at body temperature by the time the gas reaches the trachea. As a consequence of gas exchange, the fraction of oxygen in the alveolus decreases and the fraction of carbon dioxide in the alveolus increases. Because of the changes in the fractions of oxygen and carbon dioxide, the partial pressures exerted by these gases also change. The partial pressure of

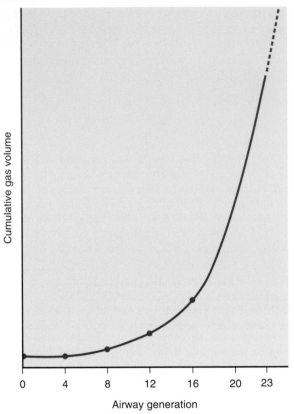

Fig. 5.1 Cumulative gas volumes in the airways with increasing generation number. The average volume of gas in the conducting airways is approximately 100 to 200 mL, whereas the average volume of gas in the terminal bronchioles, alveolar ducts, and alveoli is approximately 3000 to 4000 mL at functional residual capacity. (Modified from Leff A, Schumacker P. *Respiratory Physiology: Basics and Applications.* Philadelphia: W.B. Saunders; 1993.)

oxygen in the alveolus (P_{AO_2}) is given by the **alveolar gas equation**, sometimes also called the *ideal alveolar oxygen equation*:

$$P_{AO_2} = P_{IO_2} - \frac{P_{ACO_2}}{R}$$
$$= (P_B - P_{H_2O}) \times F_{IO_2} - \frac{P_{ACO_2}}{R}$$

where P_{IO_2} is the inspired (I) partial pressure of oxygen, which is equal to the inspired oxygen fraction (F_{IO_2}) times the difference between barometric pressure (P_B) and water vapor pressure (P_{H_2O}), P_{ACO_2} is the alveolar gas carbon dioxide tension, and R is the respiratory exchange ratio or **respiratory quotient**. Although the derivation of the alveolar gas equation is beyond the scope of this book, in its simplest terms, it represents the oxygen that is delivered to the alveolus minus the oxygen that has been consumed. In steady state, the relationship between oxygen consumption

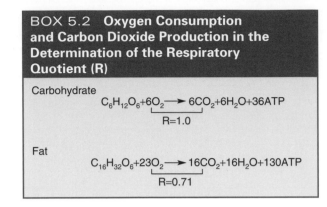

and carbon dioxide production is defined by the respiratory quotient.

The respiratory quotient is the ratio of carbon dioxide excreted ($\dot{V}_{CO_2}$) to the oxygen taken up ($\dot{V}_{O_2}$) by the lungs.

$$R = \frac{\dot{V}_{CO_2}}{\dot{V}_{O_2}}$$

It is the number of carbon dioxide molecules produced relative to the number of oxygen molecules consumed by metabolism and is dependent on a person's food intake. The respiratory quotient varies between 0.7 and 1.0 (Box 5.2). In states of exclusive fatty acid metabolism, R is 0.7, whereas in states of exclusive carbohydrate metabolism, R is 1.0. Because the respiratory quotient is rarely measured, it is estimated at 0.8 under usual circumstances, demonstrating that more oxygen is taken up than carbon dioxide is released in the alveoli. The alveolar air equation is one of the most important equations in respiratory medicine.

The partial pressures of oxygen, carbon dioxide, nitrogen, and water from ambient air to the alveolus to the blood are shown in Table 5.1.

The fraction of carbon dioxide in the alveolus is a function of the production of carbon dioxide by the cells during metabolism and the rate at which the carbon dioxide is removed or eliminated from the alveolus (i.e., alveolar ventilation) (Fig. 5.2). Even though ventilation is episodic (i.e., it occurs only during inspiration), alveolar ventilation is described as a continuous gas flow through alveoli that exchange gas with pulmonary capillary blood. The relationship between carbon dioxide production and alveolar ventilation is defined by the **alveolar carbon dioxide equation**:

$$\dot{V}_{CO_2} = \dot{V}_A \times F_{ACO_2}$$

where $\dot{V}_{CO_2}$ is the rate of carbon dioxide production by the body, $\dot{V}_A$ is the alveolar ventilation, and F_{ACO_2} is the dry fraction of carbon dioxide in alveolar gas. This relationship demonstrates that the rate of elimination of CO_2 from the alveolus is related to alveolar ventilation and the fraction of

TABLE 5.1   Total and Partial Pressures of Respiratory Gases in Ideal Alveolar Gas and Blood at Sea Level Barometric Pressure (760 mm Hg)

	Ambient Air (Dry)	Moist Tracheal Air	Alveolar Gas (R = 0.80)	Systemic Arterial Blood	Mixed Venous Blood
P_{O_2}	159	150	102	90	40
P_{CO_2}	0	0	40	40	46
P_{H_2O}, 37°C	0	47	47	47	47
P_{N_2}	601	563	571*	571	571
P_{TOT}	760	760	760	760	704†

*P_{N_2} is increased in alveolar gas by 1% because R is <1 normally.
†P_{TOT} is less in venous than in arterial blood because P_{O_2} has decreased more than P_{CO_2} has increased.

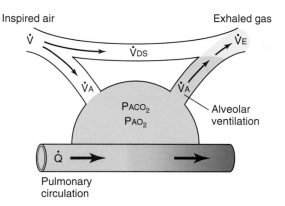

Fig. 5.2 Relationship among alveolar ventilation, dead space, and perfusion in a continuous flow model of the lung. Even though ventilation is not continuous, it is useful to view it as if it received continuous minute ventilation ($\dot{V}_E$). Alveolar ventilation ($\dot{V}_A$) is that part of the minute ventilation that reaches the alveoli and participates in gas exchange. Anatomic dead space ($\dot{V}_{DS}$) is that part of the ventilation that fills the conducting airways effectively bypassing the alveoli and thus not participating in gas exchange. $\dot{Q}$, pulmonary perfusion. (Modified from Leff A, Schumacker P. *Respiratory Physiology: Basics and Applications.* Philadelphia: W.B. Saunders; 1993.)

CO_2 in the alveolus (Fig. 5.3). Because the alveolar P_{ACO_2} is defined by the following equation:

$$P_{ACO_2} = F_{ACO_2} \times (P_B - P_{H_2O})$$

we can substitute for F_{ACO_2} in the previous equation as follows:

$$P_{ACO_2} = \frac{\dot{V}_{CO_2} \times (P_B - P_{H_2O})}{\dot{V}_A}$$

When used, both $\dot{V}_{CO_2}$ and $\dot{V}_A$ must be expressed in the same units.

This equation demonstrates a number of interesting and important relationships. The first is that there is an inverse

relationship between the partial pressure of carbon dioxide in the alveolus (P_{ACO_2}) and alveolar ventilation ($\dot{V}_A$) irrespective of exhaled CO_2. Specifically, if you double alveolar ventilation, the P_{ACO_2} will be halved, and if alveolar ventilation is halved, the partial pressure of CO_2 in the alveolus will be doubled. Second, at a constant alveolar ventilation ($\dot{V}_A$), doubling the metabolic production of carbon dioxide ($\dot{V}_{CO_2}$), such as with an increase in body temperature, will double the partial pressure of CO_2 in the alveolus (P_{ACO_2}). This relationship is specific to alveolar ventilation and not to tidal volume, of which alveolar ventilation is a part (see the discussion of dead space later in this chapter).

Clinically, this principle is used in individuals who are being mechanically ventilated and cannot self-regulate their breathing. If the partial pressure of carbon dioxide increases in their blood, it is an indication that the partial pressure of carbon dioxide in the alveolus has increased. The P_{ACO_2} (and thus, the arterial P_{CO_2}) will decrease by increasing $\dot{V}_A$. If this same individual now develops a fever and cannot increase alveolar ventilation, the arterial P_{CO_2} will increase as a result of the increase in CO_2 production.

In normal individuals, alveolar P_{CO_2} is tightly regulated to remain constant around 40 ± 2 mm Hg. Specialized chemoreceptors monitor the P_{CO_2} in arterial blood and in the brainstem with changes in minute ventilation in accordance with the level of P_{CO_2}. Increases or decreases in arterial P_{CO_2}, particularly when associated with changes in pH, have profound effects on cell functions including enzyme and transport functions. Because of this, the body tightly regulates arterial P_{CO_2}.

Because of its high diffusibility (see Chapter 8), the difference between alveolar P_{CO_2} (P_{ACO_2}) and arterial P_{CO_2} (P_{aCO_2}) is small. Alveolar P_{CO_2} is difficult to measure and arterial P_{CO_2} is easy to measure, thus $P_{ACO_2} = P_{aCO_2}$, and the two terms are used interchangeably. An increase in P_{aCO_2} either due to an increase in CO_2 production or due to a decrease in alveolar ventilation results in (respiratory) acidosis (pH < 7.35), whereas a decrease in P_{aCO_2} results in (respiratory) alkalosis (pH > 7.45) (see Chapter 9).

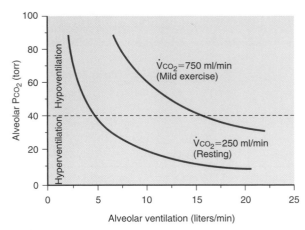

Fig. 5.3 Alveolar Pco_2 as a function of alveolar ventilation in the lung. Each line corresponds to a given metabolic rate associated with a constant production of carbon dioxide ($\dot{V}co_2$; isometabolic line). Normally, alveolar ventilation is controlled to maintain an alveolar Pco_2 of about 40 torr. During hypoventilation, the alveolar ventilation is low relative to Vco_2, and alveolar Pco_2 rises. During hyperventilation, the alveolar ventilation is excessive relative to Vco_2, and thus the alveolar Pco_2 falls. (Koeppen BM, Stanton BA, eds. *Berne and Levy's Physiology*, 7th ed. Philadelphia: Elsevier; 2018.)

Hypercapnia is an elevation in $Paco_2$ and is secondary to inadequate alveolar ventilation (hypoventilation) relative to CO_2 production. Conversely, hyperventilation is present when alveolar ventilation exceeds CO_2 production and results in a low $Paco_2$ (hypocapnia).

DISTRIBUTION OF VENTILATION

Ventilation is not evenly distributed in the lung. There are regional differences in ventilation due in large part to the effects of gravity. When an individual is in the upright position, ventilation per unit of volume is greatest in the lower regions of the lungs, compared with the upper lung regions.

The reasons for regional differences in ventilation can be best described by reexamining pleural pressures, which are not uniform throughout the chest. In the upright position, the intrapleural surface pressure is less negative in the lower, gravity-dependent regions of the chest than in the upper, nondependent regions (Table 5.2). The pleural surface pressure increases approximately +0.2 cm H_2O for every centimeter of vertical displacement from the top of the lung to the most dependent part of the lung. This pressure gradient is due to a combination of gravity and the effects of lung weight. This vertical pressure gradient creates a transpulmonary (PL) gradient (recall that $PL = PA − PPL$), and this in turn affects alveolar size (Fig. 5.4). In the upright position, alveoli near the apex of the lung are more expanded than alveoli at the base. This is because the pleural surface pressure is decreased (more negative) at the apex relative to the base because of gravity and the weight of the lung pulling down or away from the chest wall. If the pleural pressure is decreased (more negative), the static translung pressure ($PL = PA − PPL$) is increased, and the alveolar volume in this area is increased.

As inspiration begins, alveoli at the apex and at the base of the lung have different volumes and are therefore

TABLE 5.2 Pleural (PPL) and Transpulmonary (PL) (cm H₂O) Pressure at FRC at the Top and Bottom of the Lung

	TOP OF LUNG		BOTTOM OF LUNG	
Position	PPL	PL	PPL	PL
Upright	-8	8	−2	2
Supine	-4	4	0	0
Prone	-3.5	3.5	0	0

From Agostoni E. Mechanics of the pleural spaces. *Physiol Rev.* 1972;52:57–128.
FRC, functional residual capacity.

at different locations on the pressure–volume curve (see Fig. 2.2A). Alveoli at the base are at the steeper portion of the pressure–volume curve and receive more of the ventilation (i.e., they have a greater compliance). In contrast, the expanded alveoli at the apex are closer to the top of the pressure–volume curve, have a lower compliance, and thus receive proportionately less of the tidal volume.

In the absence of gravity, such as in outer space, this type of nonuniformity disappears. The effect is also less pronounced when supine compared with upright and is less when supine compared with prone. (This is because the diaphragm is pushed cephalad when supine and this affects the size of all of the alveoli.)

In addition to gravitational effects on the distribution of ventilation, there is local nonuniform ventilation among terminal respiratory units. This is caused by variable airway resistance (R) or compliance (C) and may be described by the following equation:

$$\tau = R \times C$$

in which the τ (tau) is the time constant (see Chapter 3).

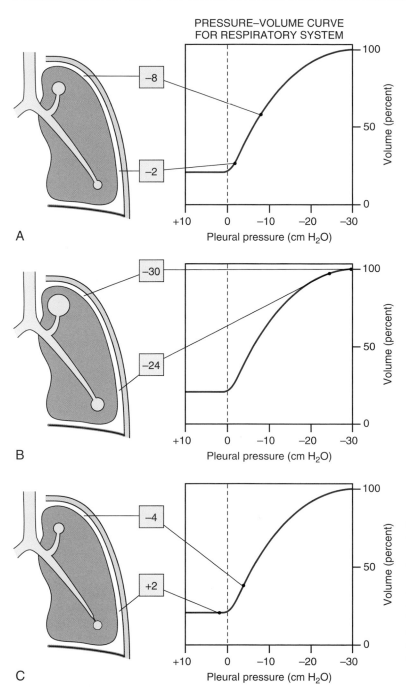

PRESSURE–VOLUME CURVE FOR RESPIRATORY SYSTEM

Fig. 5.4 The vertical transpulmonary pressure gradient in the upright lung at different lung volumes. **A,** At functional residual capacity, alveoli at the base are at the steeper portion of the pressure–volume curve and receive proportionately more ventilation. **B,** At total lung capacity, alveoli both at the base and at the apex are at the top of the pressure–volume curve and have a lower compliance. **C,** At residual volume, alveoli at the base are compressed and could even close. (Koeppen BM, Stanton BA, eds. *Berne and Levy's Physiology*, 7th ed. Philadelphia: Elsevier; 2018.)

Alveolar units with long time constants fill and empty slowly. Thus a unit with increased resistance, increased compliance, or both will take longer to fill and longer to empty (see Fig. 3.7). In normal adults, the respiratory rate is ~12 breaths per minute, with an inspiratory time of approximately 2 seconds and an expiratory time of about 3 seconds.

In normal individuals, this is sufficient time to almost reach equilibrium (Fig. 5.5). However, in the presence of an increased resistance (or an increased compliance), equilibrium is not reached. This contributes to the air trapping seen in diseases associated with increased resistance (e.g., chronic bronchitis) or increased compliance (e.g., emphysema).

TESTS OF DISTRIBUTION OF VENTILATION

Several methods have been used to examine the distribution of ventilation in humans. One of these is the single-breath nitrogen test. The subject exhales to residual volume and then takes a single maximal inspiration of 100% O_2. During the subsequent exhalation, the nitrogen concentration of the exhaled air is measured. Air (100% O, 0% nitrogen) initially exits from the conducting airways; the nitrogen concentration then begins to rise as alveolar emptying occurs. Finally, there is a plateau concentration of nitrogen as only alveoli containing nitrogen empty (Fig. 5.6).

Understanding the single-breath nitrogen test is an exercise in pulmonary physiology and the distribution of ventilation. At RV, the alveoli in the dependent portions of the lung are at a smaller volume than those in the apical portion. Thus the apical alveoli contain a larger volume of nitrogen. As the subject inhales 100% oxygen, the apical alveoli receive proportionately less oxygen than the more dependent alveoli that are located at the steeper part of the pressure–volume curve. Therefore the nitrogen concentration is higher in the apical alveoli and there is a gradual decrease in nitrogen concentration toward the base, which contains the most diluted gas. At the end of inspiration, the trachea and upper airways contain only oxygen.

As exhalation begins, the gas in the trachea and upper airways exits first, and this gas has no nitrogen. Thus phase I shows 0% nitrogen. As exhalation continues, alveolar gas begins to mix with the dead space oxygen, and the nitrogen concentration begins to slowly rise (phase II). Phase III consists entirely of alveolar gas. Initially, the gas comes predominantly from the dependent alveolar regions, where the nitrogen concentration is the lowest. As exhalation proceeds, increasing amounts of gas come from the apical regions, where nitrogen concentrations are highest. During phase III there is a gradual increase in nitrogen concentration; the normal slope of this phase is 1% to 2.5% nitrogen per liter exhaled.

The onset of phase IV is associated with an abrupt increase in nitrogen concentration. This occurs when dependent lung units have completely emptied, and more of the final portion of exhalation comes from the apical regions with the highest concentration of nitrogen. The onset of phase IV has been said to indicate the onset of airway closure in the dependent regions of the lung, and it is often called the **closing volume**. Phase IV normally begins with approximately 15% of the vital capacity remaining to be exhaled. This increases

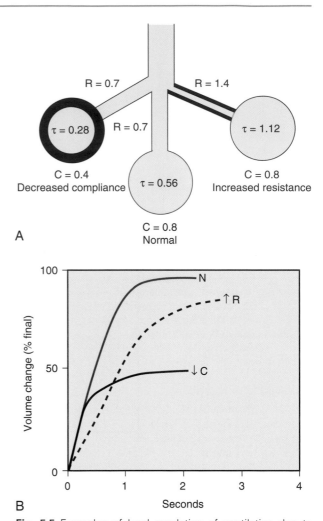

Fig. 5.5 Examples of local regulation of ventilation due to variation in resistance (R) or compliance (C) of individual lung units. **A,** In the unit at the center, the normal lung has a time constant (τ) of 0.56 second. This unit reaches 97% of final equilibrium in 2 seconds, the normal inspiratory time (N, shown in the graph in B). The unit at the right has a twofold increase in resistance; hence, its time constant is doubled. This unit is underventilated and fills more slowly, reaching only 80% equilibrium during a normal breath. The unit on the left has reduced compliance (stiff), which acts to reduce its time constant. This unit fills faster than the normal unit but receives only half the ventilation of a normal unit. **B,** Volume–time curve for normal lung (N), for lung with increased resistance (R) and for lung with decreased compliance (C). (Koeppen BM, Stanton BA, eds. *Berne and Levy's Physiology*, 7th ed. Philadelphia: Elsevier; 2018.)

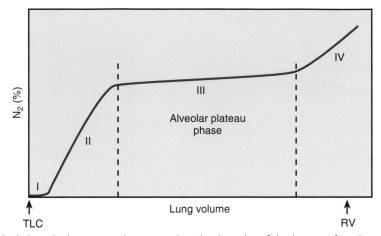

N_2 (%)

III

Alveolar plateau
phase

II

IV

I

Lung volume

TLC

RV

Fig. 5.6 The single-breath nitrogen washout curve is a simple and useful pulmonary function test of regional ventilation distribution. It clearly shows that all lung units do not have the same ventilation-to-perfusion ratio. The well-ventilated units (short time constant) empty faster than less well-ventilated units (long time constant). The portion of the curve up to the first vertical dashed line (phase I and II) represents the washout of dead space air mixed with alveolar gas. In phase III, the long alveolar plateau (between the vertical dashed lines) rises slowly (<2%) if ventilation distribution is relatively uniform, as shown here. The final phase (phase IV), after the second vertical line, shows very late, slowly emptying alveoli. This phase is accentuated with age. (Koeppen BM, Stanton BA, eds. *Berne and Levy's Physiology*, 7th ed. Philadelphia: Elsevier; 2018.)

to 25% in older individuals. With disease, both the slope of phase III and the location of the phase IV slope increase. This occurs because the normal pattern of gas distribution, including the vertical gradient of nitrogen concentration, is abolished. Disease occurs unevenly throughout the lung; regions with greater disease with high resistance empty less completely and hence receive less oxygen; in addition, they empty more slowly, and this results in the elevated slope of phase III (Fig. 5.7). Today phase IV has proved to be less sensitive than previously thought, but phase III is an excellent index of nonuniform ventilation.

DEAD SPACE

Anatomic Dead Space

Alveolar ventilation is less than tidal volume and minute ventilation because part of every breath fills and remains in the conducting airways and does not reach the alveoli. This air within the conducting airways does not participate in gas exchange. The volume of air present in the conducting airways is called the **anatomic dead space** (V_{DS}). The volume of air in the anatomic dead space is determined by the anatomy (size and number) of the

conducting airways. When the letter V is used to denote volume, the letters T, DS and A are used to denote tidal, dead space, and alveolar volume, respectively. Again, a "dot" above the letter V denotes volume per unit of time (n). Thus

$$V_T = V_{DS} + V_A$$

Therefore

$$V_T \times n = V_{DS} \times n + V_A \times n$$

Or

$$\dot{V}_E = \dot{V}_{DS} + \dot{V}_A$$

where $\dot{V}_E$ is the exhaled minute volume and $\dot{V}_{DS}$ and $\dot{V}_A$ are the dead space and alveolar ventilation per minute, respectively.

In the normal adult, at functional residual capacity (FRC), the volume of gas contained in the conducting airways is approximately 100 to 200 mL, compared with the 3000 mL of gas in the entire lung (see Fig. 5.1). With each tidal breath (approximately 500 mL), fresh gas moves first into the conducting airways and then into the alveoli. The ratio of the volume of the conducting airways (dead space) to tidal volume describes the fraction of each

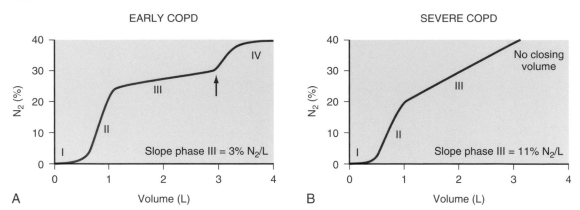

Fig. 5.7 Single-breath nitrogen washout curve in an individual with early **(A)** and severe **(B)** chronic obstructive pulmonary disease (COPD). Closing volume is noted by the arrow in A. (Modified from Hyatt RE, Scanlon PD, Nakamura M, eds. *Interpretation of Pulmonary Function Tests: A Practical Guide,* 4th ed. Rochester, MN: Scientific Publications; 2014.)

breath that is wasted in "ventilating" the conducting airways. This volume (V_{DS}) is related to the tidal volume (V_T) and to the exhaled ventilation (V_E) in the following way:

$$V_{DS} = \frac{V_{DS}}{V_T} \times V_E$$

As can be seen, dead space ventilation (V_{DS}) varies inversely with tidal volume (V_T). The larger the tidal volume, the smaller the dead space ventilation.

Normally, dead space ventilation represents 20% to 30% of the minute ventilation. This dead space is called the anatomic dead space because it is due to wasted ventilation of airways that do not and cannot participate in gas exchange (see Fig. 5.2).

Physiologic Dead Space Ventilation

Imagine a diseased lung in which some alveoli are not perfused but continue to be ventilated. These ventilated but not perfused areas of the lung, in a sense, act just like the conducting airways that are also ventilated but do not participate in gas exchange. The total volume of gas in each breath that does not participate in gas exchange is called the **physiologic dead space** ventilation. It includes the anatomic dead space and the dead space secondary to ventilated, but not perfused, alveoli or alveoli overventilated relative to the amount of perfusion. Thus the physiologic dead space is always as large as the anatomic dead space, and in the presence of disease it may be considerably larger. In healthy individuals the physiologic dead space normally represents 25% to 30% of the minute ventilation.

CLINICAL BOX

Emphysema is associated with destruction of alveolar walls and the pulmonary capillary bed. As a result, emphysema is associated with a marked increase in the physiologic dead space. What would happen to alveolar ventilation in someone with emphysema whose dead space increased from 25% to 50% of their ventilation? (Assume that tidal volume is 500 mL.)

$$V_D = \frac{V_D}{V_T} \times TV$$
$$= 0.25 \times 500 \, mL = 125 \, mL \text{ under normal conditions and so}$$

$$V_A = 500 \, mL - 125 \, mL = 375 \, mL$$

In this individual with emphysema,

$$V_D = 0.50 \times TV = 250 \, mL$$

$$V_A = 500 \, mL - 250 \, mL = 250 \, mL$$

For people with emphysema to achieve the same alveolar minute ventilation (which in this case would be 375 mL/breath × 12 breaths per minute or 4.5 L/min), they would need to either increase their respiratory frequency to 18 breaths per minute or increase their tidal volume from 500 mL to 675 mL/breath (or some combination). Either of these options is associated with increased work of breathing and over time could progress to respiratory muscle fatigue.

CLINICAL BOX: MEASUREMENTS OF DEAD SPACE

Dead space is not often measured clinically. However, dead space can be determined in two ways: using Bohr's dead space equation, originally described by the physiologist Christian Bohr at the turn of the 19th century; or using Fowler's method.

Fowler's method and Bohr's equation do not measure exactly the same thing. Fowler's method measures the volume of the conducting airways down to the level where rapid dilution of inspired gas occurs with gas already in the lung. Thus Fowler's method measures anatomic dead space. In contrast, Bohr's equation measures the volume of the lung that does not eliminate CO_2. Thus Bohr's equation measures physiologic dead space. In normal individuals, there is little difference between anatomic and physiologic dead space. In people with lung disease, however, the difference can be large.

Bohr's Dead Space Equation

Bohr's equation measures the P_{CO_2} in alveolar gas and in mixed expired gas (P_{ECO_2}) (Fig. 5.8). The dilution of CO_2 in mixed expired gas (P_{ECO_2}) relative to alveolar gas is measured and is a function of the amount of wasted ventilation relative to the minute ventilation. This is because conducting airways and ventilated but not perfused alveoli do not contribute to the CO_2 in expired gas. Exhaled gas is collected in a bag over a period of time, and the P_{CO_2} in the arterial blood (which is equal to the P_{ACO_2}) and in the bag (P_{ECO_2}) is measured. Any volume of CO_2 in the P_{ECO_2} must come from both ventilated and perfused alveoli, because ambient air contains negligible amounts of CO_2. The dead space ventilation as a function of the tidal volume ($\dot{V}_{DS}/\dot{V}_T$) is described by the following equation:

$$\frac{\dot{V}_{DS}}{\dot{V}_T} = 1 - \frac{P_{ECO_2}}{P_{ACO_2}}$$

This equation can be derived from Boyle's law as follows:

$$P_1 V_1 = P_2 V_2 \text{ (Boyle's law)}$$

where P_1 is the partial pressure of CO_2 in the bag (P_{ECO_2}) and V_1 is the exhaled tidal volume (V_T). Because all of the CO_2 was generated in alveoli that were perfused, P_2 is the arterial (alveolar) partial pressure of CO_2 and V_2 is the alveolar ventilation (V_A); that is,

$$P_{BCO_2} \cdot V_T = P_{ACO_2} \cdot V_A$$

Alveolar ventilation cannot be measured directly, but $V_A = V_T - V_{DS}$. Substituting for V_A,

$$P_{ECO_2} \cdot V_T = P_{ACO_2} \cdot (V_T - V_{DS})$$

Dividing by V_T,

$$P_{ECO_2} = P_{ACO_2} - \frac{V_{DS}}{V_T} \times P_{ACO_2}$$

Solving for V_{DS}/V_T,

$$V_{DS}/V_T = 1 - \frac{P_{BCO_2}}{P_{ACO_2}}$$

Fowler's Method

Dead space ventilation also can be measured using Fowler's method (Fig. 5.9). The subject takes a single breath of 100% oxygen and then exhales into a tube that continuously measures the nitrogen concentration in the exhaled gas. As the subject exhales, the volume of the anatomic dead space empties first. This volume comprises 100% oxygen and 0% nitrogen. As the alveoli begin to empty, the oxygen level falls and the nitrogen level begins to rise. Finally, an almost uniform gas concentration of nitrogen is seen, representing entirely alveolar gas. This phase is called the alveolar plateau. The volume with initially 0% nitrogen plus half of the rising nitrogen volume is equal to the anatomic dead space.

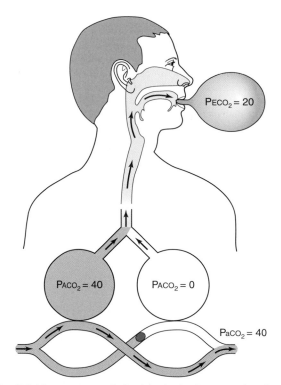

Fig. 5.8 Measurement of physiologic dead space using the dilution of carbon dioxide in mixed expired gas (P_{ECO_2}) and Bohr's dead space equation. In this example, dead space is 50% (0.5). (Redrawn from Leff A, Schumacker P. *Respiratory Physiology: Basics and Applications*. Philadelphia: W.B. Saunders; 1993.)

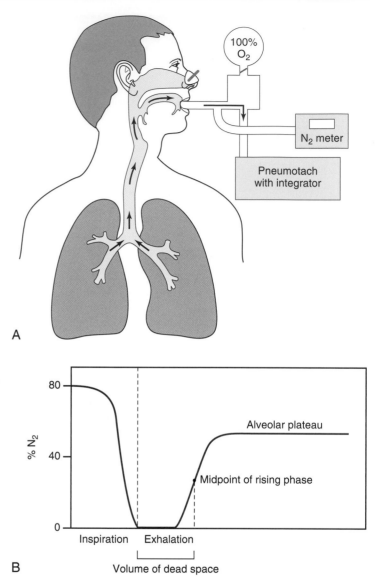

Fig. 5.9 Fowler's method for measuring anatomic dead space. **A,** The subject takes a single breath of 100% oxygen, holds his breath for a second, and then exhales. Nitrogen concentration is measured continuously during a steady rate of expiratory gas flow. **B,** At the beginning of exhalation, gas empties from the conducting airways that have been filled with 100% oxygen. Thus the nitrogen concentration in the exhaled air is 0. As gas begins to empty from alveoli, the nitrogen concentration rises and then plateaus when only gas from previously filled alveoli empties. The volume of gas exhaled to the midpoint of the rising phase of the exhaled nitrogen concentration trace is the anatomic dead space. (Modified from Levitzky M. *Pulmonary Physiology*, 8th ed. New York: McGraw-Hill; 2013.)

AGING

Aging affects both the structure and the function of the respiratory system. Lung growth, best measured by the forced expiratory volume after 1 second (FEV_1), occurs throughout childhood and reaches a peak or maximum level at approximately 18 years of age in women and 21 years of age in men. Lung function then declines, with a loss in FEV_1 of approximately 30 mL/year (Fig. 5.10). This loss occurs due to the progressive loss of alveolar elastic recoil combined with costal cartilage calcification, decreased intervertebral space, and greater spinal curvature.

FRC increases with age in association with the decrease in elastic recoil and dynamic compression. Expiratory muscle strength also decreases and the combination results in decreased expiratory airflow rates. Airway closure occurs in dependent airways. As a result, there is greater ventilation to the apices of the lung—regions that are normally less well ventilated. This results in decreased arterial oxygen

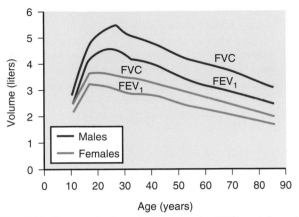

Fig. 5.10 Changes in forced vital capacity (FVC) and forced expiratory volume after 1 second (FEV_1) with age in normal men and women. Peak lung function occurs around 18 years of age for women and 21 years of age for men. (Redrawn from Knudson RJ, Slatin RC, Lebowitz MD, Burrows B. The maximal expiratory flow–volume curve. Normal standards, variability and the effects of age. *Am Rev Respir Dis*. 1976;113:587–600.)

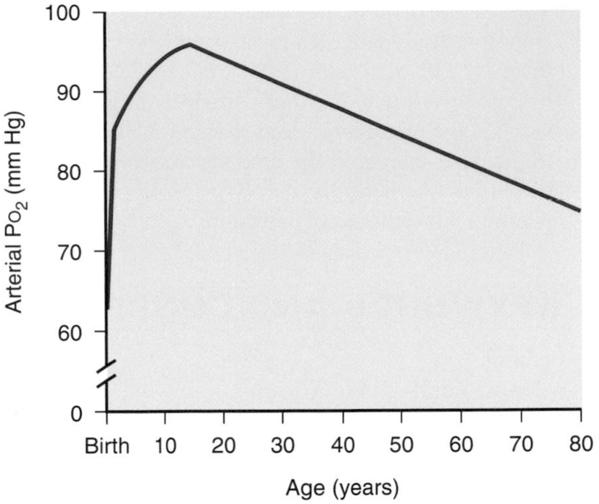

Fig. 5.11 Effect of age on arterial levels of oxygen. (Data from Mansell A, Bryan C, Levison H. Airway closure in children. J Appl Physiol. 1972;33:711-714; Nelson NM. Neonatal pulmonary function. *Pediatr Clin North Am*. 1966;13:769-799; and Sorbini CA, Grassi V, Solinas E, Muiesan GL. Arterial oxygen tension in relation to age in healthy subjects. *Respiration*. 1968;25:3–13.)

tension (see Chapter 7) as a result of ventilation:perfusion inequality (Fig. 5.11). Finally, there is a loss of alveolar surface area and decreased pulmonary capillary blood flow, resulting in decreased diffusion capacity that also contributes to the decrease in arterial oxygen tension in older individuals.

SUMMARY

1. The sum of the partial pressures of a gas must be equal to the total pressure. The partial pressure of a gas (P_{gas}) is equal to the fraction of gas in the gas mixture (F_{gas}) times the total pressure (P_{tot}).
2. By the time inspired gas reaches the trachea, it is fully saturated with water vapor, which exerts a pressure of 47 mm Hg at body temperature and dilutes the partial pressures of nitrogen and oxygen.
3. The conducting airways do not participate in gas exchange, and therefore the partial pressures of oxygen, nitrogen, and water vapor remain unchanged in the airways until the gas reaches the alveolus.
4. The partial pressure of oxygen in the alveolus is given by the alveolar air equation. This is the partial pressure of oxygen in the ideal situation—that is, in the absence of disease.
5. The respiratory quotient is defined as the ratio of carbon dioxide production to oxygen consumption. It is 0.8 under usual circumstances.
6. The relationship between carbon dioxide production and alveolar ventilation is defined by the alveolar carbon dioxide equation. There is an inverse relationship between the partial pressure of carbon dioxide in the alveolus (Pco_2) and alveolar ventilation (V_A) irrespective of exhaled CO_2. In normal individuals, the alveolar $Paco_2$ is tightly regulated to remain constant at about 40 mm Hg.
7. There are regional differences in ventilation due in large part to the effects of gravity. In an individual in the upright position (compared with the supine position), alveoli at the apex of the lung are larger and less compliant and receive less of each tidal volume breath than alveoli at the base or dependent portion of the lung.
8. Alveolar units in the lung with long time constants ($\tau = R \times C$) fill and empty slowly.
9. In the single-breath nitrogen test, the slope of phase III is an index of nonuniform ventilation.

10. The volume of air in the conducting airways is called the anatomic dead space. Dead space ventilation ($\dot{V}_{DS}$) varies inversely with tidal volume (V_T). The total volume of gas in each breath that does not participate in gas exchange is called the physiologic dead space. It includes the anatomic dead space and the dead space secondary to ventilated but not perfused alveoli or alveoli overventilated relative to the amount of perfusion.

11. Dead space ventilation can be measured using Bohr's equation and Fowler's method.

12. Aging results in a loss of lung elastic recoil, decreased expiratory muscle strength, airway closure in dependent lung units, decreased chest wall compliance, decreased arterial oxygen tension, loss of alveolar surface area, and decreased pulmonary capillary blood flow with decreased diffusion capacity.

KEYWORDS AND CONCEPTS

Aging lung
Alveolar carbon dioxide equation
Alveolar gas equation
Alveolar plateau
Alveolar ventilation
Anatomic dead space
Bohr's dead space equation
Boyle's law
Carbon dioxide production
Dalton's law
Dead space
Distribution of ventilation
Fowler's method

Gas fraction
Gas tension
Minute ventilation
Oxygen consumption
Partial pressure
Physiologic dead space
Pressure-volume curve
Respiratory quotient
Single-breath nitrogen test
Tidal volume (V_T, or TV)
Time constant (τ)
Torr
Water vapor pressure

SELF-STUDY PROBLEMS

1. If the dead space is 150 mL and the tidal volume increases from 500 to 600 mL, with the same minute ventilation, what is the effect on dead space ventilation?

2. A patient is breathing into a spirometer at a tidal volume of 500 mL and a respiratory frequency of 12 breaths per minute. The inspired gas is switched to 100% O_2 at the end of a full exhalation (residual volume), and the nitrogen concentration is monitored at the lips during the next exhalation. The nitrogen concentration is zero for the first 130 mL and then increases to a constant level of 50% at 170 mL of exhaled gas and remains at this level for the duration of exhalation. What is the dead space?

3. At Pike's Peak (445 mm Hg), what is the partial pressure of inspired air? Of air in the conducting airways?

4. What is the effect of an increased Pa_{CO_2} on alveolar P_{O_2}?

5. If alveolar ventilation is held constant, what is the effect of increased CO_2 production on alveolar P_{O_2}?

6. What is the effect of standing on your head on the distribution of ventilation?

ADDITIONAL READINGS

Agostoni E. Mechanics of the pleural space. *Physiol Rev.* 1972;52:57–128.

Anthonisen NR, Fleetham JA. Ventilation. Total, alveolar, and dead space. In: Farhi LE, Tenney SM, eds. *Gas Exchange. Handbook of Physiology, Section 3: The Respiratory System.* vol. 4. Bethesda: American Physiological Society; 1987.

Broaddus VC, Mason RJ, Ernst JD, King Jr TE, Lazarus SC, Murray JF, Nadel JA, Slutsky AS, eds. *Murray & Nadel's Textbook of Respiratory Medicine.* 6th ed. Philadelphia: WB Saunders; 2016.

Burrows B, Lebowitz MD, Camilli AE, et al. Longitudinal changes in forced expiratory volume in one second in adults: methodological considerations and findings in healthy nonsmokers. *Am Rev Respir Dis.* 1986;133:974–980.

Ferrannini E. The theoretical basis of indirect calorimetry: a review. *Metabolism.* 1988;37:287–301.

Gattinoni L, Vagginelli F, Carlesso E, et al. Decrease in Pa_{CO_2} with prone position is predictive of improved outcome in acute respiratory distress syndrome. *Crit Care Med.* 2003;31:2727–2733.

Lucangelo U, Blanch L. Dead space. *Intensive Care Med.* 2004;30:576–579.

Lum L, Saville AL, Venkataraman ST. Accuracy of physiologic dead space measurement in intubated pediatric patients using a metabolic monitor: comparison with the Douglas bag method. *Crit Care Med.* 1998;26:760–764.

Mummery HJ, Stolp BW, deL Dear G, et al. Effects of age and exercise on physiological dead space during simulated dives at 2.8 ATA. *J Appl Physiol.* 2003;94:507–517.

Shadick NA, Sparrow D, O'Connor GT, et al. Relationship of serum IgE concentration to level and rate of decline of pulmonary function; the Normative Aging Study. *Thorax.* 1996;51:787–792.

6

The Pulmonary Circulation

OBJECTIVES

1. Describe the anatomy, function, physiology, and regulation of the two circulations in the lung.
2. Describe the distribution of pulmonary blood flow.
3. Explain pulmonary vascular resistance in alveolar and extraalveolar vessels and the effect of lung volume on these resistances.
4. List the anatomic components of the alveolar–capillary network.
5. Describe lymphatic flow and its components.
6. Explain the mechanisms of pulmonary edema formation.

The systemic circulation is composed of the vascular system supplied by the left ventricle that pumps blood into the aorta for distribution to the rest of the body. In contrast, the pulmonary circulation is composed of the vascular system that conducts blood from the right side of the heart through the lungs. These two vascular systems exist in parallel, and both receive the entire cardiac output each minute.

The lung is the only organ in the body that receives blood from two separate sources. The pulmonary circulation brings deoxygenated blood from the right ventricle to the gas-exchanging units. At the gas-exchanging units, oxygen is transported across the alveolar and capillary endothelium into the red blood cell, and carbon dioxide is transferred from the blood into the alveolus before it is returned to the left atrium for distribution to the rest of the body. The second blood supply is the bronchial circulation, which arises from the aorta and provides nourishment to the lung parenchyma. The blood supply to the lung is unique in its dual circulation and its ability to accommodate large volumes of blood at low pressure.

PULMONARY BLOOD FLOW

Pulmonary blood flow consists of the entire output of the right ventricle. All of the mixed venous blood from all of the tissues in the body is pumped out of the right ventricle into the pulmonary circulation. As a result, pulmonary blood flow is equal to cardiac output—about 3.5 L/min/m² of body surface area at rest and as much as 25 L/min/m²

during exercise. At rest, the volume of blood contained in the lung (from the main pulmonary artery to the left atrium) is approximately 500 mL, or 10% of the circulating blood volume. Of this 500 mL, 70 mL of blood is contained in the pulmonary capillary bed. Approximately 280 billion capillaries supply the approximately 300 million alveoli, resulting in a surface area for gas exchange of 70 to 80 m².

The pulmonary capillary bed has the largest surface area of any vascular bed in the body. Many of these pulmonary capillaries are closed at rest and open periodically during periods of increased pulmonary blood flow. The network of capillaries is so dense that it may be considered to be a sheet of blood interrupted by small, vertical, connective-tissue supporting posts (see Fig. 1.8). At rest, it takes a red cell about 4 to 5 seconds to travel through the pulmonary circulation, with 0.75 second of this time spent in the pulmonary capillaries. The pulmonary capillaries have diameters of about 6 μm, slightly smaller than the diameter of a red blood cell (8 μm). Thus red blood cells must change their shape as they pass through the pulmonary capillaries. This shape change ensures the smallest possible distance between oxygen in the alveolus and the hemoglobin in the red cell.

During exercise, cardiac output and thus pulmonary blood flow can increase to as much as 25 L/min/m² and the pulmonary capillary volume increases and approaches about 200 mL. The increase in blood volume in the lung that occurs as a result of the increase in cardiac output during exercise occurs through two different processes (Fig. 6.1). First, closed or compressed capillary segments

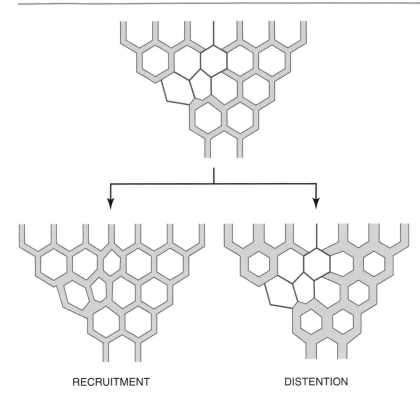

RECRUITMENT

DISTENTION

Fig. 6.1 There are two processes responsible for increased pulmonary capillary volume with exercise in the lung. At rest, many pulmonary capillaries are not perfused; with exercise and increased pulmonary blood flow, previously closed capillaries can fill with blood (recruitment) secondary to an increase in perfusion pressure or already-open capillaries can increase in volume (distention). Both processes occur during exercise and neither results in a significant increase in pulmonary vascular resistance. (Modified from Levitzky MG. *Pulmonary Physiology*, 8th ed. New York: McGraw-Hill; 2013.)

are recruited and open as the increase in cardiac output raises the pulmonary vascular pressure. Second, previously open capillaries enlarge as their internal pressure rises. Enlargement of open capillaries also occurs in individuals with left-sided heart failure, which is associated with an elevated left atrial pressure and an increase in pulmonary capillary volume.

The pulmonary veins are situated within loose interlobular connective tissue septae and receive blood from many lung units. They return blood to the left atrium through conventional and supernumerary branches. Because of their large numbers and thin walls, the pulmonary veins provide a large reservoir for blood, and these veins can either increase or decrease their capacitance to provide a constant left ventricular output in the face of a variable pulmonary arterial flow.

Pulmonary arteries and veins with diameters larger than 50 μm contain smooth muscle and are innervated through the sympathetic branch of the autonomic nervous system. Their extensive sensory innervation, located in the outer connective tissue layer (adventitia) of the vessel wall, can be stimulated by changes in vascular pressure (stretch) and various chemical substances. These vessels actively regulate their diameter and thus alter resistance to blood flow. In contrast, pulmonary arterioles and capillaries are devoid of smooth muscle.

BRONCHIAL BLOOD FLOW

The existence of a second, separate circulatory system in the lung with oxygenated blood from the systemic circulation was first observed by Frederich Ruysch in the latter half of the 17th century. This second circulatory system is the **bronchial circulation**, and it provides systemic arterial perfusion to the trachea, upper airways, surface secretory cells, glands, nerves, visceral pleural surface, lymph nodes, pulmonary arteries, and pulmonary veins (Fig. 6.2). The bronchial circulation perfuses the respiratory tract to the level of the terminal bronchioles. Lung structures distal to the terminal bronchioles, including the respiratory bronchioles, alveolar ducts, alveolar sacs, and alveoli, are directly oxygenated by diffusion from the alveolar air and receive their nutrients from the mixed venous blood in the pulmonary circulation.

Bronchial blood flow comprises only 1% to 3% of the output of the left ventricle. The bronchial arteries, usually three in number, arise either from the aorta or from the intercostal arteries and accompany the bronchial

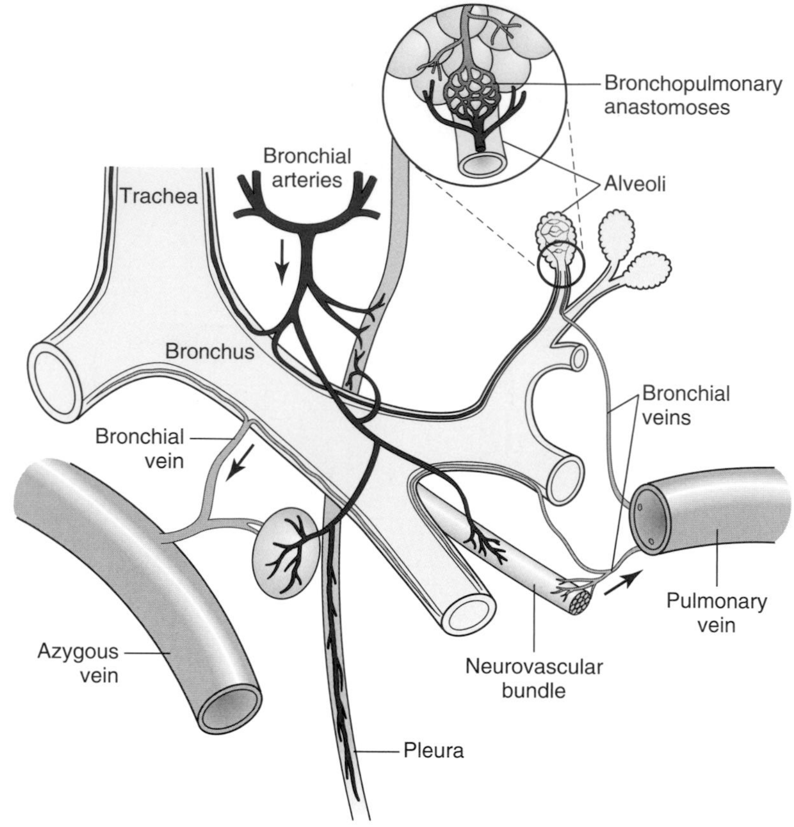

Fig. 6.2 The anatomic features of the bronchial circulation. The bronchial circulation supplies blood to the trachea and airways to the level of the terminal bronchioles as well as to the pulmonary blood vessels, visceral pleura, hilar lymph nodes, and vagus nerve and its branches. Inset depicts a bronchopulmonary anastomosis. Venous drainage in the lung is to both the right side of the circulation via the azygos and hemiazygos veins and to the left side of the circulation via the pulmonary veins (Redrawn from Deffebach ME, Charan NB, Lakshminarayan S, Butler J. The bronchial circulation: small but a vital attribute of the lung. *Am Rev Respir Dis.* 1987;135:463.)

tree and divide with it (see Fig. 1.9). The pressure in the bronchial arteries is equal to the systemic pressure and is therefore much higher than the pressure in the pulmonary circulation.

The return of venous blood from the capillaries of the bronchial circulation to the heart occurs either through true bronchial veins or through bronchopulmonary veins. True bronchial veins are present in the area of the hilum and flow into the azygos, hemiazygos, or intercostal veins before entering the right atrium. The bronchopulmonary veins are formed through a network of tributaries composed of both bronchial and pulmonary circulatory vessels, which anastomose and form vessels with an admixture of blood from both circulatory systems (see Fig. 6.2). Blood from these anastomosed vessels returns to the left atrium through pulmonary veins. It is estimated that about two-thirds of the total bronchial circulation is returned to the heart via the pulmonary veins and this anastomosis route. This deoxygenated blood, which mixes with oxygen-enriched blood in the pulmonary veins, contributes to the small

alveolar–arterial oxygen difference in normal individuals (see Chapter 7).

The physiologic function of the bronchial circulation remains somewhat of an enigma; lung transplant studies have shown that adult lungs can function normally in the absence of a bronchial circulatory system. Thus in healthy individuals, these anastomoses are probably of little importance. They may, however, be important in neonates and young children in bringing nutrients to the developing lung and in disease states in which reciprocal changes in flow in the two circulations provide a steady supply of nutrients. For example, in individuals with a **pulmonary embolus**, the bronchial circulation increases to the areas of the lung normally supplied by the pulmonary arteries; as a result, **pulmonary infarction** (death of the lung tissue) rarely occurs even with large pulmonary emboli. Similarly, in individuals who have undergone **lung transplantation** in which the bronchial circulation has been removed, necrosis (death) of the airway cells and other structures supplied by the bronchial circulation does not occur because of an increase in pulmonary circulation to these areas.

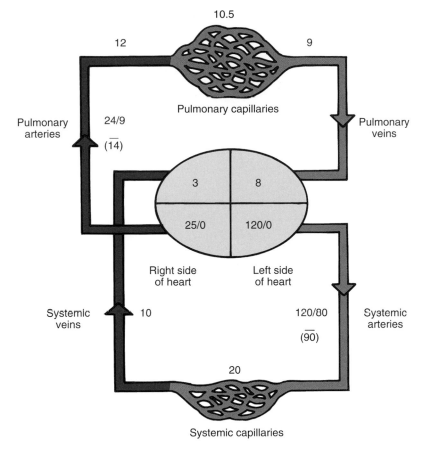

Fig. 6.3 Schematic representation of the phasic and mean pressures within the systemic and pulmonary circulations in a normal, resting human adult lying supine (dorsal recumbency). The units are millimeters of mercury (mm Hg) for easy comparison. The driving pressure in the systemic circuit is the difference between the pressure in the aorta (Pao) and the pressure in the right atrium (PRA), and is represented as (Pao – PRA) = 90 – 3 = 87 mm Hg, whereas the driving pressure in the pulmonary circuit is the differences between the pressure in the pulmonary artery (PPA) and the pressure in the left atrium (PLA), which is represented as (PPA – PLA) = 14 – 8 = 6 mm Hg. Cardiac output must be the same in both circuits in the steady state because they are in series; thus the resistance to flow through the lungs is less than 10% than the rest of the body. Note also that the pressures in the left heart chambers are higher than those in the right heart. Any congenital openings between the right and left sides of the heart favor left-to-right flow. (From Koeppen BM, Stanton BM, eds. *Berne and Levy's Physiology,* 7th ed. Philadelphia: Elsevier; 2018.)

PRESSURES AND FLOWS IN THE PULMONARY CIRCULATION

The pulmonary circulation begins in the right atrium. Deoxygenated blood from the right atrium enters the right ventricle via the tricuspid valve and is then pumped under low pressure (9–24 mm Hg) into the pulmonary artery through the pulmonic valve (Fig. 6.3). The main pulmonary artery, also known as the pulmonary trunk, is about 3 cm in diameter; it branches quickly (~5 cm from the right ventricle) into the right and left main pulmonary arteries, which supply blood to the right and left lungs, respectively. The arteries of the pulmonary circulation are the only arteries in the body that carry deoxygenated blood. The deoxygenated blood passes through a progressively smaller series of branching vessels (vessel diameters: arteries >500 μm, arterioles 10–200 μm, capillaries <10 μm) ending in a complex, mesh-like network of capillaries with very thin walls and large internal diameters relative to their wall thickness. The sequential branching pattern of the pulmonary arteries follows a pattern similar to airway branching, such that there are supporting vascular structures for each airway (see Fig. 1.9). The pulmonary circulatory system functions to (1) reoxygenate the blood and remove CO_2, (2) aid in maintenance of fluid balance in the lung, and (3) distribute the metabolic products of the lung.

Oxygenation of red blood cells occurs in the alveolus where the pulmonary capillary bed and the alveoli come together in the alveolar wall in a configuration that achieves optimal gas exchange. Gas exchange occurs through this **alveolar–capillary network.**

Oxygenated blood leaves the alveolus through a network of small pulmonary venules (15–500 μm in diameter) and veins, which quickly coalesce to form larger pulmonary veins (>500 μm in diameter) in which the oxygenated blood returns to the left atrium of the heart. In contrast to arteries, arterioles, and capillaries, which closely follow the branching patterns of the airways, venules and veins run quite distant from the airways.

Unlike systemic arteries, the arteries of the pulmonary circulation are thin-walled with minimal smooth muscle. This has important physiologic consequences, including less resistance to blood flow. Pulmonary arteries are also more distensible and compressible than systemic arterial vessels, and they are seven times more compliant. This highly compliant state requires much less work (lower pressures throughout the pulmonary circulation) for blood flow through the pulmonary circulation compared with the more muscular, noncompliant arterial walls of the systemic circulation. Furthermore, the vessels in the pulmonary circulation, under normal circumstances, are in a dilated state and have larger diameters compared with similar arteries in the systemic circulation. All of these factors contribute to a very compliant, low-resistance circulatory system, which aids in the flow of blood through the pulmonary circulation via the relatively "weak" pumping action of the right ventricle, which is less muscular than the left ventricle. The pressure gradient differential for the pulmonary circulation from the pulmonary artery to the left atrium is only 6 mm Hg (14 mm Hg in the pulmonary artery minus 8 mm Hg in the left atrium) (see Fig. 6.3). It is almost 15 times less than the pressure gradient differential of 87 mm Hg present in the systemic circulation (90 mm Hg in the aorta minus 3 mm Hg in the right atrium).

PULMONARY VASCULAR RESISTANCE

Four factors influence blood flow in the lung: **pulmonary vascular resistance** (PVR), gravity, alveolar pressure, and the arterial to venous pressure gradient. Blood flows through the pulmonary circulation in a pulsatile manner following the pressure gradient in this low resistance system. PVR cannot be measured directly but is most often calculated using Poiseuille's law, in which R equals the difference in pressure between the beginning of the tube (P_1) and the end of the tube (P_2) divided by the flow ($\dot{Q}$); that is,

$$R = \frac{P_1 - P_2}{\dot{Q}}$$

In the pulmonary circulation, PVR is the change in pressure from the pulmonary artery (P_{PA}) to the left atrium (P_{LA}) divided by the flow ($\dot{Q}_T$), which is the cardiac output; that is,

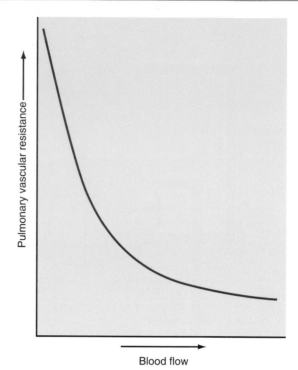

Fig. 6.4 Effect of pulmonary blood flow on pulmonary vascular resistance. With exercise, pulmonary blood flow increases and pulmonary vascular resistance decreases due to distention and recruitment of pulmonary vessels. (Data from Borst HG, et al. Influence of pulmonary arterial and left atrial pressure on pulmonary vascular resistance. *Circ Res.* 1956;4:393.)

$$PVR = \frac{P_{PA} - P_{LA}}{\dot{Q}_T}$$

Under normal circumstances, with normal cardiac output,

$$PVR = \frac{14 \text{ mm Hg} - 8 \text{ mm Hg}}{6 \text{ L/min}}$$
$$= 1.0 \text{ mm Hg/L/min}$$

This resistance is approximately 10 times less than the resistance in the systemic circulation. As previously mentioned, the low resistance in the pulmonary circulation system has two unique features, recruitment and distention, which allow for increased blood flow on demand with little or no increase in PVR (Fig. 6.4). All of the available vessels are not utilized under normal resting conditions; this allows for compensation and recruitment of new vessels upon increased demand, such as during exercise, with little or no increase in pulmonary artery pressure. The

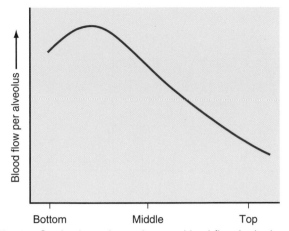

Fig. 6.5 Gravity-dependent pulmonary blood flow in the lung. In general, blood flow to alveoli at the bottom of the lung is greater than blood flow at the top at total lung capacity when an individual is in the upright position, even though at the very bottom of the lung, there is a small decrease in blood flow per alveolus. (Redrawn from Hughes JMB, Glazier JB, Maloney JE, West JB. Effect of lung volume on the distribution of pulmonary blood flow in man. *Respir Physiol.* 1968;4:58.)

distensibility of the blood vessels in the pulmonary circulation enables the vessels to increase their diameter with only a minimal increase in pulmonary arterial pressure.

At rest, about one-third of the resistance to blood flow is located in the pulmonary arteries, one-third is located in the pulmonary capillaries, and one-third is located in the pulmonary veins. In contrast, in the systemic circulation, most (70%) of the resistance to blood flow is located in the highly muscular systemic arterioles.

GRAVITY AND EFFECTS ON PULMONARY BLOOD FLOW

Because the pulmonary circulation is a low-pressure/low-resistance system, it is influenced by gravity much more dramatically than is the systemic circulation. This gravitational effect contributes to an uneven distribution of blood flow in the lung. In an upright individual, under normal resting conditions, there is a linear increase in blood flow from the apex of the lung (lowest flow; can approach zero under various conditions) to the base of the lung, where it is greatest but with no difference anterior to posterior (Fig. 6.5). Similarly, when a person is supine, blood flow is less in the uppermost (anterior) regions and greater in the lower (posterior) regions but equal in the apical and basal regions of the lung. Under conditions of stress, such as exercise, the difference in blood flow in the

upright position in the apical and basal regions becomes less, due mainly to the increase in flow and the increase in arterial pressure.

Upon leaving the pulmonary artery, blood must travel up to the apex of the lung, against gravity, in the upright position. It is estimated that for every 1 cm increase in height above the heart, there is a corresponding decrease in hydrostatic pressure relative to the change in height. Thus a change of 1 cm in height is equivalent to a change in hydrostatic pressure of 0.74 mm Hg, and a segment of lung that is 10 cm above the heart will have a decrease in arterial pressure of 7.4 mm Hg. At this point, the arterial pressure would be 6.6 mm Hg (arterial pressure at level of the heart equals 14 mm Hg minus 7.4 mm Hg). Conversely, a segment of lung 5 cm below the heart will experience an increase in arterial pressure of 3.7 mm Hg and thus have an arterial pressure of 17.7 mm Hg. The effect of gravity on blood flow affects arteries and veins equally. It is obvious from these two examples that there are wide variations in arterial and venous pressures from the apex to the base of the lung. These variations influence not only flow but also ventilation/perfusion relationships (see Chapter 7).

In addition to the arterial pressure (Pa) and venous pressure (Pv) gradients, differences in the pulmonary alveolar pressure (PA) influence blood flow in the lung. Blood flow in the lung has been divided into three zones based on the different physiologic aspects of function in each zone or region (Fig. 6.6). Zone 1 represents the apex, where it is possible to have no blood flow. This could occur at the very top of the lung where Pa is so low that it can be exceeded by PA. The capillaries collapse because of the greater external PA that prevents blood flow. Under normal conditions, this zone does not exist; however, this state may be reached during positive-pressure mechanical ventilation or if a physiologic alteration sufficiently decreases Pa. Under conditions of decreased arterial pressure, the blood flow rises only to the level at which the arterial and alveolar pressures are equal; above this, there is no flow.

Under normal circumstances, and when a person is in the upright position, most of the lung functions in what is referred to as Zones 2 and 3. In Zone 2, which comprises the upper one-third of the lung, Pa is greater than PA, which also is greater than Pv. Because PA is greater than Pv, the greater external PA partially collapses the downstream capillaries, causing a "damming" effect before the blood flows to the venous system. This phenomenon is often referred to as the "waterfall effect." In Zone 3, Pa is greater than Pv, which is greater than PA, and blood flow in this area follows the pressure gradients. Because the effect of gravity is equal on both arteries and veins, there is no change in the pressure differential at the base

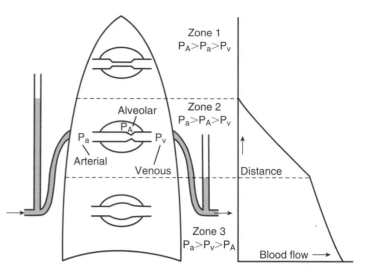

Fig. 6.6 Model depicting the uneven distribution of blood flow in the lung, based on the pressures affecting the capillaries. (From West JB, Dollery CT, Naimark J. Distribution of blood flow in isolated lung: relation to vascular and alveolar pressure. *J Appl Physiol.* 1964;19:713.)

of the lung compared with the apex. Flow is increased in the basal area due to an increase in transmural pressure, which has the effect of distending the vessels and thus lowering resistance.

EFFECTS OF PRESSURE CHANGES ON EXTRAALVEOLAR AND ALVEOLAR VESSELS

Changes in alveolar and intrapleural pressure influence pulmonary blood flow, but the effects are different depending on the location of the vessels. The vessels in the pulmonary circulation can be divided into three categories—extraalveolar, alveolar, and microcirculation. These three categories of pulmonary vessels are not well defined anatomically, but they have marked differences in physiologic properties that change under various conditions such as stress and exercise.

The extraalveolar vessels are generally larger vessels (arteries, arterioles, veins, and venules); these vessels are not influenced by alveolar pressure changes but are affected by intrapleural and interstitial pressure changes (Fig. 6.7). As the transmural pressure gradient (which is equal to the pressure inside minus the pressure outside the vessel) increases, the vessel diameter increases and resistance decreases. Changes in either the intrapleural pressure or the interstitial pressure as a result of changes in lung volume and the retractive force generated by elastin (radial traction) greatly influence vessel caliber. For example, at high lung volumes, the decrease in pleural pressure increases the transmural pressure and increases the caliber of (dilates) extraalveolar vessels, resulting in a decrease in resistance. In contrast, at low lung volumes, an increase in

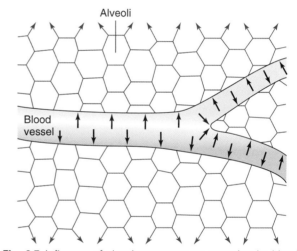

Fig. 6.7 Influence of alveolar pressure on extraalveolar blood vessels. By virtue of their location, extraalveolar blood vessels are not influenced directly by alveolar pressure. The extraalveolar blood vessels are, however, tethered to the surrounding alveoli, and thus their caliber changes with changes in lung volume. Resistance to blood flow is higher at low lung volumes because the traction on the vessel walls is decreased. (Redrawn from Leff A, Schumacker P. *Respiratory Physiology Basics and Applications.* Philadelphia: W.B. Saunders; 1993.)

pleural pressure decreases transmural pressure and has a constricting effect with an increase in resistance.

Alveolar vessels include the capillaries within the interalveolar septa. These vessels are very sensitive to shifts in alveolar pressure but not to changes in pleural or interstitial pressure (Fig. 6.8). During inspiration, alveoli increase in volume; this

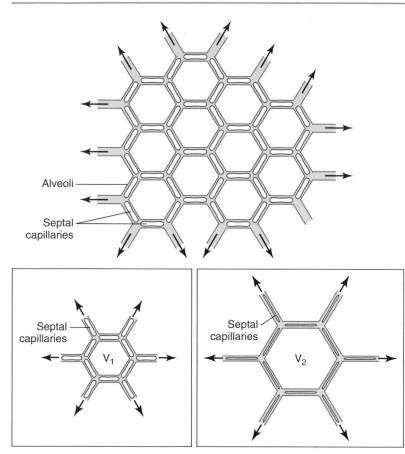

Alveoli

Septal
capillaries

Septal
capillaries

V_1

Septal
capillaries

V_2

Fig. 6.8 Influence of alveolar pressure on intraalveolar or septal capillaries. These capillaries are very thin-walled and lack significant structural features. Their size and shape are highly dependent on the pressures across their walls (inside-outside pressure difference). As a result, increases in alveolar pressure secondary to increases in lung volume distort and compress these capillaries and increase their resistance to blood flow. (Redrawn from Levitzky MG. *Pulmonary Physiology*, 8th ed. New York: McGraw-Hill; 2013.)

increase is associated with elongation and compression of the vessels located in the interalveolar septae. As a result, at high lung volumes the resistance to blood flow within alveolar vessels increases; similarly, at low lung volumes compression is less and resistance to blood flow decreases.

It should be clear from the previous discussion that changes in lung volume affect PVR through their influence on alveolar and extraalveolar vessels. Thus at end inspiration the fully distended, air-filled alveoli apply pressure on the alveolar capillaries, increasing PVR. This stretching effect during inspiration has the opposite effect on the larger extraalveolar vessels, which increase in diameter due to radial traction and elastic recoil influences. During exhalation, the deflated alveoli apply the least resistance, and PVR is diminished.

The resistances of the alveolar and extraalveolar vessels are additive at any lung volume because the alveolar and extraalveolar vessels exist in series with each other. This results in the U-shaped curve of the total pulmonary vascular resistance (Fig. 6.9). Total PVR is lowest near FRC and increases at both high and low lung volumes.

With positive-pressure mechanical ventilation, there is both an increase in alveolar pressure and a decrease in the transmural pressure gradient in the extraalveolar vessels. This results in compression of both the extraalveolar and the alveolar capillaries and can block blood flow to the area. This can create Zone 1 blood flow.

The **pulmonary microcirculation** is a term used to describe the small vessels—usually pulmonary capillaries, but arterioles and venules to some extent—that participate in liquid and solute exchange in the maintenance of fluid balance in the lung.

THE ALVEOLAR–CAPILLARY NETWORK

Gas exchange in the lung occurs in the alveolar–capillary unit. The alveolar–capillary unit results from the sequential branching pattern of the pulmonary arteries, which culminates with the branching of the small arterioles into the alveolar wall. This unique pattern establishes a dense, mesh-like network of capillaries and alveoli with little structure other than the thin epithelial lining cells

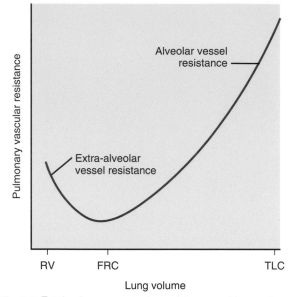

Fig. 6.9 Total pulmonary vascular resistance and lung volume. Total pulmonary vascular resistance is the sum of the resistances of the extraalveolar and the alveolar or septal capillaries. At low lung volumes, resistance increases because of the increased resistance originating from the extraalveolar vessels, whereas at total lung capacity (TLC), resistance increases because of the increase in resistance in the alveolar vessels. Total pulmonary vascular resistance is lowest at functional residual capacity (FRC). RV, residual volume. (Modified from Levitzky MG. *Pulmonary Physiology*, 8th ed. New York: McGraw-Hill; 2013.)

of the alveolus, the endothelial cells of the vessels, and their supportive matrix. There can be nearly 1000 pulmonary capillaries per alveolus, resulting in an alveolar–capillary network with a surface area of approximately 70 m² (about the size of a tennis court) (see Fig. 1.5). The structural matrix and the tissue components of this alveolar–capillary network are composed of type I alveolar epithelial cells, capillary endothelial cells, and their respective basement membranes that are organized back to back (Fig. 6.10). The distance for gas exchange through this basement membrane barrier is only about 1 to 2 μm in thickness. Surrounded mostly by air, this network creates an ideal environment for gas exchange. Red blood cells pass through this network in less than 1 second, sufficient time for CO_2 and O_2 gas exchange.

In addition to gas exchange, this network also functions in transcapillary exchange and fluid regulation within the lung. Solvents and solutes move across the capillary endothelial wall by diffusion, filtration, and/or pinocytosis. Diffusion is the most important means for solute transfer across the capillary endothelium; small molecules such as

water, NaCl, urea, and glucose move freely; their net movement is limited only by the rate at which blood flow transports them. Thus their transport is **flow-limited**. For larger molecules, diffusion across the capillary pores (clefts) limits their exchange; for these large molecules, exchange is **diffusion-limited**. Lipid-soluble molecules such as O_2 and CO_2 move across the capillary wall through pores by diffusion and directly through the capillary endothelium. O_2 diffuses across both the arterioles and venules. At low blood flow rates, this gas exchange may limit the supply of O_2 to the tissue. Pinocytosis is capable of moving large (30-nm) lipid-insoluble molecules between the blood and interstitial space.

Capillary filtration is regulated by the hydrostatic and osmotic forces across the endothelium. An increase in the intracapillary hydrostatic pressure favors the movement of fluid from the vessel to the interstitial space. Conversely, an increase in the concentration of osmotically active particles within the vessel favors movement of fluid into the vessels from the interstitial space.

All capillaries in the body have a variable degree of leakiness. At the pulmonary capillary level, the balance between hydrostatic pressure and oncotic pressure results in a small net movement of fluid (liquid, electrolytes, and protein) out of the vessels into the interstitial space. Fluids that leak into the interstitial space are inhibited from entering the airspace by the alveolar epithelium (type I and type II epithelial cells) that establishes a tight restrictive barrier and thus contains them in the interstitium. This barrier is highly advantageous because any fluid in the airspace will interfere with gas diffusion.

The alveolar–capillary network is also fragile and susceptible to a wide variety of injurious agents and events. The type I cell is the site of gas diffusion from the air into the capillaries but is quite susceptible to injury, perhaps because of its thin, elongated shape and large surface area. In certain disease states, such as interstitial lung diseases, the type I cell dies, leaving a denuded alveolar epithelium that is associated with increased permeability. The cuboidal-shaped type II epithelial cell then proliferates and differentiates into type I cells in an attempt to restore the normal lung architecture.

THE PULMONARY LYMPHATIC SYSTEM

Fluid that leaks out of the vascular compartment enters the interstitium surrounding the capillaries. From there it travels to the alveolar corners and then to the peribronchial interstitial space surrounding the bronchi and small arteries. Fluid then enters the lymphatic system, which is responsible for removing fluid from of the lung. The terminal lymphatic vessels are a closed-end network of highly permeable lymph capillaries. They lack tight junctions

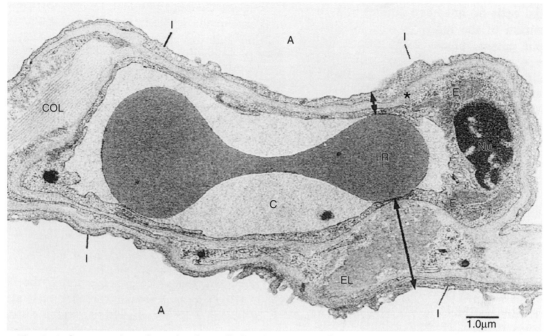

Fig. 6.10 Cross section of an alveolar wall showing the path for oxygen and carbon dioxide diffusion. The thin side of the alveolar wall barrier (short double arrow) consists of type I epithelium (I), interstitium (*) formed by the fused basal laminae of the epithelial and endothelial cells, capillary endothelium (E), plasma in the alveolar capillary (C), and finally by the cytoplasm of the red blood cell (R). The thick side of the gas-exchange barrier (long double arrow) has an accumulation of elastin (EL), collagen (COL), and matrix that jointly separate the alveolar epithelium from the alveolar capillary endothelium. As long as the red blood cells are flowing, oxygen and carbon dioxide diffusion probably occurs across both sides of the gas-exchange barrier. A, Alveolus; Nu, nucleus of the capillary endothelial cell. (Human lung specimen, transmission electron microscopy.) (From Koeppen BM, Stanton BM, eds. *Berne and Levy's Physiology*, 7th ed. Philadelphia: Elsevier; 2018.)

between endothelial cells and are anchored to connective tissue by fine filaments. Skeletal muscle contraction distorts the filaments and opens spaces between the endothelial cells. Blood capillary filtrate and the protein and cells that have passed from the vascular to the interstitial space enter the lymphatic capillaries. Lymph flows in an extensive system of one-way (monocuspid) valves, aided by skeletal muscle and lymphatic vessel contraction through thin-wall vessels of increasing diameter, and finally enters the subclavian veins at the junction with the internal jugular veins. The thoracic duct, which is the largest lymphatic vessel in the body, drains the lower extremities and the gastrointestinal tract and liver.

Fluid in the interstitium is removed from the lung by the lymphatic system and enters the circulation via the vena cava in the area of the hilum. In normal adults, it is estimated that an average of 30 mL of fluid/hour is returned to the circulation via this route. In 24 hours, a person's total plasma volume flows through the lymphatic system.

Approximately one-fourth to one-half of the circulating plasma proteins are returned by the lymphatics to the blood. This is the system for returning albumin to the circulation. The lymphatic system also filters lymph through the lymph nodes and removes foreign particles such as bacteria.

The Starling equation describes the movement of liquid across the capillary endothelium:

$$\text{Flux (flow in mL/min)} = \text{Kfc}\left[(\text{Pjv} - \text{Pis}) - \sigma(\pi\text{jv} - \pi\text{is})\right]$$

Where
Kfc = capillary filtration coefficient
Pjv = intravascular (capillary) hydrostatic pressure
Pis = interstitial hydrostatic pressure
σ = reflection coefficient (reflects the permeability of the membrane to protein)
πjv = intravascular colloid osmotic pressure
πis = interstitial colloid osmotic pressure

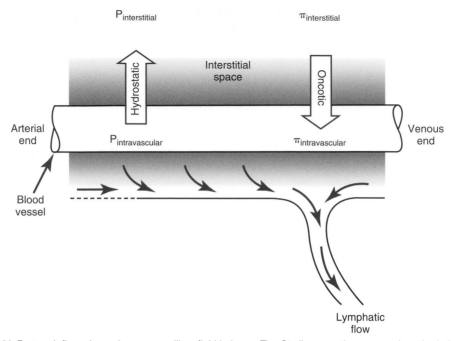

Fig. 6.11 Factors influencing pulmonary capillary fluid balance. The Starling equation summarizes the balance of forces favoring fluid flux into or out of the pulmonary vessels. Normally there is a net flux of fluid out of the vessels, which are drained from the interstitial space by the lymphatic system. (From Koeppen BM, Stanton BM, eds. *Berne and Levy's Physiology*, 7th ed. Philadelphia: Elsevier; 2018.)

In principle, the Starling equation illustrates the forces creating the net flux of fluid out of the pulmonary capillaries (Fig. 6.11). However, in practice it is not possible to actually calculate this flux. Many of the parameters needed cannot be measured. For instance, the Kfc is dependent on the number of capillaries actually being perfused, which is impossible to determine.

PULMONARY EDEMA

Increases in extravascular fluid accumulation in the lung can occur resulting in a condition called **pulmonary edema**. This fluid accumulation can occur either because of an increase in outward fluid filtration or because of a decrease in fluid removal. Causes of pulmonary edema have been categorized on the basis of the Starling equation.

Increased capillary permeability resulting in increased outward fluid filtration can occur when the integrity of the capillary endothelium is destroyed. For example, the capillary endothelium can be damaged by infections, toxins, and oxygen toxicity.

Under normal conditions, the capillary hydrostatic pressure is 10 mm Hg. Increases in capillary hydrostatic pressure result in greater outward fluid filtration. If the rate of outward fluid filtration exceeds lymphatic drainage, fluid accumulates in the interstitium. This is the most common cause of pulmonary edema. It is seen in individuals with left-sided cardiac dysfunction from cardiac infarction, left ventricular failure, or mitral valve stenosis. As pressures in the left atrium rise, the pulmonary capillary hydrostatic pressure increases and more fluid leaks into the interstitium.

The other major and common cause of pulmonary edema is a decrease in colloid osmotic pressure of the plasma. This can occur in individuals who are hypoproteinemic or after overzealous administration of intravenous fluids. Less common causes of pulmonary edema are listed in Table 6.1.

ACTIVE REGULATION OF BLOOD FLOW

Although the passive mechanisms of blood flow regulation discussed earlier in this chapter represent the major factors influencing blood flow in the lung, there are also several active mechanisms of blood flow regulation in the lung. Although the smooth muscle around the pulmonary vessels is much thinner than the musculature around the systemic vessels, it is sufficient to have a measurable effect on vessel

TABLE 6.1   Factors Predisposing to Pulmonary Edema

Factors	Clinical Problems
Starling Equation	
Increased capillary permeability (K_r; σ)	Adult respiratory distress syndrome
	Oxygen toxicity
	Inhaled or circulating toxins
Increased capillary hydrostatic pressure (P_c)	Increased left atrial pressure resulting from left ventricular infarction or mitral stenosis from left ventricular infarctio or mitral stenosis
	Overadministration of intravenous fluids
Decreased interstitial hydrostatic pressure (P_k) Too rapid evacuation of pneumothorax	Too rapid evacuation of pneumothorax or hemothorax
Decreased colloid osmotic pressure (πpt)	Protein starvation
	Dilution of blood resulting in urinary protein loss (proteinuria)
	Renal problems resulting in urinary protein loss (proteinuria)
Other Etiologies	
Insufficient pulmonary lymphatic drainage	Tumors
	Interstitial fibrosing diseases
Unknown etiology	High-altitude pulmonary edema
	Pulmonary edema after head injury (neurogenic pulmonary edema)
	Drug overdose

Source: Reproduced with permission from Levitzky MG, Cairo JM, Hall SM. *Introduction to Respiratory Care.* Philadelphia: Saunders; 1990.

caliber. This is especially true in capillaries in which blood flow depends chiefly on the contractile state of the arterioles. This contractile state is determined by the contraction and relaxation of the smooth muscle in the precapillary vessel (arteriole) and the transmural pressure gradient (discussed previously). In contrast, true capillaries are devoid of smooth muscle and are incapable of active contraction. Changes in their diameter are passive and are caused by alterations in precapillary and postcapillary resistance.

Low and high oxygen levels have a major effect on pulmonary capillary blood flow. Hypoxic vasoconstriction occurs in small arterial vessels in response to decreased arterial Po_2. The response is local and is believed to be a protective response by shifting the blood flow from the hypoxic areas to normal areas in an effort to enhance gas exchange. Isolated, local hypoxia does not alter PVR; it is estimated that approximately 20% of the vessels need to be hypoxic before a change in PVR can be measured. Low levels of inspired oxygen due to exposure to high altitudes will have a greater and general effect and can increase PVR (see Chapter 12). High concentrations of inspired oxygen can dilate pulmonary vessels and decrease PVR.

In addition to alterations in oxygen, there are a wide range of factors and mediators that can influence vessel caliber (Box 6.1). Several of these mediators warrant further discussion.

BOX 6.1   Compounds With Active Regulatory Properties in Pulmonary Blood Flow

Pulmonary Vasoconstrictors
- Low Pao_2
- Thromboxane A_2
- α-Adrenergic catecholamines
- Angiotensin
- Leukotrienes
- Neuropeptides
- Serotonin
- Endothelin
- Histamine
- Prostaglandins
- High CO_2

Pulmonary Vasodilators
- High Pao_2
- Prostacyclin
- Nitric oxide
- Acetylcholine
- Bradykinin
- Dopamine
- β-Adrenergic catecholamines

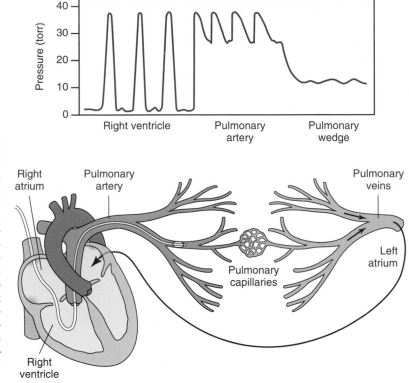

Fig. 6.12 Measurement of pulmonary capillary pressures in the lung. The right side of the heart is catheterized and a water-filled balloon is floated out into the pulmonary artery. The tip of the catheter is wedged into a branch of the pulmonary artery. When the balloon is inflated, all blood flow ceases; the pressure recorded at the balloon tip (pulmonary capillary wedge pressure) is approximately equal to the pressure in the left atrium. The recording of the various pressures as the catheter is advanced can be used to measure pulmonary artery pressure and right ventricular pressure and is useful in the intensive care unit to distinguish between pulmonary and cardiac disease. (Redrawn from Leff A, Schumacker P. *Respiratory Physiology: Basics and Applications.* Philadelphia: W.B. Saunders; 1993.)

Endothelin is a potent vasoconstrictor that is released by pulmonary endothelial cells in response to shear stress and hypoxia. Increased levels of endothelin are thought to play a major role in the development of pulmonary hypertension; the recent development of endothelin antagonist drugs represents a major advance in the treatment of this progressive group of diseases.

Thromboxane A$_2$, a product of arachidonic acid metabolism, is one of the most potent vasoconstrictors of airway and vascular smooth muscle. It is released from white blood cells, macrophages, and platelets.

The capillary endothelium is also capable of producing potent vasodilators. One of these is endothelium-derived relaxing factor, which has been shown to be the gas **nitric oxide (NO)**. NO is formed and released by the endothelium in response to acetylcholine, adenosine triphosphate (ATP), serotonin, bradykinin, histamine, and substance P. Most of these vasoconstricting and vasodilating factors are released by local cells or by inflammatory cells. They have a short half-life and their effect is usually local.

MEASUREMENT OF PULMONARY VASCULAR PRESSURES

The pressures in the pulmonary circulation can be measured during a right heart catheterization (Fig. 6.12). In this procedure, a small, fluid-filled catheter (tube) is inserted into a vein and advanced toward the heart. A balloon at the tip of the catheter is inflated with air; as a result, the catheter is carried with the blood into the right atrium and then into the right ventricle. The catheter, which is connected to a pressure transducer, records the pressure in the right atrium and right ventricle. The catheter is then passed through the pulmonic valve and floated into the pulmonary trunk, where pressure measurements are again made. Finally, the catheter lodges in a pulmonary vessel and occludes that vessel. The balloon at the tip of the catheter is inflated, and all blood flow to the area ceases.

The pressure that is measured at the point of occlusion approximates the pressure in the left atrium because there is a static column of blood in the area. The left atrial pressure measured by inflating the balloon around the tip of the catheter in the pulmonary artery and occluding blood flow is called the **pulmonary capillary wedge pressure** (see Fig. 6.12). This measurement is particularly useful in sorting out cardiac from pulmonary causes of pulmonary edema. It is, however, an invasive procedure and can be done only in the cardiac catheterization laboratory or in specially equipped intensive care units.

This same catheter, however, when equipped with a temperature sensor near the distal tip, can also be used to measure pulmonary blood flow, and thus cardiac output. In this procedure, called **thermodilution**, ice-cold water is injected into the right atrium, and the temperature is measured by the sensor located in the pulmonary artery. The temperature–time curve is integrated, and the volume and temperature of the injected bolus is recorded and used to determine the cardiac output. It can be seen that small decreases in the temperature of the fluid noted by the sensor reflect high cardiac outputs because energy is conserved and the drop in temperature reflects a rapid movement of the fluid bolus with little time to warm to body temperature. The computations are complex and computer programs are used to generate the results.

CLINICAL BOX

Infants born with certain types of congenital heart disease (e.g., Tetralogy of Fallot, a congenital heart disease associated with a ventricular septal defect, an overriding aorta, pulmonary valve stenosis and right ventricular hypertrophy) are cyanotic because of a marked decrease in pulmonary blood flow. In the case of tetralogy of Fallot, deoxygenated blood flows through the ventricular septal defect to the left ventricle, bypassing the lung. In 1945 a procedure was developed for children with this condition that revolutionized pediatric cardiology. Named after the cardiologist (Helen Taussig) and the surgeon (Alfred Blalock) who performed the first one on an infant, the Blalock-Taussig (BT) shunt is a surgically created connection between a systemic artery and the pulmonary artery. It currently uses a graft to connect the subclavian artery to the pulmonary artery to augment pulmonary blood flow (see Figure alongside). The procedure itself, however, was developed by a young African American surgical technician named Vivien Thomas in an experimental animal laboratory at Johns Hopkins. His groundbreaking work in this area was not recognized until 1976 when Mr. Thomas was bestowed an honorary Doctor of Laws degree from Johns Hopkins instead of a medical degree for which he was not eligible because of he was African American. Today BT shunts are short-term palliative procedures that are sometimes performed before full correction of the defect.

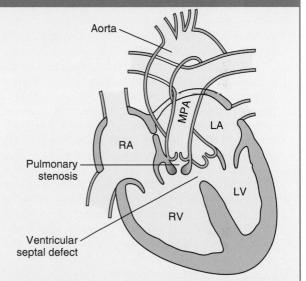

Anatomy of Tetralogy of Fallot. Features include pulmonary valve stenosis, ventricular septal defect (VSD), and an overriding aorta. As a result, right ventricular pressure increases and deoxygenated blood is shunted across the VSD into the left ventricle. LA, left atrium; LV, left ventricle; MPA, main pulmonary artery; RA, right atrium; RV, right ventricle.

SUMMARY

1. The lung is the only organ in the body with two separate blood supplies. The first is the pulmonary circulation, which brings deoxygenated blood from the right ventricle to the gas-exchanging units. In these units, oxygen is picked up and carbon dioxide is removed before the blood returns to the left atrium for distribution to the rest of the body.
2. The second blood supply is the bronchial circulation, which arises from the aorta and provides nourishment to the lung parenchyma.

3. The pulmonary circulation is a low-pressure, low-resistance system with a driving pressure almost 16 times less than that of the systemic circulation.

4. The arteries of the pulmonary circulation are the only arteries that carry deoxygenated blood.

5. The recruitment of new capillaries and the distensibility of pulmonary capillaries are unique features of the lung and allow for stress adjustments, as in the case of exercise. The arteries of the pulmonary circulation are thin-walled with minimal smooth muscle. They are seven times more compliant than systemic vessels and are easily distensible.

6. Pulmonary vascular resistance is the change in pressure from the pulmonary artery (Ppa) to the left atrium (Pla) divided by the flow (Qt), or cardiac output. This resistance is approximately 10 times less than in the systemic circulation.

7. In the upright position, under normal resting conditions, there is a linear increase in blood flow from the apex of the lung (lowest flow; can approach zero under various conditions) to the base of the lung, where it is the greatest.

8. The lung classically has been divided into three zones. Zone 1 represents the apex region, where it is possible to have no blood flow. In Zone 2, which constitutes the upper one-third of the lung, arterial pressure (Pa) is greater than alveolar pressure (Pa), which is greater than venous pressure (Pv). In Zone 3, Pa is greater than Pv, which is greater than Pa, and blood flow in this area follows the pressure gradients.

9. The extraalveolar vessels are generally larger vessels (arteries, arterioles, veins, and venules) that are not influenced by alveolar pressure changes but are affected by intrapleural and interstitial pressure changes. Alveolar vessels are the capillaries within the interalveolar septa and are sensitive to shifts in alveolar pressure but not to changes in pleural or interstitial pressure. *Pulmonary microcirculation* is a term used to describe small vessels that participate in liquid and solute exchange in the maintenance of fluid balance in the lung.

10. The alveolar–capillary network is composed of a dense mesh-like network of capillaries and alveoli separated only by their basement membranes.

11. The balance between hydrostatic and osmotic forces regulates fluid filtration, resulting in a net outward movement of fluid into the interstitium.

12. The lymphatics clear fluid from the interstitium. The fluid volume moved through the lymphatics in 24 hours is equal to an individual's total plasma volume, and one-quarter to one-half of the total plasma proteins are returned to the circulation through the lymphatics in 24 hours.

13. Pulmonary edema occurs when there is an increase in extravascular fluid accumulation in the lung, either because of an increase in outward fluid filtration or because of a decrease in fluid removal.

14. Hypoxic vasoconstriction occurs in small arterial vessels in response to decreased Po_2. Local hypoxia does not alter pulmonary vascular resistance (PVR). Important vasoconstrictors are endothelin and thromboxane A_2; nitric oxide (NO) is a potent vasodilator of the pulmonary endothelium.

KEYWORDS AND CONCEPTS

Alveolar vessels
Alveolar–capillary network
Blalock-Taussig shunt
Bronchial circulation
Capillary filtration
Cardiac output
Cystic fibrosis
Diffusion
Endothelin
Exercise
Extraalveolar vessels
Hemoptysis
Hypoxic vasoconstriction
Lung transplantation

Nitric oxide
Pulmonary capillary wedge pressure
Pulmonary circulation
Pulmonary edema
Pulmonary embolus
Pulmonary infarction
Pulmonary lymphatic system
Pulmonary microcirculation
Pulmonary vascular resistance
Starling equation
Tetralogy of Fallot
Thermodilution
Thromboxane A_2

SELF-STUDY PROBLEMS

1. What is the relationship between lung volume and vascular resistance in the entire lung? In the alveolar vessels? In the extraalveolar vessels?
2. What is the distribution of pulmonary blood flow in individuals in outer space under zero-gravity conditions?
3. How would a drop in pulmonary artery pressure affect the distribution of blood flow in the three zones of the lung?
4. What is the effect of high altitude on pulmonary artery pressure?
5. During cardiac catheterization, what is the effect of oxygen on pulmonary artery pressure and pulmonary vascular resistance?

ADDITIONAL READINGS

Bongartz G, Boos M, Scheffler K, Steinbrich W. Pulmonary circulation. *Eur Radiol.* 1998;8:698–706.

Broaddus VC, Mason RJ, Ernst JD, et al. *Murray and Nadel's Textbook of Respiratory Medicine.* 6th ed. Philadelphia: Elsevier Saunders; 2016.

Glenny RW. Blood flow distribution in the lung. *Chest.* 1998;114:8S–16S.

Leff AR, Schumacker PT. *Respiratory Physiology: Basics and Applications.* Philadelphia: WB Saunders; 1993.

Murray JP. *The Normal Lung.* 2nd ed. Philadelphia: WB Saunders; 1986.

Weibel ER. *The Pathway for Oxygen: Structure and Function of the Mammalian Respiratory System.* Cambridge, MA: Harvard University Press; 1984.

Weir EK, Archer SL. The mechanism of acute hypoxic pulmonary vasoconstriction: the tale of two channels. *FASEB J.* 1995;9:183–189.

7

Ventilation (V̇), Perfusion (Q̇), and Their Relationships

OBJECTIVES

1. Describe the significance of a normal ventilation/perfusion ratio ($\dot{V}/\dot{Q}$).
2. Characterize the $\dot{V}/\dot{Q}$ at the apex and at the base of the lung in upright individuals.
3. Calculate the alveolar–arterial oxygen difference ($AaDo_2$) and describe how to use it.
4. List the four major causes of hypoxemia and describe their anatomy and physiology.
5. List the two major causes of hypercarbia and describe their anatomy and physiology.
6. Distinguish pathophysiologic processes associated with hypoxemia using 100% oxygen.

Although ventilation and pulmonary blood flow (perfusion) are important individual components in the primary function of the lung, the relationship between ventilation and perfusion—specifically the ratio of ventilation to perfusion, defined as $\dot{V}/\dot{Q}$, is the major determinant of normal gas exchange. Before reading about ventilation–perfusion relationships, review ventilation (Chapter 5) and perfusion (Chapter 6).

VENTILATION/PERFUSION RATIO

Both ventilation ($\dot{V}$) and lung perfusion ($\dot{Q}$) are essential elements in the normal functioning of the lung, but they are insufficient to ensure normal gas exchange. For example, consider the situation in which blood is perfusing an area of the lung that has no ventilation (Fig. 7.1). Overall ventilation and overall perfusion in the lung may be normal, but in this specific area of the lung, normal gas exchange does not occur because there is no ventilation. Thus, without ventilation, the blood entering and leaving the area would be unchanged and would remain deoxygenated. Similarly, imagine an area of the lung with normal ventilation but no perfusion. Gas entering and leaving the alveoli in this area would be unchanged; that is, it would not participate in gas exchange because there is no blood flow to the area.

The ventilation/perfusion ratio ($\dot{V}/\dot{Q}$) is the ratio of ventilation to blood flow. It can be defined for a single alveolus, for a group of alveoli, or for the entire lung. At the level of a single alveolus, it is defined as the alveolar ventilation ($\dot{V}A$) divided by the capillary blood flow ($\dot{Q}c$). At the level

of the lung, it is defined as the total alveolar ventilation divided by the cardiac output.

In normal individuals, alveolar ventilation and blood flow are uniformly distributed to the gas-exchanging units with slightly less alveolar ventilation relative to pulmonary blood flow. At rest, in normal individuals, alveolar ventilation is ~4.0 L/min and pulmonary blood flow is ~5.0 L/min. Thus, in the normal lung, the overall ventilation/perfusion ratio is ~0.8; however, there is a wide range of ventilation/perfusion ratios in different lung units (Fig. 7.2). If ventilation and blood flow are mismatched, impairment of both O_2 and CO_2 transfer occurs. When ventilation exceeds perfusion, then $\dot{V}/\dot{Q}$ is greater than 1; when perfusion exceeds ventilation, $\dot{V}/\dot{Q}$ is less than 1.

Ventilation–perfusion mismatching occurs with increasing age (see Fig. 7.2) and with various lung diseases. In individuals with cardiopulmonary disease, mismatching of pulmonary blood flow and alveolar ventilation is the most frequent cause of systemic arterial hypoxemia.

A normal ventilation/perfusion ratio does not mean that ventilation and perfusion to that lung unit are normal; it simply means that the relationship between ventilation and perfusion is normal. For example, in the presence of a lobar pneumonia, ventilation to the affected lobe is decreased. If perfusion to this area remained unchanged, perfusion would be in excess of ventilation—an example of an abnormal ventilation/perfusion ratio ($\dot{V}/\dot{Q} < 1$). However, as a result of decreased ventilation to this area, hypoxic vasoconstriction occurs in the pulmonary arterioles supplying this lobe. The result is a decrease

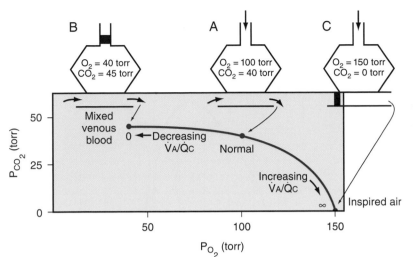

Fig. 7.1 Alveolar O_2 and CO_2 levels in relation to the ventilation/perfusion ratio ($\dot{V}/\dot{Q}$). **A,** Normally ventilated and perfused alveoli. **B,** $\dot{V}/\dot{Q}$ equal to 0 secondary to absent ventilation. O_2 and CO_2 levels in the alveolus are equal to those in the mixed venous blood. **C,** $\dot{V}/\dot{Q}$ equal to infinity secondary to absent perfusion. Note that in this alveolar unit the O_2 and CO_2 levels are equal to those in ambient air because no gas exchange occurs. (Modified from West JB. Ventilation–perfusion relationships. *Am Rev Respir Dis.* 1977;116:919.)

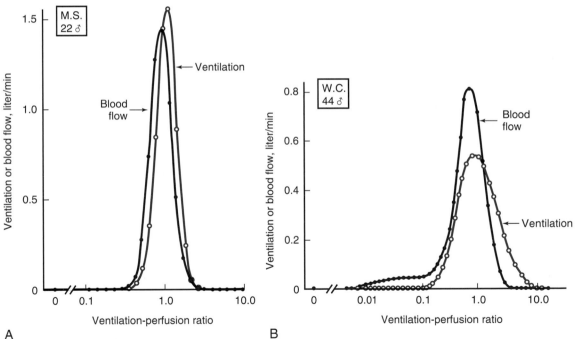

Fig. 7.2 Distribution of ventilation and blood flow in a young man **(A)** and in an older man **(B)**. In Panel A, both distributions are positioned about a ventilation/perfusion ratio ($\dot{V}/\dot{Q}$) close to 1.0; the curves are symmetric on a log scale with no areas of high or low ventilation/perfusion ratios, and there is no shunt (i.e., $\dot{V}/\dot{Q} = 0$). In Panel B, there are areas where perfusion exceeds ventilation and the $\dot{V}/\dot{Q}$ is less than 1 and areas where ventilation exceeds perfusion and the $\dot{V}/\dot{Q}$ is greater than 1, but there are no areas of shunt ($\dot{V}/\dot{Q} = 0$). (Redrawn from Wagner PD, Laravuso RB, Uhl RR, West JB. *J Clin Invest.* 1974;54:54.)

VENTILATION-PERFUSION RELATIONSHIPS

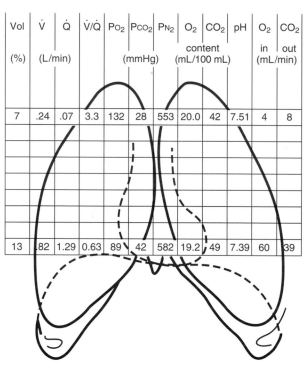

Vol (%)	V̇ (L/min)	Q̇ (L/min)	V̇/Q̇	Po₂	Pco₂	Pn₂ (mmHg)	O₂ content	CO₂ content (mL/100 mL)	pH	O₂ in	CO₂ out (mL/min)
7	.24	.07	3.3	132	28	553	20.0	42	7.51	4	8
13	1.82	1.29	0.63	89	42	582	19.2	49	7.39	60	39

Fig. 7.3 Regional differences in gas exchange down the normal lung. Only the apical and basal values are shown for clarity. (From Koeppen BM, Stanton BM, eds. *Berne and Levy's Physiology*, 7th ed. Philadelphia: Elsevier; 2018.)

in perfusion to the affected area and a more "normal" ventilation/perfusion ratio. However, neither the ventilation nor the perfusion to this area is normal (both are decreased); but the relationship between the two is (approaches) "normal."

REGIONAL DIFFERENCES IN VENTILATION AND PERFUSION

Because of regional differences in ventilation and perfusion, due largely to gravity and structural effects, even in the normal lung, V̇/Q̇ in different areas of the lung is greater than or less than the "ideal" normal value of 0.8. In the upright position, going from the top to the bottom of the lung, ventilation increases more slowly than blood flow increases. As a consequence, the V̇/Q̇ at the top of the lung is high (increased ventilation relative to blood flow in the pulmonary circulation), whereas the V̇/Q̇ at the bottom of the lung is "abnormally" low. This relationship between ventilation and perfusion is shown in Fig. 7.3. The important point here is that although the overall V̇/Q̇ in the normal lung is 0.8, it is composed of a wide range of localized ventilation/perfusion ratios (Fig. 7.4).

ALVEOLAR–ARTERIAL DIFFERENCE

In a perfect situation, there would be no difference between alveolar O_2 and arterial O_2. Even in normal individuals, a small difference in alveolar and arterial O_2 occurs. The difference between the alveolar O_2 (PAO_2) and the arterial Po_2 (Pao_2) is called the **AaDo₂**. An increase in the AaDo₂ is one of the hallmarks of abnormal O_2 exchange. The small difference between alveolar and arterial O_2 is not the result of imperfect gas exchange, but rather is due to a small number of veins (carrying deoxygenated blood) that bypass the lung and empty directly into the arterial circulation. The **thebesian vessels** of the left ventricular myocardium drain directly into the left ventricle (rather than into the coronary sinus in the right atrium), whereas some bronchial veins and mediastinal veins drain into pulmonary veins (**bronchopulmonary anastomoses**; see Fig. 6.2). This results in venous blood admixture and a decrease in arterial Pao_2 (this is an example of an **anatomic shunt**; see later in this chapter). It is estimated that approximately 2% to 3% of the cardiac output is shunted in this way.

Clinically, the effectiveness of gas exchange is measured using the partial pressures of oxygen and carbon dioxide in arterial blood. This can be done by obtaining

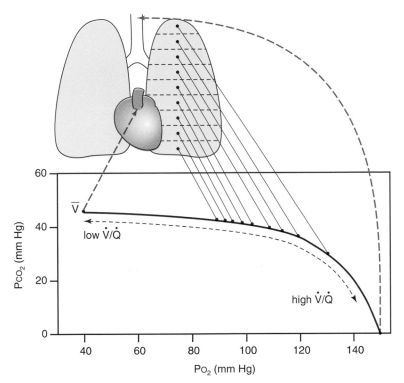

Fig. 7.4 The regional distribution of ventilation/perfusion ratios (V̇/Q̇s) in the lung. At the apex of the lung, perfusion is decreased, resulting in a V̇/Q̇ that is greater than 1 with higher alveolar oxygen (Po_2) and lower alveolar carbon dioxide (Pco_2) values. Toward the base of the lung, perfusion is greater than ventilation, resulting in a V̇/Q̇ that is less than 1 with lower alveolar Po_2 and higher alveolar Pco_2 values. V, mixed venous blood. (Redrawn with permission from West JB. Ventilation–perfusion relationships. *Am Rev Respir Dis.* 1977;116:919.)

TABLE 7.1   *Causes of Hypoxemia

Cause	Arterial Pao_2	$AaDo_2$	Arterial Pao_2 Response to 100% O_2
Anatomic shunt	Decreased	Increased	No Change in Pao_2
Decreased Fio_2	Decreased	Normal	Increased Pao_2
Physiologic shunt	Decreased	Increased	Blunted Pao_2
Low ventilation/perfusion ratio	Decreased	Increased	Increased Pao_2
Hypoventilation	Decreased	Normal	Increased Pao_2

*Diffusion abnormalities are an extremely uncommon cause of decreased arterial Pao_2 at rest but have greater significance during exercise; when associated with decreased Pao_2, the $AaDo_2$ is increased.
$AaDo_2$, alveolar–arterial oxygen difference; Fio_2, fraction of inspired oxygen; Pao_2, partial pressure of arterial oxygen.

a sample of arterial blood usually by inserting a needle into either the radial or the brachial artery (other peripheral arteries can also be used) and measuring the Pao_2 and $Paco_2$. By knowing the barometric pressure (P_B), the fraction of oxygen in the inspired air, the water vapor pressure (PH_2O), the alveolar CO_2 (which is equal to the arterial CO_2), and the respiratory quotient (estimated at 0.8, see Chapter 5), the alveolar Pao_2 can be calculated using the **alveolar air equation**. The difference between the calculated alveolar Pao_2 and the measured arterial Pao_2 is the $AaDo_2$. In normal individuals breathing room air, the $AaDo_2$ is less than 15 mm Hg. It rises approximately 3 mm Hg per decade of life. For this reason, an

$AaDo_2$ less than 25 mm Hg is considered the upper limit of normal.

Abnormalities in arterial Po_2 can occur in the presence or absence of an abnormal $AaDo_2$. The relationship between Pao_2 and the $AaDo_2$ is useful in determining the cause of an abnormal Pao_2 and in predicting response to therapy (particularly supplemental oxygen administration). Thus the $AaDo_2$ should be calculated as part of every arterial blood gas analysis. This information can then be used to determine the cause of an abnormal arterial O_2. Causes of a reduction in arterial Pao_2 (arterial hypoxemia) and its effect on $AaDo_2$ are shown in Table 7.1. Each cause is discussed in greater detail later.

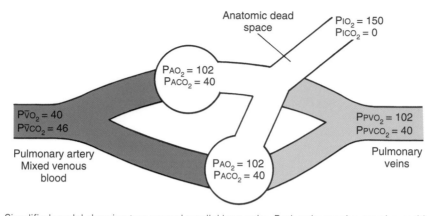

Fig. 7.5 Simplified model showing two normal parallel lung units. Both units receive equal quantities of fresh air and blood flow for their size. The blood and alveolar gas partial pressures (P) are normal values in a resting person. Pao$_2$, partial pressure of arterial oxygen; Paco$_2$, partial pressure of arterial carbon dioxide; Pao$_2$, partial pressure of alveolar oxygen; Paco$_2$, partial pressure of alveolar carbon dioxide; Pio$_2$, partial pressure of inspired oxygen; Pico$_2$, partial pressure of inspired carbon dioxide; Ppvo$_2$, partial pressure of pulmonary venous oxygen; Ppvco$_2$, partial pressure of pulmonary venous carbon dioxide. (From Koeppen BM, Stanton BM, eds. *Berne and Levy's Physiology*, 7th ed. Philadelphia: Elsevier, 2018.)

ARTERIAL BLOOD GAS ABNORMALITIES

Arterial hypoxemia is present when the arterial Po$_2$ is below the normal range. In general, an arterial Po$_2$ of less than 80 mm Hg in an adult breathing room air at sea level is abnormal. Hypoxia occurs when there is insufficient oxygen to carry out normal metabolic functions, and thus hypoxia and hypoxemia mean different things but are frequently used interchangeably. Hypercarbia is defined as an increase in arterial Pco$_2$ above the normal range (≥45 mm Hg) and hypocapnia is a lower than normal arterial Pco$_2$ (usually less than 35 mm Hg).

VENTILATION/PERFUSION RATIO IN A SINGLE ALVEOLUS

A useful way to examine the interaction and relationship between ventilation and perfusion is the two-lung unit model first described by Comroe in 1962. In Fig. 7.5, ventilation is divided between two alveoli, each of which is supplied by a part of the cardiac output. When there is uniform ventilation, half of the inspired gas goes to each of the alveoli; when there is uniform perfusion, half of the cardiac output goes to each alveolus. In this normal unit, the V̇/Q̇ in each of the alveoli is the same and equals 1. The alveoli are perfused by mixed venous blood that is deoxygenated and contains increased Pco$_2$. Alveolar O$_2$ is higher than mixed venous O$_2$, and this provides a gradient for the

movement of oxygen into the blood. In contrast, mixed venous CO$_2$ is increased relative to alveolar CO$_2$, and this provides a gradient for the movement of CO$_2$ into the alveolus. Note that in this ideal model, there is no alveolar–arterial O$_2$ difference.

ANATOMIC SHUNT

Now imagine that a certain amount of mixed venous blood bypasses the gas exchange unit and goes directly into the arterial blood (Fig. 7.6). In this instance alveolar ventilation and the distribution and composition of alveolar gas are normal. The distribution of the cardiac output is changed, however. Some of it goes through the pulmonary capillary bed supplying the two gas exchange units, whereas the rest bypasses the gas exchange units and goes directly into the arterial blood. The blood that bypasses the gas exchange unit is said to be "shunted," and because it is deoxygenated blood, it is called a **right-to-left shunt**. Most anatomic shunts occur within the heart and occur when deoxygenated blood from the right atrium or ventricle crosses the septum and mixes with blood from the left atrium or ventricle. The effect of this right-to-left shunt is to mix deoxygenated blood with oxygenated blood, and it results in varying degrees of arterial hypoxemia.

An important feature of an anatomic shunt is that the hypoxemia cannot be abolished by giving the individual 100% oxygen to breathe. This is because the blood that

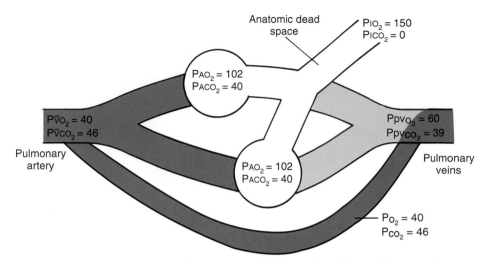

Fig. 7.6 Right-to-left shunt. Alveolar ventilation is normal, but a portion of the cardiac output bypasses the lung and mixes with oxygenated blood. The Pao_2 will vary depending on the size of the shunt. (See Fig. 7.5 for definitions of the abbreviations.) (From Koeppen BM, Stanton BM, eds. *Berne and Levy's Physiology*, 7th ed. Philadelphia: Elsevier; 2018.)

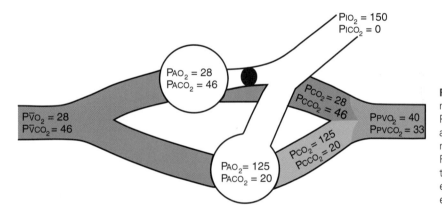

Fig. 7.7 Physiologic shunt (venous admixture). Notice the marked decrease in Pao_2 compared with Pco_2. The alveolar–arterial oxygen difference ($AaDo_2$) is 85 mm Hg $Ppvo_2 = 40$, $Ppvco_2 = 33$. (See Fig. 7.5 for definitions of other abbreviations.) (From Koeppen BM, Stanton BM, eds. *Berne and Levy's Physiology*, 7th ed. Philadelphia: Elsevier; 2018.)

bypasses ventilation is never exposed to the enriched oxygen, so it continues to be deoxygenated. In contrast, the nonshunted blood is exposed to the enriched oxygen. Because normally hemoglobin in the blood that perfuses the ventilated alveoli is almost fully saturated, the arterial Pao_2 increases slightly but most of the added O_2 is in the form of dissolved O_2, which is not an effective way to substantially increase Pao_2 (see Chapter 8).

An anatomic shunt does not usually cause an increase in $Paco_2$ even though the shunted blood has an elevated level of CO_2. This is because central chemoreceptors respond to any increase in CO_2 in the blood with an increase in ventilation (see Chapter 10). This increase in ventilation reduces the arterial $Paco_2$ to the normal range. In the presence of severe hypoxemia, the $Paco_2$ is below the normal range because the increased respiratory drive secondary to the hypoxemia further increases ventilation and decreases $Paco_2$ below the normal range.

PHYSIOLOGIC SHUNT

Many lung diseases cause a blockage in ventilation to one of the lung units (Fig. 7.7). As a result, all of the ventilation now goes to the other lung unit, and the perfusion is equally distributed between both of the lung units. The lung unit without ventilation but with perfusion has a $\dot{V}/\dot{Q}$ of zero. The blood perfusing this unit is mixed venous blood; because there is no ventilation, there is no gas exchange in the unit, and the blood leaving this unit remains mixed venous. This is called a **physiologic**

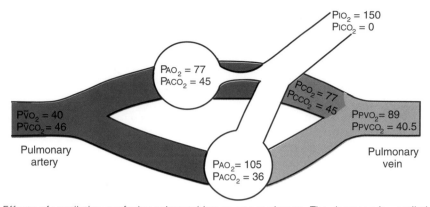

Fig. 7.8 Effects of ventilation–perfusion mismatching on gas exchange. The decrease in ventilation to the one lung unit could be due to mucus obstruction, airway edema, bronchospasm, a foreign body, or a tumor. P_{O_2}, partial pressure of oxygen; P_{CO_2}, partial pressure of pulmonary capillary O_2; $P\bar{v}_{O_2}$, partial pressure of mixed venous oxygen; $P\bar{v}_{CO_2}$, partial pressure of mixed venous carbon dioxide; P_{CCO_2}, partial pressure of pulmonary capillary CO_2. (See Fig. 7.5 for definitions of other abbreviations.) (From Koeppen BM, Stanton BM, eds. *Berne and Levy's Physiology*, 7th ed. Philadelphia: Elsevier; 2018.)

shunt (or venous admixture); it is similar in its effect to an anatomic shunt; that is, deoxygenated blood bypasses a gas-exchanging unit and admixes with arterial blood. In this instance however, the problem is a reduction in ventilation to an area of the lung that is being perfused. Clinically, **atelectasis** is the most common cause of a physiologic shunt ($\dot{V}/\dot{Q} = 0$). Atelectasis occurs when there is obstruction to ventilation of a gas-exchanging unit with subsequent loss of volume and can be caused by a mucus plug, airway edema, a foreign body, or a tumor in the airway.

VENTILATION–PERFUSION MISMATCHING

Ventilation–perfusion mismatching is the most common cause of arterial hypoxemia in patients with disorders affecting the respiratory system. In most cases, the composition of mixed venous blood, the total volume of blood flow (cardiac output), and the distribution of blood flow are normal. However, the same total alveolar ventilation is now distributed unevenly between the gas exchange units (Fig. 7.8). Because blood flow is equally distributed, the unit with the decreased ventilation has a $\dot{V}/\dot{Q}$ less than 1, and the unit with the increased ventilation has a $\dot{V}/\dot{Q}$ greater than 1. This causes variation in the alveolar and end-capillary gas compositions. Both arterial oxygen and arterial carbon dioxide will be abnormal in the blood that has come from the unit with the decreased ventilation ($\dot{V}/\dot{Q} = <1$). The unit with the increased ventilation ($\dot{V}/\dot{Q} = >1$) will have a lower Pa_{CO_2} and a higher Pa_{O_2} because it is being overventilated. The actual Pa_{O_2} and Pa_{CO_2} values will vary

depending on the relative contribution of each of these units to the arterial blood.

In this instance there will be a difference in the alveolar–arterial oxygen gradient (AaD_{O_2}). This difference occurs because the relative overventilation of one unit does not fully compensate (either by adding extra O_2 or by removing extra CO_2) for the disturbances created by underventilating the other unit. The failure to compensate is greater in the case of O_2 than in that of CO_2, owing to the flatness of the upper part of the oxyhemoglobin dissociation curve compared with the CO_2 dissociation curve (see Chapter 8). In other words, increased ventilation raises Pa_{O_2} but adds little extra O_2 content to the blood, whereas the steeper slope of the CO_2 curve allows more CO_2 to be eliminated when ventilation increases. This is because hemoglobin is close to being 100% saturated in these overventilated areas, whereas CO_2 moves by diffusion, and as long as a CO_2 gradient is maintained, CO_2 diffusion will occur.

HYPOVENTILATION

Alveolar oxygen is determined by a balance between the rate of oxygen removal (determined by the blood flow through the lung and the metabolic demands of the tissues) and the rate of oxygen replenishment by ventilation. If ventilation decreases, then PA_{O_2} will decrease and Pa_{O_2} will subsequently decrease. In addition, there is a direct relationship between alveolar ventilation and Pa_{CO_2}. When ventilation is halved, alveolar and thus arterial carbon dioxide doubles (see Fig. 5.3). This process of decreased ventilation is called **hypoventilation**. Hypoventilation always decreases Pao_2 (except when the subject breathes an enriched source of oxygen) and increases $Paco_2$.

One of the hallmarks of hypoventilation is a normal $AaDo_2$. This occurs when gas exchange and perfusion to the alveolus are normal; that is, the lung is functioning normally. The problem is that there is a decreased rate of ventilation to the unit. There are few instances of "pure" hypoventilation because, as ventilation decreases, areas of atelectasis develop, and atelectasis creates areas with ventilation/perfusion ratios of zero and an increase in the $AaDo_2$.

DIFFUSION ABNORMALITIES

Abnormalities in the diffusion of oxygen across the alveolar–capillary barrier may also result in arterial hypoxemia. Because equilibration between alveolar and capillary oxygen and carbon dioxide occurs rapidly and in a fraction of the time it takes for red blood cells to go through the pulmonary capillary network, **diffusion equilibrium** almost always occurs in normal subjects, even during exercise when transit time through the lung of red blood cells increases significantly. An alveolar–arterial oxygen difference that has been attributable to incomplete diffusion (**diffusion disequilibrium**) has been observed in normal individuals only during exercise at high altitudes (≥10,000 feet). Diffusion disequilibrium is an unusual and uncommon cause of hypoxemia. Even in individuals with abnormal diffusion capacities, diffusion disequilibrium at rest is unusual. In contrast, abnormalities of diffusion are more likely to affect arterial blood gas composition during exercise, and the effects are magnified at higher altitudes.

Alveolar capillary block, or thickening of the air–blood barrier, is not nearly as common a cause of decreased diffusion capacity as is a reduction in the volume of pulmonary capillary blood. In this disorder, the mechanism of hypoxemia is different. As capillaries are progressively destroyed or obstructed, previously unperfused capillaries are progressively recruited until finally the velocity of blood flow through the remaining vessels increases. (Recall that the lung "accepts" the entire cardiac output; flow remains normal even with destruction of capillaries until all capillaries have been recruited. At this point, flow through the remaining capillaries increases.) When this process is severe, the time available for gas exchange in these patients at rest may be similar to that observed in normal individuals during exercise. In these individuals who are experiencing increased flow at rest, during exercise, the short transit time prevents equilibration.

DISEASES ASSOCIATED WITH HYPOXIA

There are several types of congenital heart disease that cause **cyanosis** (a bluish discoloration of the lips and fingers that occurs when 5 g of reduced hemoglobin are present). In most of these disorders, anatomic shunts are the mechanism of hypoxemia. The most common of the cyanotic congenital heart diseases is Tetralogy of Fallot (see Chapter 6, Clinical Box), characterized by pulmonary valve stenosis and a ventricular septal defect (a hole in the wall between the right and left ventricles). As a result, the pressure in the right ventricle increases to supersystemic levels, and deoxygenated blood is shunted from the right ventricle to the left ventricle (anatomic shunt) bypassing the lung.

Guillain-Barré syndrome is an acute neuromuscular disease associated with ascending muscle weakness. When respiratory muscles are involved, particularly the diaphragm, minute ventilation (tidal volume × frequency) decreases, Pao_2 decreases, and $Paco_2$ increases. Guillain-Barré syndrome thus causes hypoxemia through hypoventilation.

Asthma is a chronic inflammatory lung disease characterized by exacerbations interspersed with periods of inactive disease. When the disease is inactive, pulmonary function tests and arterial blood gases are normal. During an exacerbation, there is evidence of airway inflammation, bronchospasm, and airway edema. This results in airflow obstruction, areas of poor ventilation (V̇/Q̇ mismatch), and hypoxemia.

MECHANISMS OF HYPERCARBIA

There are two major mechanisms for the development of hypercarbia (excess carbon dioxide in the blood): hypoventilation and wasted ventilation. As previously noted, there is a direct relationship between alveolar ventilation and alveolar carbon dioxide (see Fig. 5.3). When ventilation is halved, alveolar and thus arterial Pco_2 doubles. Hypoventilation always decreases Pao_2 (except when the subject breathes an enriched source of oxygen) and increases $Paco_2$.

Wasted ventilation occurs when there is a marked reduction in pulmonary blood flow in the presence of normal ventilation (V̇/Q̇ = >1 → ∞). This most often occurs because of obstruction of blood flow by a **pulmonary embolus**. In the presence of a pulmonary embolus, there is absent pulmonary blood flow to areas with normal ventilation (V̇/Q̇ = ∞). In this situation, the ventilation is "wasted" because it fails to oxygenate any of the mixed venous blood, and the ventilation to the now perfused lung is less than ideal (i.e., there is relative "hypoventilation" to this area because this area now receives all of the pulmonary blood flow with "normal" ventilation). If compensation did not occur, the $Paco_2$ would increase and the Pao_2 would decrease. Compensation after a pulmonary embolus, however, begins almost immediately with a shift in the distribution of ventilation to areas being perfused. As a result, changes in $Paco_2$ and Pao_2 are minimized.

EFFECT OF 100% OXYGEN ON ARTERIAL BLOOD GAS ABNORMALITIES

One of the ways that a right-to-left shunt can be distinguished from other causes of hypoxemia is by having an individual breathe 100% oxygen through a non-rebreathing facemask for approximately 15 minutes. When a person is breathing 100% oxygen, all of the nitrogen in the alveolus is replaced by oxygen. Thus alveolar oxygen can be derived using the alveolar air equation:

$$P_{AO_2} = 1.0 \left(P_B - P_{H_2O}\right) \times Paco_2/1.0 \,^*$$
$$= 1.0 \left(760 - 47\right) \times 40/1.0$$
$$= 663 \text{ mm Hg}$$

In the normal lung, the alveolar oxygen rapidly increases and provides the gradient for oxygen transfer into the capillary blood. This is associated with a marked increase in arterial oxygen (see Table 7.1). Similarly, during the 15- to 20-minute period of breathing enriched oxygen, even areas with very low ventilation/perfusion ratios will develop a high alveolar oxygen pressure as the nitrogen is replaced by oxygen; in the presence of normal perfusion to these areas, there is a gradient for gas exchange and the end capillary gas is highly enriched in oxygen. In contrast, in the presence of a right-to-left shunt, oxygenation is not corrected because mixed venous blood continues to flow through the shunt and mix with blood that has perfused normal units. The poorly oxygenated blood from the shunt lowers the arterial oxygen level and maintains (and even augments) the $AaDo_2$. An elevated $AaDo_2$ value during a properly conducted 100% O_2 study signifies the presence of a right-to-left shunt; the magnitude of the difference can be used to quantify the proportion of the cardiac output that is shunted.

EFFECT OF CHANGING CARDIAC OUTPUT

Changes in cardiac output are the only nonrespiratory factor that affects gas exchange. Decreasing cardiac output causes a decrease in O_2 content and an increase in CO_2 content in mixed venous blood. Increasing the cardiac output has the opposite effect. This change in O_2 and CO_2 content will have little effect on Pao_2 and $Paco_2$ in individuals with

*On 100% oxygen, the respiratory quotient is equal to 1 (Appendix C).

normal lungs unless cardiac output is extremely low. In the presence of lung disease secondary to ventilation-perfusion mismatching or in the presence of an anatomic shunt, the composition of mixed venous blood will have a significant effect on Pao_2 and $Paco_2$ levels. For any level of V̇/Q̇ abnormality, a decrease in cardiac output is associated with an increasingly abnormal Pao_2.

EFFECT OF VENTILATION–PERFUSION REGIONAL DIFFERENCES

Up to this point we have examined regional differences in ventilation and in perfusion and in the relationship between ventilation and perfusion. We have also examined the effect of various physiologic abnormalities (shunts, V̇/Q̇ mismatch, and hypoventilation) on arterial oxygen and carbon dioxide levels. Before leaving this area, however, it should be apparent to the student that because there are ventilation–perfusion differences in different regions of the lung, end-capillary blood coming from these regions will have different oxygen and carbon dioxide levels. These differences are shown in Fig. 7.9 (also see Fig. 7.3) and demonstrate the complexity of the lung. First, recall that the volume of the lung at the apex is larger than the volume at the base. As previously described, ventilation and perfusion are less at the apex than at the base, but the differences in perfusion are greater than the differences in ventilation. Thus the V̇/Q̇ is high at the apex and low at the base, and the V̇/Q̇ decreases from the apex to the base of the lung. This difference in ventilation/perfusion ratios is associated with a difference in Pao_2 and $Paco_2$ between the apex and the base; that is, the P_{AO_2} is higher and the $Paco_2$ is lower in the apex than in the base. This results in differences in end-capillary contents for these gases, with a lower Po_2 and consequently a lower oxygen content for end-capillary blood at the base compared with the apex. In addition, there is significant variation in the pH of the end capillaries in these areas because of the variation in carbon dioxide content in the presence of a constant base excess (see Chapter 9).

Because of the decreased blood flow at the apex, the oxygen consumed and the carbon dioxide produced are also decreased in this area. Because the carbon dioxide produced is more closely linked to ventilation, and the oxygen consumed is more closely linked to perfusion, the carbon dioxide produced is higher because ventilation relative to perfusion is higher. As a result, the respiratory quotient (CO_2 produced/O_2 consumed) is higher at the apex than the base. During exercise when blood flow to the apex increases and becomes more uniform in the lung, the differences between the apex and the base of the lung diminish.

VENTILATION

Intrapleural pressure
more negative

Greater transmural
pressure gradient

Alveoli larger,
less compliant

Less ventilation

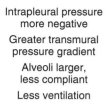
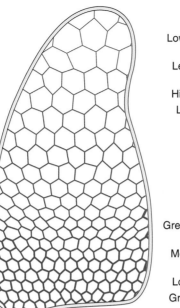

PERFUSION

Lower intravascular
pressures

Less recruitment,
distention

Higher resistance

Less blood flow

Intrapleural pressure
less negative

Smaller transmural
pressure gradient

Alveoli smaller,
more compliant

Greater ventilation

Greater intravascular
pressures

More recruitment,
distention

Lower resistance

Greater blood flow

Fig. 7.9 Regional differences in ventilation *(left)* and perfusion *(right)* in the normal, upright lung. (Redrawn from Levitzky MG. *Pulmonary Physiology,* 8th ed. New York: McGraw-Hill; 2013.)

SUMMARY

1. Regional differences in ventilation and perfusion are due in large part to the effects of gravity and structure.
2. The alveolar air equation is used to calculate the alveolar–arterial oxygen difference ($AaDo_2$), the most useful measurement of abnormal arterial oxygen. In normal individuals breathing room air, the $AaDo_2$ is less than 25 mm Hg.
3. The ventilation/perfusion ratio ($\dot{V}/\dot{Q}$) is defined as the ratio of ventilation to blood flow. In the normal lung, the average ventilation/perfusion ratio is approximately 0.8. When ventilation exceeds perfusion, the ventilation/perfusion ratio is greater than 1 ($\dot{V}/\dot{Q} = >1$); when perfusion exceeds ventilation, the ventilation/perfusion ratio is less than 1 ($\dot{V}/\dot{Q} = <1$).
4. The ventilation/perfusion ratio at the top of the lung is high (increased ventilation relative to very little blood flow in the pulmonary circulation), whereas the ventilation/perfusion ratio at the bottom of the lung is low.
5. There are four mechanisms of hypoxemia: anatomic shunt, physiologic shunt, ventilation–perfusion mismatching, and hypoventilation.
6. There are two mechanisms of hypercarbia: increase in dead space and hypoventilation.
7. Changes in cardiac output are the only nonrespiratory factors that affect gas exchange.

KEYWORDS AND CONCEPTS

Alveolar air equation
Alveolar–arterial oxygen difference ($AaDo_2$)
Alveolar capillary block
Anatomic shunt
Asthma
Atelectasis
Bronchopulmonary anastomoses
Cardiac output
Cyanosis
Diffusion disequilibrium

Guillain-Barré syndrome
Hypoventilation
Physiologic shunt
Pulmonary embolus
Right-left shunt
Tetralogy of Fallot
Thebesian veins
Ventilation/perfusion ratio ($\dot{V}/\dot{Q}$)
Wasted ventilation

SELF-STUDY PROBLEMS

1. How can you distinguish between the four causes of hypoxemia?
2. What factors determine alveolar P_{AO_2} in a single alveolus?
3. What is responsible for the greater decrease in P_{aO_2} compared with P_{aCO_2} in the presence of ventilation–perfusion inequality?

ADDITIONAL READINGS

Bongartz G, Boos M, Scheffler K, Steinbrich W. Pulmonary circulation. *Eur Radiol.* 1998;8:698–706.

Comroe Jr JH, et al. *The Lung. Clinical Physiology and Pulmonary Function Tests.* 2nd ed. Chicago: Year Book Medical Publishers, Inc; 1962:1–390.

Cutaia M, Rounds S. Hypoxic pulmonary vasoconstriction: Physiologic significance, mechanism and clinical relevance. *Chest.* 1982;97:706–718.

Glenny RW. Blood flow distribution in the lung. *Chest.* 1998;114:8S–16S.

Henig NR, Pierson DJ. Mechanisms of hypoxemia. *Respir Care Clin N Am.* 2000;6:501–521.

Lenfant C. Measurement of ventilation/perfusion distribution with alveolar arterial differences. *J Appl Physiol.* 1963;18:1090–1094.

Milic-Emili J, Henderson JA, Dolovich MB, et al. Regional distribution of inspired gas in the lung. *J Appl Physiol.* 1966;21:749–759.

Weir EK, Archer SL. The mechanism of acute hypoxic pulmonary vasoconstriction: the tale of two channels. *FASEB J.* 1995;9:183–189.

West JB, Dollery CT, Naimark A. Distribution of blood flow in isolated lung: relation to vascular and alveolar pressures. *J Appl Physiol.* 1964;19:713–724.

West JB. State of the art: ventilation-perfusion relationships. *Am Rev Respir Dis.* 1977;116:919–943.

Oxygen and Carbon Dioxide Transport

OBJECTIVES

1. Explain diffusion limitation and perfusion limitation and their importance in gas exchange
2. Apply Fick's law to the alveolar–capillary surface.
3. Describe the diffusion of oxygen and carbon dioxide across the alveolar–capillary membrane.
4. Describe the structure and function of hemoglobin in gas exchange.
5. Explain the oxyhemoglobin dissociation curve, factors that shift the curve, and the effect of these shifts on oxygen uptake and oxygen delivery.

6. Understand the differences between oxygen content, oxygen saturation, and Pao_2.
7. Outline the effect of carbon monoxide on oxygen content, oxygen saturation, Pao_2, and stimulation of peripheral chemoreceptors.
8. Describe oxygen consumption.
9. Describe the four types of tissue hypoxia.
10. Explain carbon dioxide production, metabolism, diffusion, and the carbon dioxide dissociation curve.

The maintenance of cell integrity and normal organ function is dependent on energy expenditure. The major source of energy in cells and organs is provided by the intracellular metabolism of oxygen (O_2) (**oxidative metabolism**). During oxidative metabolism, molecular oxygen is consumed within the mitochondrial electron transport system, and adenosine triphosphate (ATP) is generated. Energy is subsequently produced by the hydrolysis of ATP to adenosine diphosphate (ADP) and inorganic phosphate.

O_2 is carried in the blood from the lungs to the tissues in two forms: physically dissolved in the blood and chemically combined to hemoglobin. As O_2 is transported into the tissue, carbon dioxide (CO_2), the by-product of cellular metabolism, is transported from the tissues to the blood and then to the lungs by the pulmonary circulation. CO_2 is carried in three forms: physically dissolved in blood, as bicarbonate, and chemically combined to blood proteins as carbamino compounds. O_2 loading and unloading and CO_2 loading and unloading not only occur simultaneously but also facilitate each other both in the lung and in the tissues. Specifically, the uptake of O_2 into the tissues enhances the elimination of CO_2 from the tissues into the blood (Fig. 8.1). Similarly, the uptake of O_2 into the blood through the pulmonary capillaries is facilitated by the simultaneous unloading of CO_2 by the blood. To understand the mechanisms involved in the transport of these gases, three

processes must be considered: gas diffusion, O_2 and CO_2 transport processes, and O_2 and CO_2 delivery processes.

GAS DIFFUSION

Diffusion is the passive thermodynamic flow of molecules between regions with different partial pressures. Diffusion of a gas is defined as the net movement of gas molecules from an area in which the particular gas exerts a higher partial pressure to an area in which the gas exerts a lower partial pressure. Diffusion is different from "bulk flow," which occurs in the conducting airways. In bulk flow, gas movement occurs when there are differences in total pressure with molecules of different gases moving together along the pressure gradients. In diffusion, different gases move according to their individual pressure gradients. In diffusion, gas transport is random, occurs in all directions, and is temperature dependent. Net movement, however, is dependent on the difference in the individual gas's partial pressure. Diffusion continues until there is no longer a pressure gradient. In the lung and the tissues, diffusion is the major mechanism of gas movement. It is important both for gas movement within the alveoli (air → air) as well as for gas movement across the alveoli into the blood (air → liquid) and for gas movement from the blood into the tissue (liquid → tissue).

101

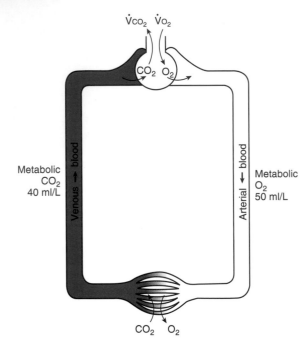

Fig. 8.1 Oxygen and carbon dioxide transport occur in both arterial and venous blood. However, the extracted or utilized oxygen is present in arterial blood, where it is transferred from arterial capillaries to the tissue. Only approximately 25% of transported oxygen is actually taken up by the tissue. The source of exhaled carbon dioxide is venous blood; it is expired via the pulmonary capillaries. The flow rates for oxygen ($\dot{V}o_2$) and carbon dioxide ($\dot{V}co_2$) shown are for 1 L of blood. The ratio of CO_2 production to O_2 consumption is the respiratory quotient, R, which at rest is about 0.80. (From Koeppen BM, Stanton BM, eds. *Berne and Levy's Physiology*, 7th ed. Philadelphia: Elsevier; 2018.)

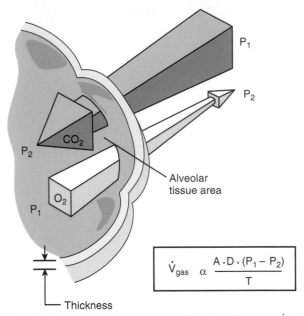

$$\dot{V}_{gas} \; \alpha \; \frac{A \cdot D \cdot (P_1 - P_2)}{T}$$

Fig. 8.2 Fick's law states that the diffusion of a gas ($\dot{V}_{gas}$) across a sheet of tissue is directly related to the surface area of the tissue (A), the diffusion constant of the specific gas (D), and the partial pressure difference of the gas on each side of the tissue ($P_1 - P_2$) and is inversely related to tissue thickness (T). (From Koeppen BM, Stanton BM, eds. *Berne and Levy's Physiology*, 7th ed. Philadelphia: Elsevier; 2018.)

O_2 is delivered to the alveoli by bulk flow in the conducting airways. The inspired gas velocity decreases as the alveoli are approached because of the dramatic increase in cross-sectional area of the airways due to the multiple bifurcations (Bernoulli principle, see Fig. 3.9). Once in the alveolus, gas movement occurs by diffusion. The process of gas diffusion is passive, non–energy-dependent, and similar whether in a gas or liquid state. O_2 moves through the gas phase in the alveoli according to its own pressure gradient, crosses the approximate 1-μm alveolar–capillary interface, and enters the blood. In moving from a gas phase in the alveolus to a liquid phase in the blood, O_2 obeys Henry's law (Appendix C), where the amount of gas absorbed by a liquid is determined by the gas pressure and solubility. Both O_2 and CO_2 maintain their molecular characteristics in blood, and both establish a partial pressure in the blood, according to Henry's law. It is this partial pressure that is measured in an arterial blood gas sample. O_2 and CO_2 in the blood are then carried out of the lung by bulk flow and distributed to the tissues in the body. In the tissues, O_2 diffuses out of the blood, across the interstitium, and into the tissue cell and its mitochondrial membrane.

The rate of diffusion of O_2 and CO_2 through the alveolar–capillary barrier and through the capillary–tissue barrier is governed by Fick's law of diffusion (Appendix C), which states that the diffusion of a gas ($\dot{V}_{gas}$) across a sheet of tissue is directly related to the surface area, the diffusion constant of the gas (which is related to the solubility of the gas and inversely to the square root of the molecular weight of the gas and the gas gradient across the tissue and indirectly related to the thickness of the tissue [Fig. 8.2]). A number of interesting and important concepts arise from these two equations. Normally, the thickness of the alveolar–capillary diffusion barrier is only 0.2 to 0.5 μm. The thickness of the barrier, however, is increased in diseases such as interstitial fibrosis and interstitial edema, and the increased thickness of the alveolar–capillary barrier interferes with diffusion. Increased partial pressure of oxygen in the alveoli increases O_2 transport by increasing the pressure gradient, and this is why supplemental O_2 therapy is used to treat many lung diseases. At the blood capillary–tissue barrier (liquid → tissue), Fick's equation demonstrates that the major rate-limiting step for diffusion from the air to the tissue is at the liquid–tissue interface. This is because at this step, the tissue thickness from the capillaries to the mitochondria is far greater than in the alveolus.

The diffusion constants for CO_2 and O_2 favor CO_2 diffusion. This is because the solubility of CO_2 in blood is about 24 times the solubility of O_2. CO_2, however, has a higher molecular weight. When both the solubility and the molecular weight are considered together, CO_2 diffuses about 20 times more rapidly through the alveolar–capillary membrane than O_2. Clinically, this is demonstrated in patients with lung diseases resulting in changes in diffusion in which decreases in blood O_2 occur much earlier than CO_2 increases in blood.

PERFUSION LIMITATION

On average, a red blood cell spends between 0.75 and 1.2 seconds in the pulmonary capillaries. Some red blood cells spend more time than this, and others spend less. Depending on the initial concentration of a gas in inspired air and how rapidly it is removed by the pulmonary capillaries, different gases will have different alveolar partial pressures. This is illustrated in Fig. 8.3 for nitrous oxide (N_2O), O_2, and carbon monoxide (CO). The major factors responsible for the difference in the shapes of these relationships are the solubility of the gases in the alveolar–capillary membrane and the solubility of the gases in the blood and their ability to chemically bind to hemoglobin.

Different gases have different solubility factors, which result in different diffusion coefficients. Gases such as N_2O, nitrogen, and helium have low solubility, whereas ether has high solubility (Fig. 8.4). In general, when the solubility of a gas in the membrane is large, gas will diffuse at a faster rate through the membrane. This is because the highly soluble gas will become dissolved in the barrier more readily than the insoluble gas. N_2O, ether, and helium move through the alveolar–capillary barrier easily, are insoluble in blood, and do not combine chemically with blood. As a result, the partial pressure gradient across the alveolar–capillary barrier is rapidly abolished (see Fig. 8.3). From that point on, no further gas transfer occurs and there is no net diffusion. For these gases, equilibration between alveolar gas and blood occurs rapidly (significantly less than the 0.75 second that the red blood cell spends in the capillary bed) and is driven by the difference in partial pressure. This type of gas exchange is **perfusion-limited** because blood leaving the capillary has reached equilibrium with alveolar gas. As illustrated in Fig. 8.3, the partial pressure of N_2O peaks quickly and is maximal by 0.1 second, at which point no further N_2O is transferred.

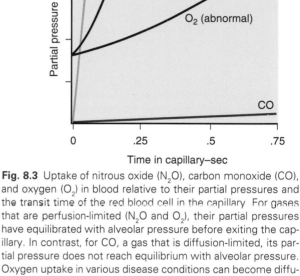

Fig. 8.3 Uptake of nitrous oxide (N_2O), carbon monoxide (CO), and oxygen (O_2) in blood relative to their partial pressures and the transit time of the red blood cell in the capillary. For gases that are perfusion-limited (N_2O and O_2), their partial pressures have equilibrated with alveolar pressure before exiting the capillary. In contrast, for CO, a gas that is diffusion-limited, its partial pressure does not reach equilibrium with alveolar pressure. Oxygen uptake in various disease conditions can become diffusion-limited. (From Koeppen BM, Stanton BM, eds. *Berne and Levy's Physiology*, 7th ed. Philadelphia: Elsevier; 2018.)

DIFFUSION LIMITATION

In contrast, the partial pressure of CO in the pulmonary capillary blood rises very slowly compared with N_2O and O_2 (see Fig. 8.3). This is because carbon monoxide has a low solubility in the alveolar–capillary membrane but a high solubility in blood. As a result, equilibration between alveolar gas and blood occurs slowly (significantly greater than the 0.75-second transit time of the red blood cell in the capillary). However, CO solubility varies with CO partial pressure. At partial pressures below 1 to 2 torr, CO solubility is high, whereas at partial pressures greater than 2 torr, CO solubility is small because CO content increases only by adding dissolved CO. For CO, equilibration is not reached during the transit time, resulting in only a minimal increase in the partial pressure. Even though there is only a small increase in partial pressure, if you measured the CO content in the blood (milliliters of CO/milliliters blood) it would be rising rapidly. The reason for this rapid rise is that CO binds chemically with hemoglobin with an affinity that is about 10 times that of oxygen for hemoglobin. The CO that is combined with the hemoglobin does

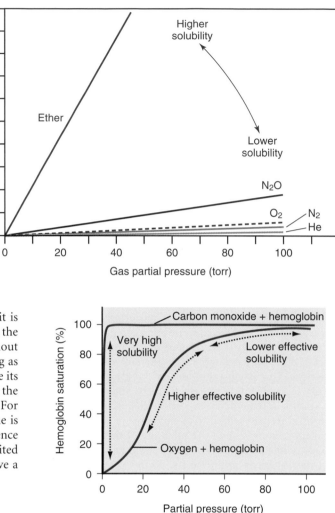

Fig. 8.4 Relationship between the content of dissolved gas and its partial pressure in blood. The solubility of the gas in the liquid is the slope of the line. A linear relationship (i.e., constant solubility at a given temperature) is seen for gases that do not combine chemically with the liquid. Note the high solubility of ether and the very low solubility of oxygen. (Redrawn from Leff A, Schumacker P. *Respiratory Physiology: Basics and Applications.* Philadelphia: W.B. Saunders; 1993.)

not contribute to the partial pressure of CO because it is no longer physically dissolved in the blood. As a result, the partial pressure gradient for CO is maintained throughout the capillary bed, and exchange of CO is still occurring as the red blood cell leaves the end of the capillary because its rate of equilibration is slow relative to the time spent in the capillary. This type of gas transfer is **diffusion-limited**. For CO, this occurs because its solubility in the membrane is low, whereas its solubility in blood is high. In the absence of red blood cells, CO uptake would be perfusion-limited because now both the "blood" and the membrane have a similar low solubility to CO.

DIFFUSION OF O_2 AND CO_2

O_2 (and CO_2 and CO) combines chemically with blood. As a result, the relationship between gas content in the blood and partial pressure is nonlinear (Fig. 8.5). The slope of the relationship for any gas is its **effective solubility**. The effective solubility of oxygen varies with partial pressure and is greatest at lower partial pressures. O_2 has a relatively low solubility in the membrane of the blood–gas barrier but a high effective solubility in blood because of its combining with hemoglobin. O_2 does not combine with hemoglobin as quickly as CO binds, and so the partial pressure of O_2 in the blood rises more rapidly than does the partial pressure of CO (see Fig. 8.3). Once bound to hemoglobin, O_2 no longer exerts a partial pressure, and so the partial pressure gradient across the alveolar-capillary membrane is maintained, and O_2 transfer continues. Hemoglobin, however, quickly becomes

Fig. 8.5 Oxygen and carbon monoxide content as a function of their partial pressure in blood. The effective solubility of each gas in blood is equivalent to the slope of the line at any point. Thus oxygen is highly soluble at partial pressures of 20 to 60 torr but relatively insoluble above 100 torr (where most of the hemoglobin sites are occupied). In contrast, carbon monoxide solubility is extremely large at a partial pressure of less than 1 torr. At partial pressures greater than 1 torr, carbon monoxide content increases by adding dissolved carbon monoxide only and its solubility is small. (Redrawn from Leff A, Schumacker P. *Respiratory Physiology: Basics and Applications.* Philadelphia: W.B. Saunders; 1993.)

saturated with O_2. When this happens, the partial pressure of O_2 in the blood rises rapidly and is equal to the alveolar partial pressure. At this point, no further O_2 transfer from the alveolus to the equilibrated blood can occur. Thus under normal conditions, O_2 transfer from

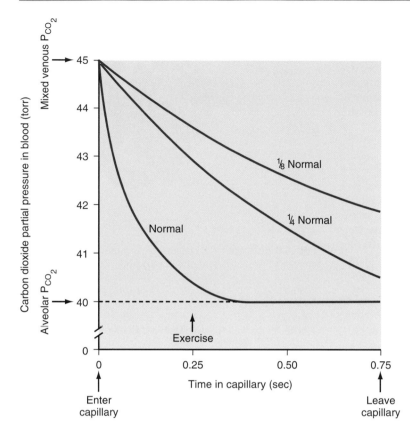

Fig. 8.6 Partial pressure of carbon dioxide as a function of the duration of time that the red blood cell spends in the capillary. Under normal conditions, the P_{CO_2} of blood entering the capillary is 46 torr and decreases to 40 torr by the time the blood leaves the capillary. When the diffusion through the alveolar-capillary barrier is reduced to one-fourth and one-eighth of normal, the P_{CO_2} approaches but is not normal by the time the blood leaves the capillary. With exercise, the time spent in the capillary is reduced to 0.25 second. This is sufficient in the normal lung but can result in an abnormal Pa_{CO_2} in the lung with abnormal diffusion. (Redrawn from Wagner PD, West JB. Effects of diffusion impairment on O_2 and CO_2 time courses in pulmonary capillaries. *J Appl Physiol.* 1972;33:62.)

the alveolus to the pulmonary capillary is perfusion-limited. That is, the rate of equilibration is sufficiently rapid (usually within 0.25 second) for complete equilibration to occur during the transit time of the red blood cell within the capillary.

DIFFUSION OF CO_2

The time course of CO_2 equilibration in the pulmonary capillary is shown in Fig. 8.6. In a normal individual, equilibrium is reached in about 0.25 second, the same time period for O_2. The effective solubility of CO_2 is higher than that of O_2 because CO_2 is more soluble in blood than O_2, and its solubility is less variable (Fig. 8.7). If the diffusivity of CO_2 is 20 times higher than that of O_2 and the solubility is higher, why is the time to equilibrium the same? It is the same because the partial pressure gradient for CO_2 is much less than the gradient for O_2, and CO_2 has a lower membrane–blood solubility ratio. As a consequence, O_2 and CO_2 take approximately the same amount of time to reach equilibration, and CO_2 transfer, like that of O_2, is usually perfusion-limited.

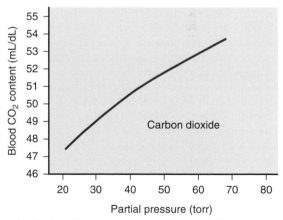

Fig. 8.7 Carbon dioxide content as a function of its partial pressure in blood. Carbon dioxide is much more soluble in blood than is oxygen (compare with Fig. 8.5 and note the steeper slope). Unlike oxygen, its solubility is relatively constant as a function of partial pressure (the solubility is the slope of the line). (Redrawn from Leff A, Schumacker P. *Respiratory Physiology: Basics and Applications.* Philadelphia: W.B. Saunders; 1993.)

Diffusion limitation for both O_2 and CO_2 could occur if the red blood cell spent less than 0.25 second in the capillary bed. Occasionally, this can be seen in very fit athletes during vigorous exercise and in healthy subjects who exercise at high altitude. It may also be present during exercise in individuals with an abnormally thickened barrier due to fibrosis or interstitial edema and at rest in individuals with severe lung disease.

OXYGEN TRANSPORT

Oxygen is carried in the blood in both the dissolved gaseous state in plasma and bound to hemoglobin (Hgb) as oxyhemoglobin ($HgbO_2$) within red blood cells. O_2 transport occurs primarily through $HgbO_2$, with a minimal contribution of dissolved O_2. For example, at a Pao_2 of 100 mm Hg, only 3 mL of O_2 is dissolved in 1 L of plasma. The contribution of hemoglobin within the red blood cell enhances the O_2-carrying capacity of blood by about 65-fold. Non–O_2-bound hemoglobin is referred to as *deoxyhemoglobin*, or reduced hemoglobin.

HEMOGLOBIN STRUCTURE

Hemoglobin has a molecular weight of 66,500 kDa and consists of four nonprotein O_2-binding heme groups and four polypeptide chains, which make up the globin protein portion of the Hgb molecule (Fig. 8.8). The four polypeptide chains of adult Hgb (hemoglobin type A, or HgbA) are composed of two alpha chains and two beta chains. Iron is present in each heme group in the reduced ferrous (Fe^{+2}) form and is the site of O_2-binding. Each of the polypeptide chains can bind one molecule of oxygen to the iron-binding site on its own heme group. Both the globin component and the heme group with its iron atom in the reduced or ferrous state must be in a proper spatial orientation for the chemical reaction with oxygen to occur.

Variations in the amino acid sequence of the globin subunits have significant physiologic consequences. For example, fetal Hgb (HgbF) is produced by the fetus to meet the oxygen demands of its specialized environment. HgbF is composed of two alpha chains and two gamma chains. This change in structure in HgbF increases its affinity for O_2 and aids in the transport of O_2 across the placenta. In addition, as discussed later in this chapter, HgbF is not affected or inhibited by the glycolysis product 2,3-diphosphoglycerate (2,3-DPG) in red blood cells, thus further enhancing O_2 uptake. During the first year of life, HgbF is replaced by HgbA.

Genetic substitutions of various amino acids result in a number of abnormal hemoglobins. These changes usually occur in the alpha and beta chains. More than 125 abnormal hemoglobins have been reported.

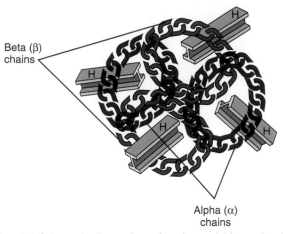

Fig. 8.8 Schematic illustration of a hemoglobin molecule showing the globin (protein) component with two alpha and two beta chains and the four iron-containing heme groups (oxygen-binding) positioned in the center of each globin portion. Each hemoglobin molecule can bind four oxygen molecules. (From Koeppen BM, Stanton BM, eds. *Berne and Levy's Physiology*, 7th ed. Philadelphia: Elsevier; 2018.)

CLINICAL BOX

The most important and most common of the genetic Hgb amino acid substitutions is sickle cell hemoglobin (HgbS), which results in the disease called **sickle cell anemia**. Sickle cell anemia is an inherited, homozygous, recessive condition in which individuals have an amino acid substitution (valine for glutamic acid) on the beta chain of the hemoglobin molecule. This creates HgbS, which when unbound (deoxyhemoglobin) forms a gel that distorts the normal biconcave shape of the red blood cell to create a crescent or "sickle" form. This change in shape increases the tendency of the red blood cell to form thrombi or clots that obstruct small vessels and results in a clinical condition known as a **sickle cell crisis**. The symptoms of this condition vary, depending on the site of the obstruction. If it occurs in the central nervous system, patients suffer a stroke. If it occurs in the lung, patients can suffer a pulmonary infarction with death of the lung tissue. Although in its homozygous form sickle cell anemia is a life-shortening clinical condition, individuals with the heterozygous form (sickle cell trait) are resistant to malaria. Thus there is a survival advantage in regions in the world where malaria is prevalent.

OXYGEN BINDING TO HEMOGLOBIN

The binding of O_2 to hemoglobin alters the light absorption characteristics of hemoglobin; this is responsible for the difference in color between oxygenated arterial blood ($HgbO_2$) and deoxygenated venous blood (Hgb). The binding of O_2 to hemoglobin is readily reversible, and this ready reversibility is a critical component that facilitates the delivery of O_2 to the tissue from the blood. The binding and dissociation of O_2 with Hgb occurs in milliseconds, which is well suited for the average capillary transit time of 0.75 second for the red blood cell.

There are ~280 million Hgb molecules per red blood cell, which provides a unique and efficient mechanism to transport O_2. Because the amount of hemoglobin present in each red blood cell is relatively equal, the amount of hemoglobin in blood is directly proportional to the percentage of blood volume occupied by red blood cells (**hematocrit**). It should be noted that **myoglobin**, the O_2-carrying and storage protein of muscle tissue, is similar to hemoglobin in structure and function except that it has only one subunit of the hemoglobin molecule; thus its molecular weight is about one-fourth that of hemoglobin. Myoglobin aids in the transfer of O_2 from blood to muscle cells and in the storage of O_2, which is especially critical in O_2-deprived conditions.

When oxygen combines with hemoglobin, the iron usually remains in the ferrous state. In a condition known as **methemoglobinemia**, compounds such as nitrites and various cyanides (released in the environment during the burning of plastics or in the workplace from photo supplies, electroplating, and mining) can oxidize the iron molecule in the heme group changing it from the reduced ferrous state to the ferric state (Fe^{+3}). Hemoglobin with iron in the ferric state is brown instead of red. Methemoglobin blocks the release of O_2 from hemoglobin, which inhibits delivery of O_2 to the tissues, a critical aspect of reversible O_2 transport. Under normal conditions, ~1% to 2% of hemoglobin-binding sites are in the ferric state. Intracellular enzymes such as glutathione reductase can reduce the methemoglobin back to the functioning ferrous state. Patients with methemoglobinemia have an absence of glutathione reductase.

DISSOLVED OXYGEN

Oxygen diffuses passively from the alveolus to the plasma, where it dissolves. In its dissolved form, O_2 maintains its molecular structure and gaseous state. It is this form that is measured clinically in an arterial blood gas sample as the Pao_2. The dissolved O_2 in blood is the product of the oxygen solubility (0.00304 mL O_2/dL · torr) times the oxygen tension (torr). In a healthy normal adult, approximately 0.3 mL of O_2 is dissolved in 100 mL blood. This is commonly expressed as 0.3 volumes percent (vol%), where the vol% is equal to the mL O_2/100 mL blood. It can be seen that the O_2 dissolved in plasma is insufficient to meet the body's O_2 demands. In particular, the resting oxygen consumption of an adult is 200 to 300 mL O_2/min. For dissolved oxygen to meet this resting O_2 consumption, a cardiac output of almost 67 L/min would be required; that is,

$$\frac{200 \text{ mL } O_2/min}{0.3 \text{ mL } O_2/100 \text{ mL blood}} = \frac{66{,}666 \text{ mL blood}}{min}$$

$$= 66.7 \text{ L/min}$$

During exercise, this cardiac output would need to further increase 10–15-fold. Normal individuals can achieve a cardiac output with vigorous exercise in the range of 25 L/min. Clearly, dissolved oxygen in the blood cannot meet the metabolic needs of the body even at rest, much less during exercise. Thus the contribution of dissolved oxygen to total O_2 transport is small. In fact, when calculating the O_2 content in blood, the dissolved O_2 is frequently ignored. This small amount of additional dissolved O_2 becomes significant, however, in individuals with severe hypoxemia being treated with high levels of inspired oxygen.

OXYGEN SATURATION

Each hemoglobin molecule can bind up to four O_2 atoms, and each gram of hemoglobin can bind up to 1.34 mL (range of 1.34 to 1.39 mL depending on methemoglobin levels) of O_2. The term **oxygen saturation** (So_2) refers to the amount of O_2 bound to hemoglobin relative to the maximal amount of O_2 (100% O_2 capacity) that can bind hemoglobin. It is equal to the O_2 content in the blood (minus the physically dissolved O_2) divided by the O_2-carrying capacity of hemoglobin in the blood times 100%.

$$\% \text{ Hgb saturation} = \frac{O_2 \text{ bound to Hgb}}{O_2 - \text{carrying capacity of Hgb}} \times 100\%$$

Both O_2 content and O_2-carrying capacity are dependent on the amount of hemoglobin in blood and both are expressed as milliliters O_2/100 milliliters blood. In contrast, hemoglobin saturation is only a percentage. Thus $HgbO_2$ saturation is not interchangeable with the O_2 content. Individuals with different Hgb levels will have different O_2 contents but can have the same hemoglobin saturation.

At 100% saturation (100% So_2), the heme group is fully saturated with oxygen. Correspondingly, at 75% So_2, three of the four heme groups are occupied by O_2. The binding of O_2 to each heme group increases the affinity of the hemoglobin molecule to bind additional O_2. Thus, when three of the heme groups are O_2-bound, the affinity of the fourth heme group to bind O_2 is increased. Because there are about 14 g Hgb/100 mL blood, the normal O_2 capacity is 18.76 mL (1 g Hgb binds 1.34 mL $O_2 \times$ 14 g Hgb) of O_2/100 mL blood. A mildly anemic individual with an Hgb concentration of 10 g/100 mL blood and normal lungs would only have an O_2 capacity of 13.40 mL O_2/100 mL blood; a severely anemic individual with an Hgb concentration of 5 g would have an O_2 capacity of 6.70 mL O_2/100 mL blood—one-third of normal.

OXYGEN CONTENT (CONCENTRATION) OF BLOOD

The O_2 content in blood is the volume of O_2 contained per unit volume of blood. The total O_2 content is the sum of the O_2 bound to hemoglobin and the dissolved O_2. The hemoglobin-bound O_2 content is determined by the concentration of hemoglobin (in g/dL), the O_2-binding capacity of the hemoglobin (1.34 mL O_2/g Hgb), and the percent saturation of the hemoglobin. The dissolved O_2 content is the product of the O_2 solubility (0.00304 mL O_2/dL · torr) times the O_2 tension (torr). Oxygen content decreases with increased CO_2 and CO and in individuals with anemia (Fig. 8.9).

As an example, consider an arterial blood gas with a Pao_2 of 60 torr and an arterial Sao_2 of 90%. The patient's hemoglobin is 14 g/dL. What would the total (Hgb-bound and dissolved) O_2 content be?

Hgb – bound O_2 content
$$= \frac{1.34 \text{ mL}}{\text{g Hgb}} \times \frac{14 \text{ g Hgb}}{\text{dL blood}} \times \frac{90\% \text{ Saturation}}{100}$$
$$= 16.88 \text{ mL/dL blood}$$

Dissolved O_2 content
$$= PaO_2 \times O_2 \text{ solubility}$$
$$= 60 \text{ torr} \times 0.00304 \text{ mL } O_2/\text{dL·torr}$$
$$= 0.18 \text{ mL } O_2/\text{dL}$$

Total O_2 content $= 16.88 \text{ mL/dL} + 0.18 \text{ mL/dL}$
$$= 17.06 \text{ mL/dL blood}$$

Oxygen content varies with changes in oxygen saturation and hemoglobin. For example, what is the oxygen content in someone receiving 30% supplemental O_2 with a Pao_2 of 95 torr and an So_2 of 97%?

Hgb°O_2 content
$$= 1.34 \text{ mL/dL} \times 14 \text{ gm/dL} \times 0.97 = 18.20 \text{ mL/dL}$$

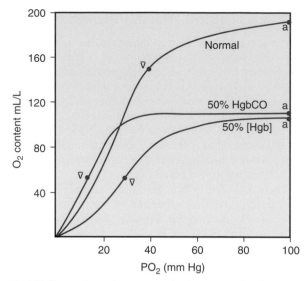

Fig. 8.9 Comparison of oxygen content curves under three conditions shows why HgbCO is so toxic to the oxygen transport system. Fifty percent [Hgb] represents a reduction in circulating hemoglobin by half; 50% HgbCO represents binding of half the circulating hemoglobin with CO. The 50% [Hgb] and 50% HgbCO curves show the same decreased oxygen content in arterial blood. However, CO has a profound effect in lowering venous Po_2. The arterial (a) and mixed venous ($\bar{v}$) points of constant cardiac output are indicated. (From Koeppen BM, Stanton BM, eds. *Berne and Levy's Physiology*, 7th ed. Philadelphia: Elsevier; 2018.)

Dissolved O_2 content
$$= 95 \text{ torr} \times 0.00304 \text{ mL } O_2/\text{dL·torr} = 0.29 \text{ mL/dL}$$

Total O_2 content
$$= 18.20 \text{ mL/dL} + 0.29 \text{ mL/dL} = 18.49 \text{ mL/dL}$$

Oxygen therapy has significantly increased the total O_2 content. Note, again, the small contribution of dissolved O_2 to the total O_2 content.

THE OXYHEMOGLOBIN DISSOCIATION CURVE

The majority of O_2 in plasma quickly diffuses into the red blood cells where it chemically binds to the heme groups of the hemoglobin molecule, forming oxyhemoglobin (HgbO_2). The chemical binding of O_2 to hemoglobin occurs in the lung and this HgbO_2 complex is the major transport mechanism for oxygen. It is also reversible at the tissue level where hemoglobin gives up its oxygen to the tissue. The number of O_2 molecules bound to hemoglobin is dependent on the partial pressure of O_2 in the blood. The

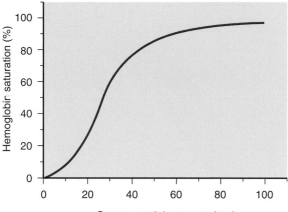

Fig. 8.10 Oxyhemoglobin dissociation curve showing the relationship between the partial pressure of oxygen in blood and the percentage of the hemoglobin binding sites that are occupied by oxygen molecules (percent saturation). Adult hemoglobin (HgbA) is about 60% saturated at a P_{O_2} of 30 torr, 90% saturated at 60 torr, and about 75% saturated at 40 torr. (From Koeppen BM, Stanton BM, eds. *Berne and Levy's Physiology*, 7th ed. Philadelphia: Elsevier; 2018.)

oxyhemoglobin dissociation curve displays the relationship between the O_2 partial pressure (P_{O_2}) in the blood and the percentage of O_2-binding sites occupied by O_2 molecules (Fig. 8.10). As the partial pressure of O_2 increases, hemoglobin saturation increases. The curve, however, is S-shaped (not linear), reflecting the change in the affinity of Hgb for O_2 with increased binding of O_2 to the heme.

The oxyhemoglobin dissociation curve demonstrates a number of interesting features. The curve begins to plateau at a P_{O_2} of about 50 mm Hg and flattens at a P_{O_2} of 70 mm Hg. At partial pressures below 60 mm Hg, O_2 readily binds to Hgb as the P_{O_2} increases (linear portion). At a P_{O_2} of 60 mm Hg, hemoglobin is 90% saturated; increases in P_{O_2} above this level will have only minor influences on hemoglobin saturation. Specifically, increasing the P_{O_2} from 60 to 100 mm Hg, will increase hemoglobin saturation only 7%. The clinical significance of the flat portion of the oxyhemoglobin dissociation curve is that a drop in P_{O_2} anywhere from 100 mm Hg to 60 mm Hg results in hemoglobin that is more than 90% saturated; this virtually assures adequate O_2 delivery to the tissues. The curve also demonstrates that increasing the P_{O_2} above 100 mm Hg has little effect on O_2 content in the blood because hemoglobin is already (almost) fully saturated. Along the steep or linear portion of the curve, blood O_2 content and thus O_2 delivery to the tissue are significantly compromised when the P_{O_2} falls below 60 mm Hg. The clinical significance of this portion of the curve is that a large amount of O_2 is released from

hemoglobin with only a small change in P_{O_2}; this facilitates the diffusion of O_2 to the tissue. The point on the curve at which 50% of the hemoglobin is saturated with O_2 (two O_2 molecules on one Hgb molecule) is called the P_{50} (Fig. 8.11). In adults at sea level, this occurs at a P_{O_2} of 27 mm Hg.

FACTORS ASSOCIATED WITH SHIFTS IN THE OXYHEMOGLOBIN DISSOCIATION CURVE

The oxyhemoglobin dissociation curve can be shifted either to the right or the left as a result of numerous clinical conditions. The curve is shifted to the right when the affinity of hemoglobin for O_2 decreases. This results in decreased hemoglobin binding O_2 at a given P_{O_2} and is seen as an increase in the P_{50}. The curve is shifted to the left when the affinity of hemoglobin for O_2 increases. This results in a lower P_{50}. A shift in the curve to the right aids in the release of O_2 into tissues and cells, whereas a shift in the curve to the left aids in the uptake/binding of O_2 to hemoglobin in the lung. Processes that shift the oxyhemoglobin dissociation curve are shown in Fig. 8.12.

The Bohr Effect

Changes in blood pH also shift the oxyhemoglobin dissociation curve. A decrease in pH shifts the curve to the right (enhancing O_2 dissociation); conversely, an increase in pH shifts the curve to the left (increasing O_2 affinity). During cellular metabolism, CO_2 is produced and released into the blood, resulting in the increased generation of hydrogen ions and a decrease in pH. This results in a shift of the dissociation curve to the right, which has a beneficial effect by aiding in the release (dissociation of O_2 from Hgb) and diffusion of O_2 into the tissue and cells. The shift to the right appears to be not only due to the decrease in pH but also a direct effect of CO_2 on hemoglobin. Conversely, as blood passes through the lungs, CO_2 is exhaled, resulting in a decrease in hydrogen ion content and an increase in pH, which results in a shift to the left in the dissociation curve. The higher hemoglobin affinity for O_2 enhances the binding of O_2 to hemoglobin. This effect of CO_2 on the affinity of hemoglobin for oxygen is known as the **Bohr effect** (named after the Danish physiologist, Christian Bohr). The Bohr effect is due in part to the change in pH that occurs as CO_2 increases and in part to the direct effect of CO_2 on hemoglobin. The Bohr effect enhances O_2 delivery to the tissue and O_2 uptake in the lungs (Fig. 8.13).

Temperature

Body temperature increases in muscles during exercise. This increase in temperature shifts the dissociation curve to the right, thus enabling more O_2 to be released in the muscles, where it is needed because of increased demand.

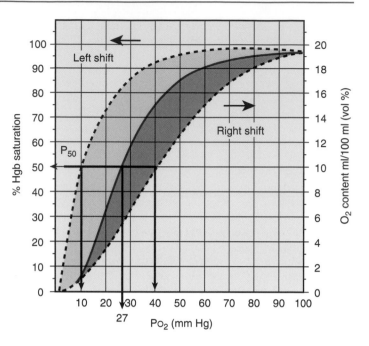

Fig. 8.11 The P_{50} represents the partial pressure at which hemoglobin is 50% saturated with oxygen. When the oxygen dissociation curve shifts to the right, the P_{50} increases. When the curve shifts to the left, the P_{50} decreases. (From Koeppen BM, Stanton BM, eds. *Berne and Levy's Physiology*, 7th ed. Philadelphia: Elsevier; 2018.)

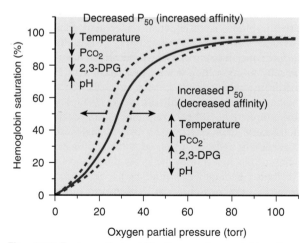

Fig. 8.12 Factors that shift the oxyhemoglobin dissociation curve. The affinity of hemoglobin for oxygen is expressed as the P_{50}. Increases in P_{CO_2}, temperature, and 2,3-diphosphoglycerate (2,3-DPG) or decreases in pH shift the oxyhemoglobin dissociation curve to the right (increased P_{50} = decreased affinity), whereas opposite changes shift the curve to the left (decreased P_{50} = increased affinity) relative to the standard value of 27 torr. (From Koeppen BM, Stanton BM, eds. *Berne and Levy's Physiology*, 7th ed. Philadelphia: Elsevier; 2018.)

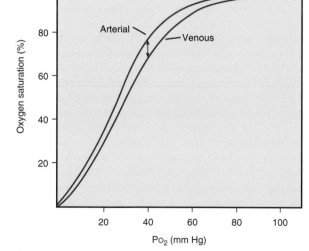

Fig. 8.13 Normal arterial and venous $HgbO_2$ equilibrium curves. In the lung, the effect of the shift to the left caused by a decrease in hydrogen ion concentration enhances oxygen uptake. In the systemic capillaries, significant O_2 unloading begins at about P_{O_2} = 70 mm Hg. The rising hydrogen ion concentration caused by the entry of CO_2 shifts the curve to the right, enhancing oxygen dissociation. The P_{50} of the arterial curve is 27 mm Hg; the P_{50} of the venous curve is 29 mm Hg. (From Koeppen BM, Stanton BM, eds. *Berne and Levy's Physiology*, 7th ed. Philadelphia: Elsevier; 2018.)

A decrease in body temperature during cold weather, especially in the extremities (lips, fingers, toes, and ears), shifts the curve to the left (higher Hgb affinity). In this instance the Pao_2 may be normal but the release of O_2 in these extremities is not facilitated. That is why these areas can display a bluish coloration with exposure to cold (known as **acrocyanosis**). Temperature also affects the solubility of O_2 in plasma. At 20°C, 50% more O_2 will be dissolved in plasma.

2,3-Diphosphoglycerate

Mature red blood cells do not have mitochondria and therefore respire via anaerobic glycolysis. During glycolysis, large quantities of the metabolic intermediary 2,3-diphosphoglycerate (2,3-DPG) are formed within the red blood cell. As 2,3-DPG levels increase in the red blood cell, the affinity of hemoglobin for O_2 decreases proportionately, thus shifting the oxyhemoglobin dissociation curve to the right. The affinity of 2,3-DPG for hemoglobin is greater than that for O_2; as a result, 2,3-DPG directly competes with O_2 for Hgb-binding sites. Conditions that increase 2,3-DPG include hypoxia, decreased hemoglobin concentration, and increased pH. Increases in 2,3-DPG with hypoxia result in greater O_2 release from hemoglobin at any Po_2, mitigating hypoxia's effects on the tissues. Red blood cells with HgbS (sickle cell trait) have increased levels of 2,3-DPG. Decreased levels of 2,3-DPG are observed in stored blood samples; this could theoretically present a problem due to the greater $HgbO_2$ affinity, which inhibits the unloading of O_2 in tissues.

Fetal Hemoglobin

As discussed previously, fetal hemoglobin has a greater affinity for O_2 than does adult hemoglobin. Fetal hemoglobin thus shifts the oxyhemoglobin dissociation curve to the left.

Carbon Monoxide

Carbon monoxide (CO) binds to the heme group of the Hgb molecule at the same site as O_2, forming carboxyhemoglobin (HgbCO). A major difference, however, as illustrated in comparing the oxyhemoglobin and carboxyhemoglobin dissociation curves, is that the affinity of CO for hemoglobin is about 200 times greater than that of O_2 (Fig. 8.14). Thus small amounts of CO greatly inhibit the binding of O_2 to hemoglobin. In addition, in the presence of CO, the hemoglobin molecules' affinity for O_2 is enhanced, which shifts the dissociation curve to the left, further inhibiting the unloading and delivery of O_2 to tissue. Thus CO prevents O_2 loading into the blood in the lungs and O_2 unloading in the tissues. As the Pco of blood approaches 1.0 torr, all of the Hgb-binding

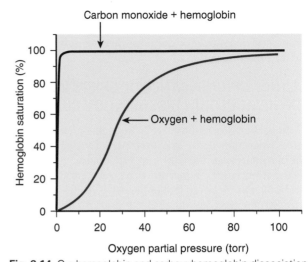

Fig. 8.14 Oxyhemoglobin and carboxyhemoglobin dissociation curves. Carbon monoxide and oxygen compete for the same binding sites on hemoglobin, but carbon monoxide has an affinity for hemoglobin that is approximately 200 times greater than O_2. Thus above a blood Pco of about 0.5 torr, all of the hemoglobin-binding sites are occupied by carbon monoxide. (From Koeppen BM, Stanton BM, eds. *Berne and Levy's Physiology*, 7th ed. Philadelphia: Elsevier; 2018.)

sites are occupied by CO, and hemoglobin is unable to bind to O_2. This situation is not compatible with life and is the mechanism of death in individuals with CO poisoning. CO is colorless, odorless, and tasteless and does not produce symptoms of breathlessness or difficulty breathing (see Chapter 10 on regulation of respiration for the reason).

In healthy individuals, carboxyhemoglobin occupies about 1% to 2% of the Hgb-binding sites; however, in cigarette smokers and in individuals who reside in high-density urban traffic areas, it can be increased to 10%.

Treatment for individuals with high levels of CO, such as after inhaling car exhaust or due to smoke inhalation in a burning building, consists of high concentrations of O_2 to displace CO from hemoglobin. Increasing the barometric pressure above atmospheric, through the use of a barometric chamber, substantially increases the oxygen tension. This increase in barometric pressure promotes the further dissociation of CO from hemoglobin.

Nitric oxide (NO) also has a great affinity (200,000 times greater than O_2) for hemoglobin and binds irreversibly to it at the same site as O_2. Endothelial cells can synthesize NO, which has vasodilatation properties and is used therapeutically as an inhalant in patients with pulmonary hypertension. Although not common, NO poisoning can occur, and one should be cautious when administering NO therapy for long periods.

CLINICAL SIGNIFICANCE OF SHIFTS IN THE OXYHEMOGLOBIN DISSOCIATION CURVE

Shifts of the dissociation curve to the right or left have little effect when they occur at oxygen partial pressures within the normal range (80–100 mm Hg; plateau part of the dissociation curve). However, at oxygen partial pressures below 60 mm Hg (steep part of the curve), shifts in the oxyhemoglobin dissociation curve can dramatically influence O_2 transport. For example, in a patient with lung disease who has a Pao_2 equal to 60 mm Hg, the Hbg saturation is 90%, which is still adequate for normal functioning. However, if the patient experiences a decrease in pH, the dissociation curve shifts to the right and the Hgb saturation could drop to less than 70%, which would significantly impair O_2 delivery.

OXYGEN DELIVERY TO THE TISSUES

As blood circulates from the lungs, it is exposed to tissues with a lower Po_2, and oxygen is released by the hemoglobin. Oxygen delivery from the lungs to the tissue varies with cardiac output (QT), the hemoglobin content of blood, and the ability of the lung to oxygenate the blood. The total O_2 delivered (Do_2) to the tissue can be calculated by multiplying the cardiac output (QT) times the O_2 content of arterial blood (Cao_2); that is,

$$DO_2 = QT \times (CaO_2) \times 10 \text{ (to change the vol\%}$$
$$\text{from mL } O_2/dL \text{ to mL } O_2/L)$$

Under normal conditions, the cardiac output is about 5 L/min and the O_2 content in arterial blood is 20 vol%; thus, under normal conditions,

$$DO_2 = 5 \text{ L/min} \times 20 \text{ vol\%} \times 10 = 1000 \text{ mL } O_2/\text{min}$$

OXYGEN CONSUMPTION

Not all of the O_2 carried in the blood is unloaded at the tissue level. The principle of conservation of mass, also known as the Fick relationship, can be applied to calculate oxygen consumption. The O_2 extracted from the blood by the tissue (that is, the O_2 consumption, or ($\dot{V}o_2$) is the difference between the arterial O_2 content (Cao_2; i.e., the amount of O_2 delivered) and the venous O_2 content (Cvo_2;

the O_2 content remaining after release to the tissues) times the cardiac output; that is,

$$\dot{V}O_2 = QT[(CaO_2 - CvO_2) \times 10]$$

Under normal conditions, when the Cao_2 is 20 vol% and the Cvo_2 is 15 vol%, the amount of O_2 actually consumed by the tissues is 5 vol% (5 mL of O_2 for each 100/mL of blood or 50 mL of O_2 for each liter of blood). With a cardiac output of 5 L/min, the total amount of O_2 consumed in 1 minute is 250 mL/min (50 mL O_2/L blood × 5 L/min).

An interesting but underused approach to understanding O_2 consumption is the **O_2 extraction ratio** (also referred to as the O_2 coefficient ratio), which is the amount of O_2 extracted by the tissue divided by the amount of O_2 delivered:

$$O_2 \text{ extraction ratio} = \frac{CaO_2 - CvO_2}{CaO_2}$$

$$= \frac{20 \text{ Vol\%} - 15 \text{ Vol\%}}{20 \text{ Vol\%}} = 0.25$$

Under normal conditions, only 25% of the O_2 that is delivered to the tissues is actually used by the tissues. This significant reserve is one of the reasons individuals are able to tolerate large changes in O_2 content. It is possible to significantly change the O_2 extraction ratio without a change in the difference between Cao_2 and Cvo_2. As shown previously, the normal O_2 extraction ratio is 0.25 with a Cao_2 and Cvo_2 difference of 5 vol%. If the Cao_2 decreases to 8 vol% with a Cvo_2 of 3 vol%, the O_2 extraction ratio now becomes 0.62 even though the Cao_2 and Cvo_2 difference remains 5 vol%.

$$\text{Abnormal } O_2 \text{ extraction}$$
$$= \frac{CaO_2 - CvO_2}{CaO_2} = \frac{8 \text{ vol\%} - 3 \text{ vol\%}}{8 \text{ vol\%}} = \frac{5 \text{ vol\%}}{8 \text{ vol\%}}$$
$$= 0.62$$

Hypothermia, relaxation of skeletal muscles, and an increase in cardiac output will reduce O_2 consumption and will decrease the O_2 extraction ratio. Conversely, a decrease in cardiac output, anemia, hyperthermia, and exercise increase O_2 consumption and will increase the O_2 extraction ratio.

TISSUE HYPOXIA

Tissue hypoxia occurs when there is insufficient O_2 available to the cells to maintain adequate aerobic metabolism to carry out normal cellular activities. Anaerobic metabolism occurs in association with the generation of increased levels of lactate and hydrogen ions and the subsequent formation

TABLE 8.1 Tissue Hypoxia

| Type of Hypoxia | Cause | MECHANISM | | | | |
		PaO_2	CaO_2	Amount O_2 Delivered	Amount O_2 Utilized	Response to 100% O_2
Hypoxic	Pulmonary disease with ↓ PaO_2	Low	Low	Low	Normal	Yes
Circulatory	Vascular disease	Normal	Normal	Low	Normal	No
	Arterial-venous shunt (malformation)					No
Anemic	CO poisoning	Normal	Low	Normal	Normal	Yes*
	Anemia					No
Histologic	Cyanide Sodium azide	Normal	Normal	Normal	Low	No

*Hyperbaric oxygen.

of lactic acid. This results in a significant decrease in the blood pH. In severe hypoxia, the body—especially the lips and nailbeds—takes on a blue-gray coloration (cyanosis) due to the lack of O_2 and the increased levels of deoxyhemoglobin. **Hypoxemia** and/or tissue hypoxia can occur (see Chapter 7). Hypoxemia refers to an abnormal Po_2 in arterial blood, which at sea level on room air is a Pao_2 less than 80 torr. Hypoxia usually occurs at a lower Po_2 and, although various mitigating circumstances can influence the absolute level at which there is insufficient O_2 for cell function, hypoxia often occurs when the Pao_2 falls below 60 torr.

As shown in Table 8.1, four major types of tissue hypoxia can occur via different mechanisms. *Hypoxic hypoxia* is the most common and occurs in lung diseases such as chronic obstructive pulmonary disease (COPD), pulmonary fibrosis, and neuromuscular diseases. As a result of these diseases, there is a decrease in Pao_2 and/or Cao_2 with a subsequent decrease in O_2 delivery to the tissues. *Circulatory (stagnate) hypoxia* is the result of diminished blood flow to an organ, usually due to vascular disease or an arterial venous shunt. *Anemic hypoxia* is caused by the inability of the blood to carry O_2 either due to low hemoglobin (anemia) or to its inability to carry O_2, as in the case of CO poisoning. *Histologic hypoxia* results when there is a block in the electron transport system in mitochondrial respiration, thus preventing the utilization of O_2 by the cell. Histologic hypoxia occurs with respiratory chain poisoning, such as with cyanide, sodium azide, and the pesticide rotenone. Similar to an anatomic shunt, neither circulatory, anemic, nor histologic hypoxia respond well to increased Fio_2.

Tissue oxygenation is directly dependent on the hemoglobin concentration and thus the number of red blood cells available in the circulation. **Erythropoiesis** (red blood cell production in the bone marrow) is controlled by the hormone *erythropoietin,* which is synthesized in the kidney by cortical interstitial cells. Although under normal conditions hemoglobin levels are stable, under conditions of decreased O_2 delivery, low hemoglobin concentrations, or low Pao_2 levels, the kidney cortical interstitial cells are stimulated to increase erythropoietin secretion, and this leads to increased production of red blood cells. Chronic renal disease can damage the cortical interstitial cells and result in their inability to synthesize erythropoietin. Anemia ensues, with decreased hemoglobin concentrations directly related to the lack of erythropoietin production. Erythropoietin replacement therapy has been shown to be effective in this condition.

CARBON DIOXIDE TRANSPORT

Carbon dioxide is carried in the blood in three ways: physically dissolved, as bicarbonate ions (HCO_3^-), and chemically bound to amino acids. By far the predominant transport mechanism of CO_2 is via HCO_3^- in red blood cells (Table 8.2). CO_2 is a by-product of tissue metabolism; approximately 200 to 250 mL of CO_2 is produced per minute. Under steady-state conditions at rest, with a cardiac output of 5 L/min, 4 to 5 mL of CO_2 must be eliminated by the lung for every 100 mL of blood.

CARBON DIOXIDE PRODUCTION, METABOLISM, AND DIFFUSION

CO_2 is critical in the maintenance of physiologic homeostasis and is a major factor in regulating hydrogen ion (H^+) concentrations in blood, cells, and other body tissues. It is also an important chemical stimulus in the regulation of respiration in normal individuals via chemoreceptors in the peripheral circulation and central nervous system

TABLE 8.2 Transport of CO_2 per Liter of Normal Human Blood		Arterial	Mixed Venous	A–V Difference*
Pco_2	mm Hg	40	46	6
Dissolved	mL/L	25	29	4
Carbamino	mL/L	24	38	14
HCO_3^-	mL/L	433	455	22
Total	mL/L	482	522	40

*Arterial-venous difference.

(see Chapter 10). The major sources of CO_2 production are in mitochondria during the aerobic cellular metabolism of glucose and in the conversion of carbohydrates to fats. Carbonic acid (H_2CO_3) is a major product of cellular metabolism and is readily metabolized to CO_2 and H_2O. During the metabolism of one glucose molecule, six CO_2 molecules are produced and six O_2 molecules are consumed (see Box 5.2). CO_2 production, which at rest is about 200 mL/min, can be increased sixfold during conditions of stress or exercise. The body has enhanced storage capabilities for CO_2 compared with O_2. Whereas Pao_2 is dependent on factors in addition to alveolar ventilation, $Paco_2$ is solely dependent on alveolar ventilation and CO_2 production. There is an inverse relationship between alveolar ventilation and $Paco_2$ (see Fig. 5.3).

The diffusion of CO_2 from the cell to the capillaries occurs through passive diffusion from higher to lower partial pressures of CO_2. When the intracellular concentration of CO_2 or its partial pressure ($Pcco_2$) exceeds the tissue concentration ($Ptco_2$), CO_2 moves out of the cell and into the surrounding tissue. Subsequently, $Ptco_2$ is increased; when it exceeds the capillary Pco_2, diffusion of CO_2 occurs from the tissue into the capillaries just before the blood enters the venous system. The CO_2 is then carried in venous blood to the lungs, where it is removed in exhaled gas. Diffusion of CO_2 occurs so readily from the alveolar lumen to the capillaries, and vice versa, that the $Paco_2$ and $Paco_2$ are equal. Under normal conditions, $Ptco_2$ is 50 mm Hg, venous Pco_2 ($Pvco_2$) is 46 mm Hg, and $Paco_2$ is 40 mm Hg. Thus under normal conditions the difference between $Paco_2$ and $Pvco_2$ is about 6 mm Hg. The blood level of CO_2 is highest on the venous side after the CO_2 has been picked up in the capillaries. In contrast to the exchange of O_2 from the arterial side of the circulatory system, CO_2 exchange occurs primarily from the venous side.

BICARBONATE

Once CO_2 diffuses through the tissue and reaches the plasma, it quickly physically dissolves and establishes a partial pressure ($Paco_2$). CO_2 readily diffuses from the plasma to the red blood cells, and an equilibrium is established between the red blood cells and plasma. The major pathway for the generation of HCO_3^- is the reaction of CO_2 with H_2O to form carbonic acid (H_2CO_3), which then readily dissociates to form bicarbonate (HCO_3^-) and free H^+ ions (Fig. 8.15); that is,

$$CO_2 + H_2O \xleftrightarrow{CA} H_2CO_3 \leftrightarrow H^+ + HCO_3^-$$

This reaction occurs slowly by chemical reaction standards (seconds) in tissue and plasma and is not thought to be of major significance in these two compartments. However, it is catalyzed within red blood cells by the enzyme **carbonic anhydrase** (CA), which speeds up the reaction time to microseconds and is the major source of HCO_3^- generation. Once formed within the red blood cells, the HCO_3^- diffuses out of the cell in exchange for Cl^-. This Cl^- exchange is referred to as the **chloride shift** (also called the Hamburger phenomenon and the anionic shift to equilibrium). The Cl^- binds to K^+, which was released by hemoglobin during the transfer of O_2 from hemoglobin to the tissue. The chloride shift maintains the electrostatic homeostasis of the cells. In addition, osmotic equilibrium is maintained in the red blood cell because water also accompanies the Cl^- movement. For this reason red blood cells are actually slightly swollen in the venous system compared with the arterial system.

This pathway of CO_2 to carbonic acid to bicarbonate is reversible. It is shifted to the right to generate more bicarbonate when CO_2 enters the blood from the tissue, and it is shifted to the left to generate more CO_2 when CO_2 is exhaled in the lungs.

The free H^+ ions are quickly buffered by binding to plasma proteins or, if within the red blood cell, the H^+ ions bind to hemoglobin to form an $H \cdot Hgb$ complex. The H^+ ion buffering is critical to keep the reaction moving toward the synthesis of HCO_3^-; high levels of free H^+ will push the reaction back in the opposite direction. This H^+ source is mainly responsible for the slightly more acidic

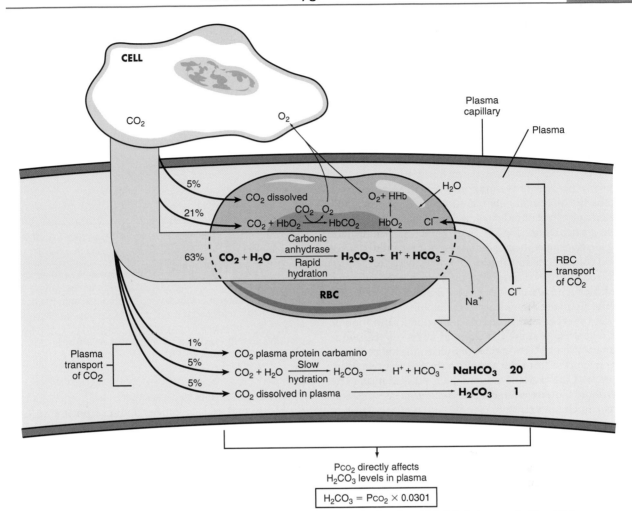

Fig. 8.15 Mechanisms of CO_2 transport. The predominant mechanism by which CO_2 is transported from the tissue cells to lung is in the form of HCO_3^-. (From Koeppen BM, Stanton BM, eds. *Berne and Levy's Physiology*, 7th ed. Philadelphia: Elsevier; 2018.)

nature of venous blood (pH 7.35) compared with arterial blood (pH 7.40).

$$CO_2 + H_2O \leftrightarrow H^+ + HCO_3^-$$
$$\updownarrow$$
$$H^+ + Hgb \leftrightarrow H\,Hgb$$

DISSOLVED CARBON DIOXIDE

Although CO_2 is 20 times more soluble than O_2 in water, the dissolved form of CO_2 still remains a small amount of the total transported CO_2. With this said, the dissolved form of CO_2 is much more important in CO_2 transport than is the dissolved form of O_2. Approximately 5% to 10% of the total CO_2 transported by blood is carried in physical solution. Also, although CO_2 transport and H^+ regulation occur simultaneously, they occur independently of each other and are controlled by different factors.

CARBAMINO COMPOUNDS

CO_2 can also combine chemically with the terminal amine groups in blood proteins to form carbamino compounds. Most of the CO_2 transported in this way is bound to the amino acids in hemoglobin because most of the protein found in blood is globin. Deoxyhemoglobin binds more CO_2 as carbamino groups than oxyhemoglobin, facilitating loading in the tissues and unloading in the lung. Approximately 5% to 10% of the CO_2 content in blood consists of carbamino compounds.

CARBON DIOXIDE DISSOCIATION CURVE

In contrast to O_2, the dissociation (removal and uptake) of CO_2 from the blood is almost directly related to the P_{CO_2}, and therefore the dissociation curve for CO_2 is linear (Fig. 8.16). When plotted on similar axes, the CO_2 dissociation curve is steeper than the oxygen dissociation curve. The degree of hemoglobin saturation with O_2 has a major effect on the CO_2 dissociation curve. Although O_2 and CO_2 bind to hemoglobin at different sites, deoxygenated hemoglobin has a greater affinity for CO_2 than oxygenated hemoglobin. The deoxygenated hemoglobin more readily forms carbamino compounds and also more readily binds free H^+ ions released during the formation of HCO_3^-. Thus deoxygenated blood (venous blood) freely takes up and transports more CO_2 than oxygenated arterial blood.

The effect of changes in oxyhemoglobin saturation on the relationship of the CO_2 content to P_{CO_2} is referred to as the **Haldane effect** and is reversed in the lung when O_2 is transported from the alveoli to the red blood cells. As a result of the Haldane effect, the CO_2 dissociation curve for whole blood is shifted to the right at greater levels of oxyhemoglobin and shifted to the left at greater levels of deoxyhemoglobin. Because of the Haldane effect, CO_2 uptake is facilitated in the presence of deoxyhemoglobin, and CO_2 unloading is facilitated in the presence of oxyhemoglobin.

In summary, the red blood cell is ideally constructed to transport O_2 and CO_2. Oxygen unloading along the

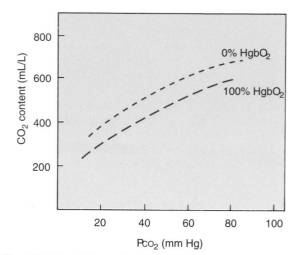

Fig. 8.16 Blood CO_2 equilibrium curves at different hemoglobin saturations (% $HgbO_2$). Venous blood can transport more CO_2 than arterial blood at any given P_{CO_2}. Compared with the hemoglobin oxygen equilibrium curve, the CO_2 curves are essentially straight lines between a P_{CO_2} of 20 and 80 mm Hg. (From Koeppen BM, Stanton BM, eds. *Berne and Levy's Physiology*, 7th ed. Philadelphia: Elsevier; 2018.)

systemic capillary is enhanced by increases in P_{CO_2} and by decreases in pH (Bohr effect), whereas CO_2 loading into the blood is enhanced by decreases in oxyhemoglobin saturation (Haldane effect). Oxygen is bound to hemoglobin when CO_2 exists in the form of HCO_3^-, which is produced in the red blood cell and transported into the plasma.

SUMMARY

1. The major source of energy in cells and organs is provided by the intracellular metabolism of oxygen (O_2) to generate ATP.
2. O_2 is carried in the blood from the lungs to the tissues in two forms: physically dissolved in the blood and chemically combined to hemoglobin.
3. Carbon dioxide (CO_2) is carried in the blood in three forms: physically dissolved in blood, chemically combined to blood proteins as carbamino compounds, and as bicarbonate.
4. Gases (nitrous oxide [N_2O], ether, helium) with a rapid rate of air-to-blood equilibration are perfusion-limited, and gases (CO) with a slow air-to-blood equilibration rate are diffusion-limited. Under normal conditions,

O_2 transport is perfusion-limited but can be diffusion-limited in certain conditions.
5. Fick's law of diffusion states that the diffusion of a gas across a sheet of tissue is directly related to the surface area of the tissue, the diffusion constant of the specific gas, and the partial pressure difference of the gas on each side of the tissue and is inversely related to tissue thickness.
6. O_2 loading and unloading and CO_2 loading and unloading not only occur simultaneously but also facilitate each other.
7. CO_2 diffuses approximately 20 times more rapidly through the alveolar–capillary membrane than does O_2.

8. O_2 binds quickly and reversibly to the heme groups of the hemoglobin (Hgb) molecule.

9. In its dissolved form, O_2 maintains its molecular structure and gaseous state. It is this form that is measured clinically in an arterial blood gas sample as the Pao_2.

10. The ability of CO_2 to alter the affinity of Hgb for O_2 (the Bohr effect) enhances O_2 delivery to tissue and O_2 uptake in the lungs.

11. Tissue hypoxia occurs when insufficient amounts of O_2 are supplied to the tissue to carry out normal levels of aerobic metabolism.

12. The major source of CO_2 production is in the mitochondria during aerobic cellular metabolism. The reversible reaction of CO_2 with H_2O to form carbonic acid (H_2CO_3) with its subsequent dissociation to HCO_3^- and H^+ is catalyzed by the enzyme carbonic anhydrase within red blood cells and is the major pathway for HCO_3^- generation.

13. The CO_2 dissociation curve from blood is linear and directly related to Pco_2.

14. There are four major types of tissue hypoxia: hypoxic hypoxia, circulatory hypoxia, anemic hypoxia, and histologic hypoxia.

15. The O_2 dissociation curve is S-shaped, not linear. In the plateau area (>60 mm Hg), increasing the Po_2 has only a minimal effect on Hgb saturation; the same is true if there is a decrease in Po_2 from 100 to 60 mm Hg. This assures adequate Hgb saturation over a large range of Po_2. The steep portion of the curve (20–60 mm Hg) illustrates that during O_2 deprivation (low Po_2), O_2 is readily released from Hgb with only small changes in Po_2, which facilitates O_2 diffusion to the tissue.

KEYWORDS AND CONCEPTS

2,3-diphosphoglycerate (2,3-DPG)
Adenosine triphosphate
Bicarbonate ions
Bohr Effect
Bulk flow
Carbamino compounds
Carbon monoxide
Carbonic anhydrase
Carboxyhemoglobin (HgbCO)
Chloride shift
CO content
CO_2 dissociation curve
CO_2 transport
Conservation of mass
Deoxyhemoglobin
Diffusion
Diffusion constant
Diffusion-limited gas exchange
Effective solubility
Erythropoiesis
Fetal hemoglobin

Fick's law of diffusion
Haldane effect
Hemoglobin
Henry's law
Hypoxemia
Hypoxia
Methemoglobinemia
Myoglobin
Nitric oxide
Nitrous oxide
O_2 content
O_2 extraction ratio
O_2 transport
Oxidative metabolism
Oxygen saturation (So_2)
Oxyhemoglobin
Oxyhemoglobin dissociation curve
Perfusion-limited gas exchange
Sickle cell anemia
Tissue hypoxia

SELF-STUDY PROBLEMS

1. What are the physiologic parameters that cause the oxyhemoglobin dissociation curve to shift?

2. How do the shifts in the oxyhemoglobin dissociation curve aid in O_2 and CO_2 uptake and delivery?

3. A patient appears to be suffering from hypoxic symptoms. An arterial blood gas reveals an Sao_2 of 98%. Is it possible for this patient to be experiencing tissue hypoxia?

4. What are the major forms in which O_2 and CO_2 are transported in the blood?

5. Using the oxyhemoglobin dissociation curve, explain why giving supplemental oxygen to increase the P_{O_2} has little effect on improving oxygen delivery in most patients and is beneficial only in patients with a Pa_{O_2} of less than 60 mm Hg.

6. What is tissue hypoxia and what are the mechanisms that cause it?

7. Explain why some gases are diffusion-limited and others are perfusion-limited and how, under certain circumstances, oxygen can be either.

ADDITIONAL READINGS

Grippi MA, Elias JA, Fishman JA, et al. *Fishman's Pulmonary Diseases and Disorders.* 5th ed. New York: McGraw Hill; 2015.

Jelkmann W. Erythropoietin: Structure, control of production and function. *Physiol Rev.* 1992;72:449–489.

Klocke RA. Carbon dioxide transport. In: Crystal RG, West JB, Barnes PJ, Weibel ER, eds. *The Lung: Scientific Foundations.* 2nd ed. New York: Lippincott Williams & Wilkins; 1997.

Leach RM, Treacher DF. Oxygen transport—2. Tissue hypoxia. *BMJ.* 1998;317:1370–1373.

*Perrella M, Bresciani D, Rossi-Bernardi L. The binding of CO_2 to human hemoglobin. *J Biol Chem.* 1975;250:5413–5418.

Reeves RB, Park HK. CO uptake kinetics of red cells and CO diffusion capacity. *Respir Physiol.* 1992;88:1.

Russell JA, Phang PT. The oxygen delivery-consumption controversy. *Am J Respir Crit Care Med.* 1994;149:433–437.

Treacher DF, Leach RM. Oxygen transport—1. Basic principles. *BMJ.* 1998;317:1302–1306.

*Weibel ER. Morphologic basis of alveolar-capillary gas exchange. *Physiol Rev.* 1973;53:257–312.

*West JB. Effect of slope and shape of dissociation curve on pulmonary gas exchange. *Respir Physiol.* 1969;8:66–85.

*These are classics.

Pulmonary Aspects of Acid–Base Balance and Arterial Blood Gas Interpretation

This chapter describes the clinical interpretation of Po_2 and Pco_2 levels in arterial blood. The partial pressures of O_2, CO_2, and pH in the blood can be measured readily. Their values show the net effect of disease on gas exchange, and thus in the assessment of lung disease the arterial blood gas measurement is the best overall test of lung function. Arterial blood gas values cannot be determined by clinical assessment alone, even by experienced clinicians. For example, cyanosis does not become apparent until the arterial oxygen falls to less than 50 torr or 80% saturation, and quality of air exchange determined by auscultation is a poor assessment of alveolar ventilation. Thus arterial blood gas measurements are an important and essential tool in caring for critically ill patients, guiding therapy, and monitoring the progression of chronic lung disease.

PRINCIPLES OF INTERPRETING ARTERIAL BLOOD GAS VALUES

Just as other laboratory tests such as chest radiographs benefit from a careful, systematic approach, so does the interpretation of arterial blood gas values. Arterial blood gases should always be interpreted in light of the patient's history and symptoms. Recall the Irish proverb: *Normal values are normal in normal people.* For example, if a patient's respiratory rate is three times normal and the measured arterial $Paco_2$ is 40 mm Hg ("normal"), it does not necessarily mean that this patient has normal lungs. Rather, this patient is maintaining normal alveolar ventilation (i.e., a

normal $Paco_2$) by markedly increasing his or her respiratory rate. As we shall see, a number of mechanisms (such as an increase in minute ventilation) can compensate for abnormalities in gas exchange and can bring the body back toward homeostasis. Normal values for arterial blood gas measurements are shown in Table 9.1.

TYPES OF ACID–BASE ABNORMALITIES

There are nine fundamental acid–base conditions: normal, acute, and chronic respiratory acidosis; acute and chronic respiratory alkalosis; acute and chronic metabolic acidosis; and acute and chronic metabolic alkalosis. Acute conditions occur over a relatively short period of time; chronic conditions occur over longer periods (hours and days) and are associated with compensation, usually by the kidney but occasionally by the lung. **Acidemia** occurs when there is an excess of hydrogen ions in the blood, and **alkalemia** occurs when there are too few hydrogen ions in the blood. Values associated with various blood gas disturbances are listed in Table 9.1.

MEASURING ARTERIAL BLOOD GASES

Obtaining an Arterial Blood Gas Sample

Arterial blood can be sampled by needle puncture of a radial artery (Fig. 9.1). Other sites, used occasionally but associated with a greater potential risk of complications,

TABLE 9.1 Normal Values and Acid–Base Disturbances*

pH Normal	7.35–7.45	**HCO$_3^-$ Normal**	22–28 mEq/L
Acidosis		*Depression*	
Mild	7.30–7.35	Mild	19–22 mEq/L
Moderate	7.25–7.30	Moderate	17–19 mEq/L
Severe	<7.25	Severe	<17 mEq/L
Alkalosis		*Elevation*	
Mild	7.45–7.50	Mild	28–31 mEq/L
Moderate	7.50–7.55	Moderate	31–35 mEq/L
Severe	>7.55	Severe	>35 mEq/L
Pao$_2$ Normal	>85 mm Hg	**Base Excess Normal**	–3 to +4 mEq/L
Hypoxemia		*Depression*	
Mild	55–85 mm Hg	Mild	–4 to –7 mEq/L
Moderate	40–55 mm Hg	Moderate	–7 to –10 mEq/L
Severe	<40 mm Hg	Severe	> –10 mEq/L
Paco$_2$ Normal	35–45 mm Hg	*Elevation*	
		Mild	+4 to +8 mEq/L
Hypercapnia		Moderate	+8 to +12 mEq/L
Mild	45–50 mm Hg	Severe	> +12 mEq/L
Moderate	50–60 mm Hg		
Severe	>60 mm Hg	**Anion Gap**	5–11 mEq/L
		AaDo$_2$†	10–25 mm Hg (on room air)
Hypocapnia			
Mild	30–45 mm Hg		
Moderate	25–30 mm Hg		
Severe	<25 mm Hg		

*For a 25-year-old adult at sea level on room air. Normal values can vary slightly in different laboratories.
†The alveolar–arterial oxygen difference (AaDo$_2$) widens with age.

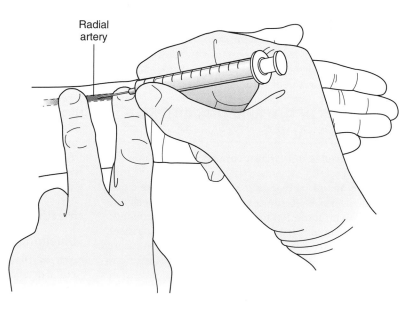

Radial artery

Fig. 9.1 Radial artery puncture. Before performing a radial artery puncture, test the adequacy of the ulnar collateral supply by compressing the radial artery and noting that the palm does not blanch. The syringe should be rinsed with sodium heparin to prevent clotting of the sample. (Redrawn from Waring WW, Jeansonne LO III. *Practical Manual of Pediatrics*, 2nd ed. St. Louis: Mosby; 1982.)

are the brachial and femoral arteries. Blood is collected into a heparinized syringe to prevent clotting. Air bubbles are expelled to prevent equilibration of the sample with ambient air, and the sample is kept on ice until analyzed. Routinely three measurements are obtained: Pao_2, $Paco_2$, and pH. Base excess (or deficit) and HCO_3^- (using the **Henderson-Hasselbach equation**) can be calculated from the measured values for Pco_2 and pH. (HCO_3^- can also be directly measured as part of serum electrolytes.) When frequent sampling of arterial blood is needed, a catheter can be inserted, most often in the radial artery.

Pulse Oximetry

Arterial puncture is uncomfortable for patients and is associated with a small but finite risk. Pulse oximetry is a noninvasive method of assessing arterial oxygenation that is now widely used in hospitalized patients. The sensor device can be clipped on the patient's finger and oxygen saturation can be displayed continuously on a monitor. Specific wavelengths of light are passed through the finger, and the oximeter measures the pulsatile absorption of light by arteriolar blood. Because oxygenated and deoxygenated hemoglobin have different patterns of light absorption, they produce different results. The major advantage of pulse oximetry is that it provides a continuous measurement.

However, this method has two major limitations: (1) the oximeter measures O_2 saturation, not Po_2; and (2) it provides no information about Pco_2 and pH.

Arterial pH

pH is the negative log of the hydrogen ion concentration. Measurement of arterial pH is the only way to determine whether the blood is too alkaline or too acid. Low pH values (<7.35) indicate acidemia or an increase in hydrogen ions; pH values greater than 7.45 indicate alkalemia, a decrease in hydrogen ions. **Acidemia** and **alkalemia** refer to conditions in the blood; acidosis and alkalosis refer to the process that causes the abnormality. Maintenance of a normal or near-normal pH in the blood is important, because arrhythmias can result when the pH falls below 7.25, and seizures and vascular collapse can occur when the pH rises above 7.55.

The acid–base status of blood can be analyzed using the **Henderson-Hasselbach equation** for the bicarbonate buffer system. This equation states that the pH in blood is equal to a constant (pK) plus the log ratio of bicarbonate to Pco_2. That is,

$$pH = pK + \log \frac{[HCO_3^-]}{0.3 \times PCO_2}$$

TABLE 9.2 Patterns of Acid–Base Disturbances

	Pco_2	pH	HCO_3^-
Respiratory Acidosis			
No compensation	↑↑	↓↓	NL
Metabolic compensation	↑↑	↓	↑↑
Respiratory Alkalosis			
No compensation	↓↓	↑↑	NL
Metabolic compensation	↓↓	↑	↓↓
Metabolic Acidosis			
No compensation	NL	↓↓	↓↓
Respiratory compensation	↓	↓	↓↓
Metabolic Alkalosis			
No compensation	NL	↑↑	↑↑
Respiratory compensation	↑	↑	↑↑

NL, normal; ↑↑ and ↓↓ represent a greater increase and decrease, respectively, than ↑ and ↓.

The pK is a constant (pK = 6.1) that is related to the dissociation of carbonic acid (H_2CO_3). The bicarbonate concentration is determined by the kidney, whereas the lung determines the Pco_2. When the HCO_3^- is constant, increases in Pco_2 result in decreases in pH, and decreases in Pco_2 result in increases in pH. As long as the ratio of bicarbonate to 0.03 Pco_2 is 20, the pH remains at 7.4. Compensatory mechanisms in the body are responsible for maintaining the ratio of HCO_3^- to 0.03 Pco_2 at 20.

RESPIRATORY ACIDOSIS AND ALKALOSIS

Respiratory effects on acid–base status center around the elimination of CO_2. The two basic respiratory alterations are respiratory acidosis and respiratory alkalosis (Table 9.2). Respiratory acidosis is associated with a decrease in pH secondary to an increase in $Paco_2$ and is due to a decrease in the elimination of CO_2 by the lungs. Increases in $Paco_2$ can be due to either increased dead-space ventilation or hypoventilation (see Chapter 7). In contrast, respiratory alkalosis is associated with an increase in pH secondary to a decrease in $Paco_2$ and is due to an increase in the elimination of CO_2 by the lungs. Excess removal of CO_2 from the blood by the lungs is called **hyperventilation**.

A respiratory acidosis can be either acute or chronic. In an individual who has been given a moderate dose of a narcotic, a respiratory depressant, minute ventilation can decrease significantly and if this occurs, arterial Pco_2 levels rise. The increase in Pco_2 occurs over minutes

---

BOX 9.1   Respiratory Causes of Acidosis and Alkalosis

Respiratory Acidosis

- Central respiratory control center depression (narcotics, anesthetics, sedatives)
- Neuromuscular disorders (muscular dystrophy, myasthenia gravis, spinal cord injury)
- Chest wall restriction (kyphoscoliosis)
- Restrictive lung disease (pulmonary fibrosis, pneumothorax, pleural effusion, extreme obesity)
- Obstructive pulmonary disease (emphysema, chronic bronchitis, upper airway obstruction, cystic fibrosis)

Respiratory Alkalosis

- Hyperventilation (anxiety, encephalitis, tumors)
- Fever
- Acute asthma
- Pulmonary embolism
- Hypoxia, high altitude
- Salicylate ingestion
- Progesterone (hyperventilation of pregnancy)

BOX 9.2   Metabolic Causes of Acidosis and Alkalosis

Metabolic Acidosis

- Drug ingestion (methanol, ethanol, ethylene glycol, ammonium chloride)
- Diarrhea
- Renal dysfunction
- Lactic acidosis (shock, acute respiratory distress syndrome, carbon monoxide)
- Ketoacidosis (diabetes, starvation, alcoholism)

Metabolic Alkalosis

- Vomiting (nasogastric suctioning)
- Diuretics
- Antacid ingestion

---

and is associated with an immediate decrease in pH (see Henderson-Hasselbach equation). There is not sufficient time for any compensatory mechanism to occur. This results in an acute, or uncompensated, respiratory acidosis.

In individuals with chronic lung disease, the changes in gas exchange in the lung occur slowly, and as disease progresses, the arterial CO_2 levels begin to rise slowly. The CO_2 combines with water to form H_2CO_3, which dissociates to form H^+ and HCO_3^-. Prompted by the increase in Pco_2 in the renal tubular cells, the kidney conserves HCO_3^- and excretes H^+ ions as H_2PO_4 or NH_4^+. The increase in plasma HCO_3^- shifts the $HCO_3^-/0.03\ Pco_2$ ratio back toward normal levels. Renal compensation, however, like all other compensatory mechanisms, is not "perfect" or complete, and thus although the pH approaches 7.4, it remains slightly less than this value. In this example, although $Paco_2$ rises, the change in pH is buffered by an increase in HCO_3^- ion. Some examples of diseases associated with respiratory acid–base balance disturbances are listed in Box 9.1.

METABOLIC ACIDOSIS AND ALKALOSIS

Respiratory alterations in acid–base status are related to changes in CO_2, and metabolic abnormalities are associated with either a gain or a loss of fixed acid or bicarbonate in the extracellular fluid. For example, with vomiting there is a loss of stomach acid; this results in a metabolic alkalosis

due to loss of fixed acid. The lung is able to quickly compensate for these metabolic abnormalities by changing ventilation, resulting in either increased or decreased elimination of CO_2. Thus a metabolic acidosis stimulates ventilation, CO_2 elimination, and a rise in pH toward normal levels, whereas a metabolic alkalosis suppresses ventilation and CO_2 elimination and the pH decreases toward the normal range. This is then followed by the slower elimination by the kidneys of excess acid or bicarbonate. For example, in individuals with uncontrolled diabetes, the increase in blood sugar is associated with an increase in ketones and the development of ketoacidosis. The pH in the blood decreases. This decrease in pH is buffered, however, by an increase in minute ventilation, resulting in a decrease in Pco_2 followed by ketone elimination in the urine. Common diseases associated with metabolic acid–base balance disorders are listed in Box 9.2.

RESPIRATORY AND RENAL COMPENSATORY MECHANISMS

Homeostasis is a process of control mechanisms that helps stabilize body systems by returning them to a more normal state. Because cells are unable to function outside of a relatively narrow pH range, homeostatic or **compensatory mechanisms** are important for cell and organ survival. Compensatory mechanisms are quickly activated to offset disturbances in acid–base balance; as a result, it is unusual to see uncompensated primary acid-base abnormalities. Changes in function in the respiratory and renal systems are the major acid–base compensatory mechanisms. The respiratory system compensates for metabolic acidosis or alkalosis by altering alveolar ventilation. The kidneys compensate for a respiratory acidosis or metabolic acidosis of nonrenal origin by excreting fixed acids and by retaining filtered bicarbonate; they compensate for a respiratory alkalosis and metabolic alkalosis of nonrenal origin by decreasing hydrogen ion excretion and bicarbonate.

Most acid–base disorders are complex, with elements of both acute (uncompensated) and chronic (compensated) changes present. In examining acid–base abnormalities, then, the question frequently arises about what is the primary abnormality and what is the compensatory response. How is it possible to sort out the primary abnormality from the compensatory response? There are two important principles to remember. The first is that compensation is rarely complete; the second is that compensatory acid–base responses rarely overcompensate.

Respiratory Compensation

The respiratory system compensates for metabolic acid-base balance disorders by altering alveolar ventilation. When CO_2 production is constant, alveolar P_{CO_2} is inversely proportional to alveolar ventilation (see Fig. 5.3). When a metabolic acidosis is present, the increased blood H^+ concentration stimulates chemoreceptors, which in turn stimulate alveolar ventilation and decrease arterial P_{CO_2}. Respiratory compensation for a metabolic alkalosis is to decrease alveolar ventilation, resulting in an increase in alveolar P_{CO_2}.

The relation between arterial levels of CO_2 and pH with and without renal compensation is demonstrated by the following two rules. For each increase of 10 mm Hg in P_{aCO_2}, the pH will fall 0.03 units if time is allowed for renal compensation, and 0.08 units if the process is acute and insufficient time for renal compensation has occurred. (Renal compensation takes around 48 hours to occur.) For example, is the following elevation in P_{aCO_2} acute or chronic?

$$\text{pH } 7.20 \, ; \; PaCO_2 \text{ 65 mm Hg}$$

If the increase in P_{aCO_2} is acute, an increase in P_{aCO_2} from 40 to 65 mm Hg will result in a decrease in pH; that is,

$$0.08 \times 25/10 \text{ mm Hg} = 0.20 \text{ units}$$

or

$$7.40 - 0.20 = 7.20$$

If the increase in P_{aCO_2} is chronic, an increase in P_{aCO_2} from 40 to 65 mm Hg will result in a decrease in pH; that is,

$$0.03 \times 25/10 \text{ mm Hg} = 0.075 \text{ units}$$

or

$$7.40 - 0.075 = 7.32$$

Therefore in this example, the elevation in P_{aCO_2} is entirely acute. Note that if the process had occurred over days, renal compensation would have occurred and the change in pH would have been smaller—that is, closer to 7.32 instead of 7.20.

Although it is useful to think about acid–base changes as either acute or chronic, with few exceptions (such as the acute administration of a respiratory depressant in the earlier example), compensation for changes in P_{CO_2} begins immediately. Examine now the following pH and P_{CO_2} combination.

$$\text{pH } 7.28 \, ; \; P_{CO_2} \text{ 70 mm Hg}$$

If the increase in P_{aCO_2} is acute, an increase in P_{aCO_2} from 40 to 70 mm Hg will result in a decrease in pH; that is,

$$0.08 \times 30/10 \text{ mm Hg} = 0.24 \text{ units}$$

or

$$7.40 - 0.24 = 7.16$$

If the increase in P_{aCO_2} is chronic, an increase in P_{aCO_2} from 40 to 70 mm Hg will result in a decrease in pH; that is,

$$0.03 \times 30/10 \text{ mm Hg} = 0.09 \text{ units}$$

or

$$7.40 - 0.09 = 7.31$$

Here the decrease is in between 7.31 and 7.16, suggesting that an increase in P_{CO_2} has occurred sometime between 24 and 48 hours. Furthermore, this is a respiratory acidosis because the P_{aCO_2} is increased to more than 40 mm Hg with a reduced pH.

RENAL COMPENSATION

The kidneys compensate for acidosis either of respiratory or nonrenal origin by excreting fixed acids and by retaining filtered bicarbonate. An increase in CO_2 inside the renal tubular cells, produced either by the tubular cell or by an increase in dissolved CO_2 in the blood, combines with water to form carbonic acid via the carbonic anhydrase reaction:

$$CO_2 + H_2O \xleftrightarrow{\text{CA}} H_2CO_3 \leftrightarrow H^+ + HCO_3^-$$

The hydrogen ions generated in this reaction are transported into the tubular lumen, and the bicarbonate is reabsorbed into the peritubular capillary (Fig. 9.2). Electrical neutrality is maintained by the exchange of sodium ions for the hydrogen ions. The hydrogen ions in the tubular lumen are buffered by tubular bicarbonate, phosphate, and other buffers and may be converted to H_2O and CO_2 by

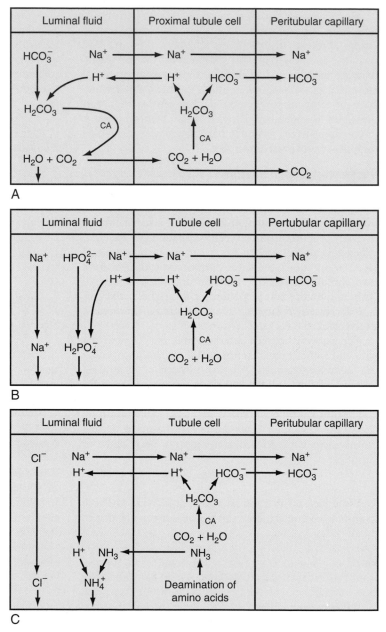

FIG. 9.2 Renal fixed acid excretion and bicarbonate retention. Approximately 90% of all filtered bicarbonate ions are reabsorbed directly or by the mechanism shown **(A)**. The remaining 10% is reabsorbed in the process of titration of tubular phosphate ions **(B)** or by the generation of ammonium ions **(C)**. (Redrawn from Levitzky MG. *Pulmonary Physiology*, 8th ed. New York: McGraw-Hill; 2013.)

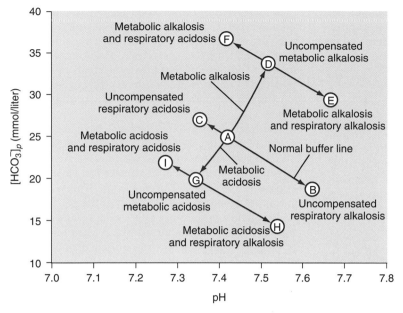

FIG. 9.3 Acid–base paths in vivo. (Redrawn from Davenport HW. *The ABC of Acid–Base Chemistry*, 6th ed. Chicago: University of Chicago Press; 1974.)

the carbonic anhydrase in the brush border of the proximal tubular cells. Approximately 90% of all filtered bicarbonate ions are reabsorbed in the proximal tubule.

The kidneys normally secrete 50 mEq of H^+ and reabsorb about 50 mEq of bicarbonate daily.

In alkalosis, the kidney decreases both hydrogen ion secretion and bicarbonate reabsorption. At plasma bicarbonate levels greater than 28 mEq/L, the kidney excretes bicarbonate.

BASE EXCESS AND ANION GAP

Two other calculated values can also be used to determine the processes responsible for the acid–base status. These are the **base excess** and the **anion gap**. Base excess can be used to determine whether a metabolic acidosis is present while the anion gap can help identify the cause of the metabolic acidosis. Base excess represents the change in buffer base (BB), which is the sum of HCO_3^- and buffer in the blood. It is the number of milliequivalents (mEq) of acid or base needed to titrate 1 L of blood to pH 7.4 at 37°C if the $Paco_2$ is held constant at 40 torr. Base excess (BE) changes from its normal value of 0 ± 3 mEq/L only with metabolic acid–base changes.

The following reaction determines the base excess:

$$CO_2 + H_2O \xrightleftharpoons{CA} H_2CO_3 \leftrightarrow H^+ + HCO_3^-$$
$$\updownarrow$$
$$H\,Buff \leftrightarrow H^+ + Buf$$

The sum of HCO_3^- and Buf is called the buffer base (BB):

Base excess (BE) = Change in buffer base (BB)

If carbon dioxide is retained and increases, then H^+, generated by the shift to the right (**Le Chatelier's principle**), moves down to be buffered; HCO_3^- concentration increases; and the buffer (Buf) concentration decreases. A respiratory change therefore results in no change in the sum (BB) of HCO_3^- and Buf; hence BE equals zero. A change in pH of 0.15 units results from a buffer base change of 10 mEq/L.

Changes in base excess can be seen graphically in the **Davenport diagram** (Fig. 9.3). The Davenport pH-HCO_3^- diagram is a graphic representation of the Henderson-Hasselbach equation. Three different buffer lines (slanting down and to the right) define the $[HCO_3^-]$ and pH responses to the addition of acid or base to plasma. The CO_2 isopleth line (slanting up and to the right) relates pH to $[HCO_3^-]$ and is shown here for a Pco_2 equal to 40 torr. Point A represents the normal situation with pH = 7.40, $[HCO_3^-]$ = 24 mEq/L, and Pco_2 = 40 mm Hg. An increase in bicarbonate concentration shifts the buffer line from CAB to DF (see Fig. 9.3). In this case the base excess, given by the vertical distance between the two buffer lines, is increased. A reduction in bicarbonate concentration displaces the buffer line from CAB to GH and results in a negative base excess, which is also called a **base deficit**.

Once a metabolic acidosis has been identified, the anion gap can be used to identify its cause. The anion gap represents the difference between the concentration of the major plasma cation (Na^+) and the major plasma anions (Cl^- and HCO_3^-); that is,

$$Anion\ gap = [Na^+] - ([Cl^-] + [HCO_3^-])$$

The rationale for this is that when acid is added to body fluids, the $[H^+]$ increases and the $[HCO_3^-]$ decreases. In addition, the concentration of the anion, which is associated with the acid, will increase. It is important to remember, however, that a real anion gap does not exist. It is just that there are anions that are not being measured. The full, correct equation should be:

$$[Na^+] + [unmeasured\ cation] = [Cl^-] + [HCO_3^-] \\ + [unmeasured\ anions]$$

Normally the anion gap ranges from 5 to 11 mEq/L, with most of this gap being made up by the negative charges on plasma proteins; an anion gap greater than 12 mEq/L is abnormal.

A change of 10 mm Hg in $Paco_2$ will result in an approximate change of 4 mEq/L in $[HCO_3^-]$ if renal compensation has occurred. If the anion of the acid is Cl^-, the anion gap will be normal (i.e., the decrease in $[HCO_3^-]$ is matched by an increase in $[Cl^-]$). Thus the metabolic acidosis associated with diarrhea or renal tubular acidosis is associated with a normal anion gap. In contrast, if the anion of the nonvolatile acid is not Cl^- (e.g., lactate), the anion gap will increase (i.e., the decrease in $[HCO_3^-]$ is not matched by an increase in the $[Cl^-]$, but rather by an increase in the concentration of the unmeasured anion). Thus the anion gap is increased in the metabolic acidosis associated with renal failure, ketoacidosis, lactic acidosis, or the ingestion of large quantities of aspirin.

ARTERIAL OXYGENATION

The arterial measurement of Po_2 reports the partial pressure of O_2 physically dissolved in blood. It is determined by the gradient for O_2 transport across the alveolar–capillary membrane, which is largely determined by the alveolar O_2. As previously described (see Chapter 5), the ideal alveolar O_2 is given by the alveolar gas equation, and the difference between the ideal alveolar O_2 and the actual arterial O_2 (the alveolar–arterial oxygen difference, or $AaDo_2$) is used to determine whether there is evidence of abnormal arterial oxygenation (see Chapter 7).

In interpreting arterial blood gas values, it is essential to know whether the individual is receiving supplemental O_2 or is on room air. One quick check of this is to add the Pao_2 and the $Paco_2$ together. The sum of the Pao_2 and $Paco_2$ with the patient breathing room air should be less than 130 mm Hg (at sea level). If it is greater than 130 mm Hg, the patient may have been on supplemental oxygen.

The fraction of inspired oxygen (Fio_2) that an individual is receiving is difficult to determine when they are receiving oxygen by nasal cannula. To convert nasal oxygen flow (L/min) to approximate Fio_2, assume a 4% increase in Fio_2 per liter of nasal flow. This is a reasonable approximation, however, only if the patient's minute ventilation (respiratory rate × tidal volume) is nearly normal. Normal values for arterial oxygen tension also decrease with age. One way to estimate the normal Pao_2 with increasing age is:

$$PaO_2 = 105 - patient's\ age/2$$

Thus the normal arterial oxygen tension of an 80-year-old individual is 65 mm Hg. It is apparent that in elderly individuals there is only a small margin between normal and what could be harmful to various organs and cells in the body

Finally, the arterial Po_2 response to 100% supplemental oxygen can be used to determine the pathophysiologic process responsible for hypoxemia (see Chapter 7). Persistent hypoxemia despite 100% oxygen or an increasing Fio_2 indicates the presence of a shunt and is frequently seen in children with cyanotic congenital heart disease.

ANALYZING ARTERIAL BLOOD GAS VALUES

A systematic approach to interpreting arterial blood gas values is useful in understanding underlying pathophysiologic abnormalities.

Step 1: Is There an Acidosis or Alkalosis?

First, examine the acid–base component of an arterial blood gas by examining the pH. If the pH is 7.45 or greater, an alkalosis, respiratory, metabolic, or both, is present. Similarly, a pH of 7.35 or less is indicative of an acidosis. A normal pH indicates normal acid–base status or a mixed disturbance that is balanced (e.g., a respiratory acidosis with a metabolic alkalosis).

Step 2: Is the Primary Disorder of Respiratory or Metabolic Origin?

Next examine the Pco_2 and its relation to the pH. An abnormal Pco_2 is greater than 45 mm Hg or less than

TABLE 9.3 Compensation Formulas for Acid–Base Disturbances

Primary Disorder	Primary Response	Compensatory Response	Chronic Response Magnitude
Respiratory acidosis	P_{CO_2}	HCO_3^-	HCO_3^- increases 3.5 mEq/L for each 10 mm Hg increase in P_{CO_2}
Respiratory alkalosis	P_{CO_2}	HCO_3^-	HCO_3^- falls 5 mEq/L for each 10 mm Hg increase in P_{CO_2}
Metabolic acidosis	HCO_3^-	P_{CO_2}	$P_{CO_2} = 1.5\,(HCO_3^-) + 8 \pm 2$
Metabolic alkalosis	HCO_3^-	P_{CO_2}	P_{CO_2} increases 6 mm Hg for each 10 mEq/L increase in HCO_3^-

Adapted from Weinberger SE. *Principles of Pulmonary Medicine*, 5th ed. Philadelphia: Elsevier; 2008.

35 mm Hg. If the pH value moves in the appropriate direction of the P_{CO_2} (i.e., increased pH with decreased P_{CO_2} or decreased pH with increased P_{CO_2}), a respiratory disorder is the primary disturbance. Similarly, if the pH value does not move in the appropriate direction of the P_{CO_2}, a metabolic disorder is the primary disturbance. Specifically, if there is an acidosis and the P_{CO_2} is greater than 45 mm Hg, the acidosis is respiratory in nature. If there is an acidosis and the P_{CO_2} is less than 40 mm Hg, the acidosis is metabolic with respiratory compensation (hyperventilation). In the same way, if there is an alkalosis and the P_{CO_2} is greater than 40 mm Hg, the alkalosis is metabolic with respiratory compensation (hypoventilation), and if there is an alkalosis and the P_{CO_2} is less than 40 mm Hg, the alkalosis is respiratory in nature.

Step 3: Is There Evidence of Respiratory or Metabolic Compensation?

The final step in analysis of acid–base balance is to determine whether the changes are acute or chronic. For a primary respiratory abnormality, calculate the change in pH that would occur if the change in P_{CO_2} were acute (0.08/10 mm Hg change in P_{CO_2}) or chronic (0.03/10 mm Hg change in P_{CO_2}). For a primary metabolic disorder, a rough guide is that the P_{aCO_2} should approximate the last two digits of the pH value (e.g., 7.25 should be associated with a P_{CO_2} of 25 mm Hg). Equations to calculate respiratory compensation for primary metabolic disorders are available but are not widely used clinically (Table 9.3).

Step 4: What Is the Alveolar–Arterial Oxygen Difference (AaDO₂)?

It is important to determine whether oxygen exchange is normal. Using the alveolar air equation, determine the ideal P_{aO_2}. Compare this value with the measured P_{aO_2}. If the difference is greater than 25 mm Hg with the patient breathing room air, there is a problem with oxygenation.

CLINICAL BOX

A 55-year-old-woman, who is in good health, is upset because she has just learned that her husband is having an affair and has gambled away all their savings. She is brought to the emergency department in an agitated and breathless state. Three possible sets of arterial blood gas measurements are given in the following table. (Assume respiratory quotient (R) = 0.8 and barometric pressure = 760 mm Hg). Which set of measurements best fits the patient's condition and history?

	Set A	Set B	Set C
pH	7.20	7.52	7.52
P_{aO_2} (mm Hg)	100	100	120
P_{aCO_2} (mm Hg)	20	20	20
HCO_{3-} (mEq/L)	0	24	24
BE (mEq/L)	−15	+1	+1

There is no previous history of lung or heart disease, and clearly this woman has experienced a major life crisis. Set A gas is consistent with metabolic acidosis with respiratory compensation; Set B gas is consistent with an acute respiratory alkalosis and a normal base deficit; Set C is most likely a laboratory error; it is unlikely that a 55-year-old woman would have an AaDO₂ = 5 mm Hg. Most likely she is experiencing an anxiety reaction (Set B).

SUMMARY

1. The arterial blood gas measurement of Pao_2, $Paco_2$, and pH is the best overall test of lung function.
2. Arterial blood gas values should always be interpreted in light of the patient's history and symptoms.
3. Pulse oximetry measures oxygen saturation continuously.
4. The Henderson-Hasselbach equation for the bicarbonate buffer system states that the pH in blood is equal to a constant (pK) plus the log ratio of bicarbonate (kidneys) to Pco_2 (respiratory system).
5. Respiratory effects on acid–base status center around the elimination of carbon dioxide, whereas renal effects center around the excretion of fixed acids and the retention of filtered bicarbonate.
6. A respiratory acidosis is associated with a decrease in pH secondary to an increase in $Paco_2$ and is due to a decrease in the elimination of CO_2 by the lungs. A respiratory alkalosis is associated with an increase in pH secondary to a decrease in $Paco_2$ and is due to an increase in the elimination of CO_2 by the lungs.
7. Compensation for metabolic abnormalities by the respiratory system occurs quickly, whereas renal compensation for respiratory abnormalities occurs over a period of 24 to 48 hours.
8. Compensation by the kidneys or lungs is rarely complete, and responses rarely overcompensate.
9. For each increase of 10 mm Hg in $Paco_2$, the pH will fall 0.03 units if time is allowed for renal compensation and 0.08 units if the process is acute and insufficient time for renal compensation has occurred.
10. The base excess represents the change in buffer base in the blood and is increased if a metabolic acidosis is present.
11. The anion gap represents the difference between the concentration of the major plasma cation (Na^+) and the major plasma anions (Cl^- and HCO_3^-) and can be used to determine the cause of a metabolic acidosis.
12. There are four steps in interpreting an arterial blood gas: (1) determine whether an acidosis or alkalosis is present, (2) determine whether the primary disorder is of respiratory or metabolic origin, (3) determine whether there is respiratory or metabolic compensation, and (4) determine the alveolar-arterial oxygen difference ($AaDo_2$).

KEYWORDS AND CONCEPTS

Acid–base balance
Alveolar ventilation
Alveolar-arterial oxygen difference ($AaDo_2$)
Anion gap
Arterial pH
Base deficit
Base excess
Bicarbonate
Buffer base
Carbonic anhydrase
Chatelier's principle
Davenport diagram

Fixed acid
Henderson-Hasselbach equation
Homeostasis
Hyperventilation
Hypoventilation
Metabolic acidosis
Metabolic alkalosis
Pulse oximetry
Renal compensation
Respiratory acidosis
Respiratory alkalosis
Respiratory compensation

SELF-STUDY PROBLEMS

1–5. Match the blood gas values and the basic defect or disease. All blood gases were drawn with the individual on room air.

a. pH = 7.40; $Paco_2$ = 40 mm Hg; Pao_2 = 110 mm Hg
b. pH = 7.34; $Paco_2$ = 60 mm Hg; Pao_2 = 60 mm Hg
c. pH = 7.25; $Paco_2$ = 25 mm Hg; Pao_2 = 110 mm Hg
d. pH = 7.50; $Paco_2$ = 30 mm Hg; Pao_2 = 50 mm Hg

e. pH = 7.47; $Paco_2$ = 45 mm Hg; Pao_2 = 80 mm Hg

1. Metabolic acidosis
2. Metabolic alkalosis
3. Laboratory error or patient on oxygen
4. Chronic hypoventilation with normal lung parenchyma
5. Hypoxemia with hyperventilation

6. A 3-month-old infant is admitted to the hospital with wheezing, vomiting, and decreased appetite. She is diagnosed with respiratory syncytial virus bronchiolitis and moderate dehydration from vomiting and decreased oral intake. Her arterial blood gas values while breathing room air are as follows: pH = 7.32; $Paco_2$ = 25 mm Hg; Pao_2 = 66 mm Hg; BE = −12 mEq/L. The best interpretation of theses blood gas values is:
   a. Metabolic acidosis, respiratory alkalosis
   b. Metabolic acidosis, respiratory acidosis
   c. Metabolic alkalosis, respiratory acidosis
   d. Metabolic alkalosis, respiratory alkalosis
   e. Respiratory alkalosis
7. A 59-year-old man is admitted to the hospital in acute respiratory distress resulting from emphysema complicated by pneumonia. He is conscious but confused, disoriented, and slow to respond to questions. He uses accessory muscles to breathe, and there is decreased chest expansion and motion of the diaphragm. The man is started on oxygen therapy using a 24% Venturi mask (Fio_2 = ~24%). An arterial blood gas analysis reveals the following values: pH = 7.33; Pao_2 = 48 mm Hg; $Paco_2$ = 67 mm Hg; HCO_3^- = 34 mEq/L. The best interpretation of these values is:
   a. Metabolic acidosis, respiratory alkalosis
   b. Metabolic acidosis, respiratory acidosis
   c. Metabolic alkalosis, respiratory alkalosis
   d. Respiratory acidosis

ADDITIONAL READINGS

Levitsky MG. *Pulmonary Physiology*. 8th ed. New York: McGraw-Hill; 2013.

Lim KG, Morgenthale TI. Pulmonary function tests, part 2: using pulse oximetry. *J Respir Dis*. 2005;26:85–88.

Morganroth ML. An analytic approach to diagnosing acid-base disorders. *J Crit Illness*. 1990;5:138–150.

Shapiro BA, Peruzzi WT, Kozelowski-Templin R. *Clinical Application of Blood Gases*. 5th ed. St. Louis: Mosby; 1994.

Weinberger SE. *Principles of Pulmonary Medicine*. 5th ed. Philadelphia: Elsevier; 2008.

Williams AJ. ABC of oxygen: assessing and interpreting arterial blood gases and acid-base balance. *BMJ*. 1998;317:1213–1216.

10

Control of Respiration

OBJECTIVES

1. Provide an overview of the three basic elements of the ventilatory control system.
2. Explain the structure and function of central chemoreceptors and peripheral chemoreceptors and their interrelationship.
3. Describe five chest wall and lung reflexes important in the control of respiration.
4. Describe the anatomy of the central respiratory control center and the relationship between the ventral and dorsal respiratory groups.

5. Describe the role of cerebrospinal fluid hydrogen ion and HCO_3^- in the regulation of respiration.
6. Explain the effects of hypoxemia, increased work of breathing, sleep, and acidosis on the ventilatory response to CO_2.
7. List three diseases associated with abnormal respiratory control.

Respiration demonstrates automaticity as well as self-modulation (voluntary). Although intermittent respiratory movements have been observed in utero, regular, automatic respiration begins at birth. Inspiration and exhalation occur automatically under the control of neurons located in the brainstem. At the same time, however, voluntary hyperventilation is easy, breath-holding is possible within limits, and the breathing pattern is modulated by the need for speech and singing.

Ventilatory control refers to the generation and regulation of rhythmic breathing by the respiratory center in the brainstem and its modification by the input of information from higher brain centers and systemic receptors. From a mechanical perspective, the goal of breathing is to minimize work; from a physiologic perspective, the goal is to maintain blood gas levels and specifically to regulate arterial P_{CO_2}. A third goal of breathing is to maintain the acid–base environment of the brain through the effects of ventilation on arterial P_{CO_2}.

OVERVIEW OF VENTILATORY CONTROL

From a functional perspective, the ventilatory control system consists of three basic elements (Fig. 10.1):
1. Sensors (peripheral and central chemoreceptors and pulmonary mechanoreceptors) that gather information and feed that information to the central controller.

2. The central controller (the respiratory control center) located in the brain that integrates and coordinates the information and sends signals to the effectors.
3. The effectors (respiratory muscles including the diaphragm) that produce changes in the ventilatory pattern.

As described in Chapter 5, alveolar ventilation is a function of respiratory rate and tidal volume. Respiratory rate is determined by the signal frequency from the central controller to the effectors, whereas tidal volume is determined by the activity of the individual nerve fibers in the effectors to their motor units, including the frequency and duration of discharges and the number of units activated.

The **respiratory control center** is located in the reticular formation of the medulla oblongata beneath the floor of the fourth ventricle. This center is not a discrete nucleus, but rather a poorly defined collection of different nuclei that generate and modify the basic rhythmic ventilatory pattern. It consists of two main parts: a **ventilatory pattern generator**, where the rhythmic pattern is generated; and an **integrator**, which processes inputs from higher brain centers and chemoreceptors and controls the rate and amplitude of the ventilatory pattern. The integrator controls the pattern generator and determines the appropriate ventilatory drive. Input to the integrator arises from higher brain centers including the cerebral cortex, hypothalamus, amygdala, limbic system, and cerebellum.

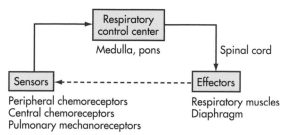

Fig. 10.1 The three major elements of the respiratory control system. Sensors, including central and peripheral chemoreceptors and pulmonary mechanoreceptors, feed information to the respiratory control center. In turn, the respiratory control center sends signals to the effectors such as the respiratory muscles and the diaphragm. Stimulation of the effectors subsequently reduces sensor activity through negative feedback.

Within the central nervous system, **central chemoreceptors** are located just below the ventrolateral surface of the medulla. These chemoreceptors detect changes in the Pco_2/pH of brainstem interstitial fluid and modulate ventilation.

Peripheral structures also provide input to the integrator and control ventilatory drive. Chemosensitive **peripheral chemoreceptors** are located on specialized cells in the aortic arch (**aortic bodies**) and at the bifurcation of the internal and external carotid arteries in the neck (**carotid bodies**). These chemoreceptors respond to changes in their local environment associated with decreases in Po_2, increases in Pco_2, and decreases in the pH of arterial blood and give afferent information to the central respiratory control center through the **vagus nerve** (aortic bodies) and the **carotid sinus nerve**, a branch of the glossopharyngeal nerve (carotid bodies), to make adjustments in alveolar ventilation that change whole body Pco_2, pH, and Po_2. Finally, the ventilatory pattern can be modulated by **pulmonary mechanoreceptors** and **irritant receptors** in the lung in response to the degree of lung inflation or the presence of an irritant in the airways.

The collective output of the respiratory control center to the motor neurons controls the **muscles of respiration** (the effectors), and it is this output that results in automatic, rhythmic respiration. The responsible motor neurons are located in the anterior horn of the spinal column. Intercostal muscles and the accessory muscles of respiration are controlled by motor neurons located in the thoracic region of the spinal column. Diaphragmatic motor neurons are situated in the cervical region of the spine and control diaphragmatic activity through the phrenic nerve.

In contrast to automatic respiration, voluntary respiration bypasses the medullary respiratory control center. It originates in the motor cortex, with information passing directly to the motor neurons in the spine through the corticospinal tracts. The respiratory muscle motor neurons thus act as the final site of integration of voluntary (corticospinal tract) and automatic (ventrolateral tract) control of ventilation. Voluntary control of these muscles competes with automatic influences at the level of the spinal motor neurons and can be demonstrated by breath-holding. At the start of a breath hold, voluntary control dominates the spinal motor neurons, but as the breath hold continues, automatic ventilatory control eventually overpowers the voluntary effort and limits the duration of the breath hold.

There are also motor neurons that innervate the muscles of the upper airway. These are located within the medulla near the respiratory control center. They innervate muscles in the upper airways through cranial nerves. When activated, they result in dilation of the pharynx and large airways at the initiation of inspiration.

THE RESPIRATORY CONTROL CENTER

Most of what is known about the control of ventilation comes from studies in animals in which focal areas of the brain have been destroyed (ablation) or in which the brainstem has been surgically cross-cut. When the brain is cross-cut between the medulla and the pons, periodic breathing is maintained even if all other afferents to the area, including the vagus nerve, are severed, demonstrating that the inherent rhythmicity of breathing originates in the medulla. If the brain is transected below this area, breathing ceases. Although no single group of neurons in the medulla has been found to be the breathing "pacemaker," there are two distinct groups of nuclei within the medulla that are involved in respiratory pattern generation (Fig. 10.2).

The first group is the **dorsal respiratory group** (DRG), which is composed of cells in the nucleus tractus solitarius located in the dorsomedial region of the medulla. These cells have the property of intrinsic periodic firing and are primarily responsible for inspiration and for the basic rhythm of ventilation. The tractus solitarius is also the primary projection site of visceral afferent fibers of the 9th cranial nerve (glossopharyngeal) and the 10th cranial nerve (vagus). These nerves provide information about Po_2, Pco_2, and pH from peripheral chemoreceptors and systemic arterial blood pressure. The vagus nerve also carries information from pulmonary mechanoreceptors. The input from the 9th and 10th cranial nerves to the DRG is thought to constitute the initial intracranial processing station for these afferent inputs. However, even when all afferent stimuli to the DRG have been abolished, the DRG continues to generate repetitive bursts of action potentials. Thus the DRG represents the breathing "pacemaker." Nuclei in this area project primarily to the contralateral spinal cord,

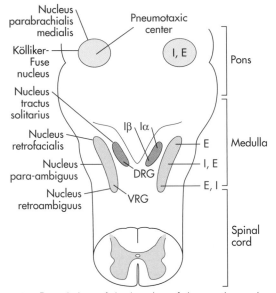

Fig. 10.2 Dorsal view of the location of the pontine and medullary respiratory neurons. DRG, dorsal respiratory group; E, expiratory; I, inspiratory; Iα and Iβ, two populations of inspiratory neurons in the DRG inhibited and excited, respectively, by lung inflation; VRG, ventral respiratory group. (Modified from Broaddus VC, Mason RJ, Ernst JD, King TE Jr, Lazarus SC, Murray JF, et al., eds. *Murray & Nadel's Textbook of Respiratory Medicine*, 6th ed. Philadelphia: W.B. Saunders; 2016.)

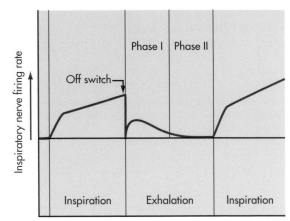

Fig. 10.3 Neural signaling of inspiratory motor neurons involves one inspiratory and two expiratory phases. Inspiration is abrupt, followed by a steady ramp-like increase in neuron firing rate. At the end of inspiration, there is an off-switch event, resulting in a rapid decline in firing rate. Exhalation begins with a paradoxical increase in inspiratory neuron firing that brakes the expiratory phase. During the second phase of exhalation, this neuron firing becomes absent. (Redrawn from Leff A, Schumacker P. *Respiratory Physiology: Basics and Applications.* Philadelphia: W.B. Saunders; 1993.)

where they serve as the principal initiators of phrenic nerve activity (supplying the diaphragm). The DRG also sends many fibers to the ventral respiratory group.

The second group of cells is the **ventral respiratory group** (VRG). The VRG is located bilaterally in the ventrolateral region of the medulla and is composed of three cell groups (the rostral nucleus retrofacialis, the caudal nucleus retroambiguus, and the nucleus para-ambiguus). The VRG contains both inspiratory and expiratory neurons. The primary function of these neurons is to drive either spinal respiratory neurons innervating the intercostal and abdominal muscles or the upper airway muscles of inspiration. Specifically, inspiratory neurons from the nucleus retroambiguus project to the contralateral external intercostals and to inspiratory and expiratory cells within the medulla, whereas expiratory neurons project to the contralateral spinal cord to drive the internal intercostals and abdominal muscles. The neurons in the nucleus para-ambiguus are primarily vagal motoneurons that innervate the laryngeal and pharyngeal muscles and are active during both inspiration and exhalation. Discharge from the cells in these areas appears to excite some cells and to inhibit other cells. The retrofacialis nucleus consists primarily of

expiratory neurons. One group of expiratory cells located most rostrally in the retrofacialis nucleus is called the **Bötzinger complex**. This is the only group of neurons in the VRG that have been demonstrated to inhibit inspiratory cells in the DRG.

Inspiration and exhalation at the level of the respiratory control center involve three phases—one inspiratory phase and two expiratory (exhalation) phases (Fig. 10.3). After a latent period of several seconds during which there is no activity, inspiration begins with an abrupt increase in discharge in a crescendo pattern from cells in the nucleus tractus solitarius, and the nucleus retroambiguus. This steady ramp-like increase in firing rate occurs throughout inspiration, during which respiratory muscle activity becomes stronger. At the end of inspiration, there is an "off-switch" event that results in a marked decrease in neuron firing, at which point inspiratory muscle tone falls to its preinspiratory level and exhalation begins. At the start of exhalation (phase I), there is a paradoxical increase in inspiratory neuron firing that slows down or "brakes" the expiratory phase by increasing inspiratory muscle tone as well as expiratory neuron firing. This inspiratory neuron firing decreases and becomes absent during phase II of exhalation.

Although many different neurons in the DRG and VRG are involved in ventilation, each cell type appears to have a specific function. For example, within the DRG there are cell populations called Iα cells, which are inhibited by lung inflation, and Iβ cells, which are excited by lung inflation. These two cell populations may be important in the **Hering-Breuer reflex**, an inspiratory-inhibitory reflex that arises from afferent stretch receptors located in the smooth muscle of the airways. Increasing lung inflation stimulates these stretch receptors and results in an early exhalation by stimulating neurons associated with the off-switch phase of inspiratory muscle control.

Two other areas located in the brainstem are also important in respiratory control. The **pneumotaxic center** is located in the upper pons in the nucleus parabrachialis medialis and the Kölliker-Fuse nucleus. Impulses from the pneumotaxic center result in premature termination of the inspiratory ramp, resulting in a shortened inspiration. As a result of a shortened inspiration, respiratory rate increases. Thus the pneumotaxic center can regulate tidal volume and respiratory rate. It appears to be important in fine-tuning respiratory rhythm.

The **apneustic center** is located in the lower pons. When the brain is sectioned just above this area, **apneusis**, or prolonged inspiratory gasps, are seen if the vagus nerves are also transected. (Apneusis does not occur if the vagus nerves are intact.) Apneusis is probably caused by a sustained discharge of medullary respiratory neurons. Its role in humans is unclear, but it may be the site of afferent information that terminates inspiration. Apneustic breathing is seen after head trauma that damages the pons, and its presence helps localize the site of injury.

Thus rhythmic breathing depends on a continuous (tonic) inspiratory drive from the dorsal respiratory group and on intermittent (phasic) expiratory inputs from the cerebrum, thalamus, cranial nerves, and ascending spinal cord sensory tracts. The DRG may drive the VRG, but contrary to early thought, reciprocal inhibition between the two groups is unlikely.

SPINAL PATHWAYS

Axons from the respiratory control center from the cortex and from other supraspinal sites descend in the spinal cord white matter to the diaphragm and to the intercostal and abdominal muscles. These descending axons are coupled with local spinal reflexes in an integrated manner. Descending axons with inspiratory activity excite external intercostal motor neurons and, at the same time, inhibit internal intercostal motor neurons by exciting spinal inhibitory interneurons. Premature infants have uncoordinated respiratory muscle activity, especially during sleep, that can result in paradoxical chest wall and abdominal motion. In addition to contributing to abnormal gas exchange, this

paradoxical motion can result in respiratory muscle fatigue and respiratory failure.

CENTRAL CHEMORECEPTORS

Chemoreceptors are receptors that respond to a change in the chemical composition of the blood or other fluid around it. Central chemoreceptors are specialized cells that are located on the ventrolateral surface of the medulla but are anatomically separate from the medullary-located respiratory control center (Fig. 10.4). These chemoreceptors are sensitive to the pH of the extracellular fluid around them. Because this extracellular fluid is in contact with the cerebrospinal fluid (CSF), changes in the pH of the CSF affect ventilation by acting on these chemoreceptors.

CSF is in part an ultrafiltrate of plasma that is secreted continuously by the choroid plexus and reabsorbed by the arachnoid villi. Because it is in contact with the extracellular fluid in the brain, CSF reflects the conditions surrounding the cells in the brain. Although the origin of CSF is the plasma, the composition of CSF is not the same as plasma because there is a barrier to free ion flow between the two sites. This barrier is termed the **blood–brain barrier**, and it separates CSF from the arterial

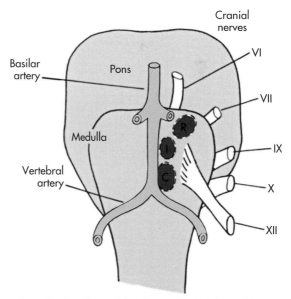

Fig. 10.4 The locations of the three CO_2 ($[H^+]$)-sensitive areas on the ventrolateral medulla. The receptor cells are not actually at the surface but are close to it. R, I, and C refer to the rostral, intermediate, and caudal receptor areas, respectively. (From Koeppen BM, Stanton BM, eds. *Berne and Levy's Physiology*, 7th ed. Philadelphia: Elsevier; 2018.)

blood. It is composed of endothelial cells, smooth muscle, and pial and arachnoid membranes, and it regulates ion flow. In addition, the choroid plexus also determines the composition of CSF.

The blood–brain barrier is relatively impermeable to hydrogen and HCO_3^- ions, but molecular CO_2 diffuses across it readily (Fig. 10.5). Because of this, alterations in arterial P_{CO_2} are rapidly transmitted to the CSF with a time constant of about 60 seconds. Thus the P_{CO_2} in the CSF parallels the arterial P_{CO_2}. It is not identical, however, because carbon dioxide is also produced by the cells of the brain as a product of metabolism. As a consequence, the P_{CO_2} in the CSF is usually a few torr higher than the P_{CO_2} in the arterial blood, and the pH is slightly more acidic (7.32–7.33) than in plasma.

In addition to being a plasma ultrafiltrate with a slightly lower pH, the P_{CO_2} of CSF is about 10 mm Hg higher than arterial P_{CO_2} and the protein content is considerably lower than plasma (15–45 mg/100 mL, compared with 6.6–8.6 g/100 mL in plasma). As a result of this lower protein

concentration, CSF has a lower buffering capacity compared with blood.

Similar to plasma, the **Henderson-Hasselbach equation** relates the pH of CSF to the bicarbonate ion concentration (HCO_3^-):

$$pH = pK + \log \frac{[HCO_3^-]}{0.3 \times PCO_2}$$

where 0.03 is the solubility coefficient of CO_2 in mmol/liter torr and pK is the negative log of the dissociation constant for carbonic acid (pK = 6.1). The Henderson-Hasselbach equation demonstrates that increases in P_{CO_2} will be associated with decreases in pH at any given bicarbonate concentration. Likewise, increases in CSF bicarbonate will result in an increase in CSF pH at any given P_{CO_2}. As a consequence of this relationship, an increase in arterial P_{CO_2} will result in an increase in CSF P_{CO_2} and a decrease in CSF pH. Compared with blood, the buffer line of CSF is lower and not as steep as the buffer line of blood (because of the

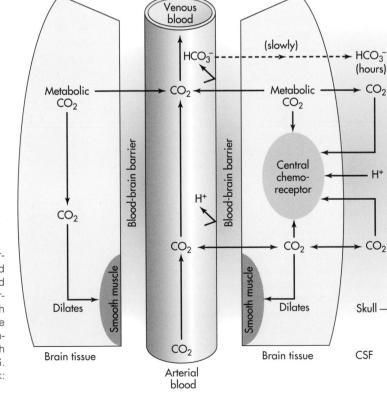

Fig. 10.5 CO_2 and the blood–brain barrier. Arterial CO_2 crosses the blood–brain barrier and rapidly equilibrates with cerebrospinal fluid (CSF) CO_2. H^+ and HCO_3^- ions cross the barrier only slowly. Arterial CO_2 combines with metabolic CO_2 to dilate smooth muscle. The pH of the CSF is lower and the P_{CO_2} is higher with little protein buffering compared with arterial blood. (Modified from Levitzky MG. *Pulmonary Physiology*, 8th ed. New York: McGraw-Hill; 2013.)

reduced buffering capacity). As a result, arterial hypercapnia leads to a greater change in hydrogen ion concentration in CSF compared with arterial blood.

An increase in H$^+$ ion concentration or Pco_2 or both results in a decrease in CSF pH that stimulates the central chemoreceptors, resulting in an increase in ventilation (Fig. 10.6). Ventilation increases almost linearly with changes in H$^+$ concentration. Thus the CO_2 in blood regulates ventilation by its effect on the pH of CSF. The resulting hyperventilation reduces Pco_2 in the blood and therefore in CSF. Increased arterial Pco_2 is also accompanied by cerebral vasodilation that enhances the diffusion of CO_2 into CSF. Although central chemoreceptors are very sensitive to changes in carbon dioxide, central chemoreceptors do not respond to hypoxia.

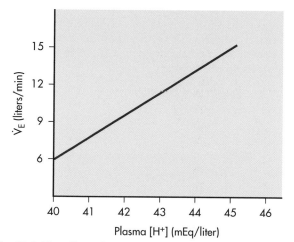

Fig. 10.6 The effect of H$^+$ concentration on minute ventilation ($\dot{V}_E$). Note that the relationship is linear. (Redrawn from Levitzky MG. *Pulmonary Physiology*, 8th ed. New York: McGraw-Hill; 2013.)

Changes in arterial pH that are not caused by changes in Pco_2 take longer to influence CSF. This is because hydrogen ions cross the blood–brain barrier too slowly to affect the central chemoreceptors. Other receptors, particularly peripheral chemoreceptors, respond to a metabolic acidosis of nonbrain origin. Alveolar ventilation increases secondary to acidotic stimulation of peripheral chemoreceptors, and arterial Pco_2 falls (Table 10.1). This results in diffusion of CO_2 out of CSF, an increase in CSF pH, and a decrease in central chemoreceptor stimulation. Over hours to days, the HCO_3^- concentration in CSF falls and the pH in the CSF returns to normal (7.32). How the HCO_3^- concentration in CSF falls in not clear. Mechanisms that have been suggested include diffusion of HCO_3^- across the blood–brain barrier, active transport of HCO_3^- out of the CSF, or decreased HCO_3^- formation as a result of carbonic anhydrase activity. That it occurs, however, is unquestioned because the pH of CSF in individuals with chronic obstructive pulmonary disease (COPD) and a chronic respiratory acidosis is nearly normal, with a CSF HCO_3^- concentration that is proportional to the increased CO_2 in the blood. Thus in CSF homeostasis, mechanisms and processes exist that regulate changes in pH and bring the system back to almost normal. The changes in CSF bicarbonate concentration, however, occur slowly over several hours, whereas the changes in Pco_2 in CSF can occur over minutes. Adjustments in ventilation attempt to maintain a normal CSF and arterial pH and Pco_2.

PERIPHERAL CHEMORECEPTORS

The carotid and aortic bodies are peripheral chemoreceptors that respond to decreases in arterial Po_2 (but not to changes in O_2 content), increases in Pco_2, and decreases in pH and transmit afferent information to the

TABLE 10.1	**Effects of Metabolic Acidosis (of Nonbrain Origin) on Arterial and Central Chemoreceptor Ventilatory Drive**					
	ARTERIAL BLOOD		**ARTERIAL CHEMO-RECEPTOR DRIVE**	**CEREBROSPINAL FLUID**		**CENTRAL CHEMO-RECEPTOR DRIVE**
	pH	Pco_2		Pco_2	pH	
Initial acidosis	↓↓	Normal	↑↑	Normal	Normal	Normal
Ventilatory compensation for arterial acidosis	↓	↓↓	↑	Normal	Normal	Normal
"Diffusion" of CO_2 from CSF to blood	↓	↓↓	↑	↑	↓	↓

↑↑ and ↓↓ imply a great increase and decrease, respectively, than ↑ and ↓.

central respiratory control center. The peripheral chemoreceptors are the only chemoreceptors that respond to decreases in P_{O_2}. Both the central and peripheral chemoreceptors respond to changes in P_{CO_2}, with the peripheral chemoreceptors being responsible for approximately 40% of the ventilatory response to CO_2. Peripheral chemoreceptors respond rapidly; in fact, they are able to respond to breath-to-breath alterations in arterial blood composition. The carotid bodies appear to exert a greater influence on the respiratory control center than the aortic bodies, which appear to have a greater influence on the cardiovascular system.

The peripheral chemoreceptors are small, highly vascularized structures located near the bifurcations of the common carotid arteries (carotid bodies) and in the arch of the aorta (aortic bodies) (Fig. 10.7). They consist of type I (glomus) cells that are rich in mitochondria and endoplasmic reticulum. They also contain several types of cytoplasmic granules (synaptic vesicles) that contain different neurotransmitters, including dopamine,

acetylcholine, norepinephrine, and neuropeptides. The type I cells are especially rich in dopamine and are the cells primarily responsible for sensing P_{O_2}, P_{CO_2}, and pH. Small increases in chemoreceptor discharge occur even with small decreases in arterial P_{O_2}, but marked increases in chemoreceptor activity occur when arterial P_{O_2} decreases to less than 75 mm Hg. Increases in ventilation result when the P_{O_2} falls below 50 to 60 mm Hg. Afferent nerve fibers synapse with type I cells and transmit information to the brainstem through the carotid sinus nerve (carotid body) and vagus nerve (aortic body). It is not known how they respond to arterial changes in P_{CO_2} and pH.

It can be seen from the preceding discussion that ventilation is regulated by changes in arterial and CSF pH and their effects on peripheral and central chemoreceptors. Homeostasis, the return toward normal ventilation, is regulated by changes in HCO_3^- transport in CSF and by renal compensatory mechanisms (Fig. 10.8). The Clinical Box illustrates this relationship.

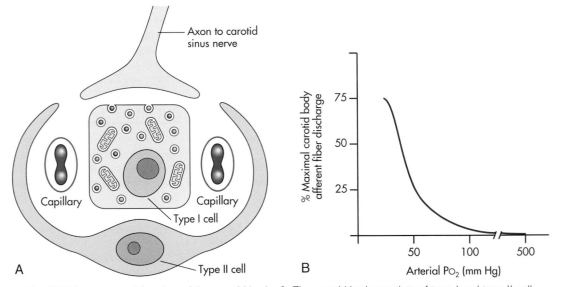

Fig. 10.7 Structure and function of the carotid body. **A,** The carotid body consists of type I and type II cells and has a rich capillary network. The type I, or glomus, cells contain large numbers of synaptic vesicles that contain neurotransmitters. These neurotransmitters are released in response to increased P_{CO_2}, decreased pH, or decreased P_{O_2} in the arterial blood. The released neurotransmitters act on adjacent nerve terminals. Signals from these nerve terminals are transmitted to the medullary respiratory control center through the carotid sinus nerve. **B,** Effect of P_{O_2} on carotid body afferent fiber discharge. There is a marked increase in activity when the arterial P_{O_2} falls below 75 mm Hg. When the P_{O_2} falls below 60 mm Hg, ventilation increases. (Modified and redrawn from Leff A, Schumacker P. *Respiratory Physiology: Basics and Applications.* Philadelphia: W.B. Saunders; 1993.)

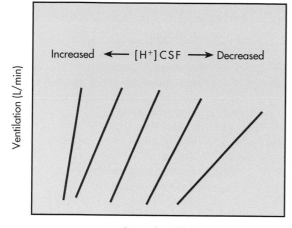

Fig. 10.8 The ventilatory response to P_{CO_2} is affected by the hydrogen ion concentration, [H^+], of the cerebrospinal fluid (CSF) and brainstem interstitial liquid. When a subject is in chronic metabolic acidosis (e.g., diabetic acidosis), the [H^+] CSF is increased and the ventilatory response to inspired P_{CO_2} is increased (steeper slope). Conversely, when a subject is in chronic metabolic alkalosis (a relatively uncommon condition), the [H^+] CSF is decreased, and the ventilatory response to inspired P_{CO_2} is decreased (reduced slope). The positions of the response lines are also shifted, indicating altered response thresholds. (From Koeppen BM, Stanton BM, eds. *Berne and Levy's Physiology*, 7th ed. Philadelphia: Elsevier; 2018.)

CHEST WALL AND LUNG REFLEXES

A number of reflexes arise from the chest wall and lung and affect ventilation and ventilatory patterns (Table 10.2). First described in 1868, the **Hering-Breuer inspiratory-inhibitory reflex** is stimulated by increases in lung volume, especially those associated with an increase in both ventilatory rate and tidal volume. It is a stretch reflex mediated by vagal fibers located within the smooth muscle of large and small airways, which, when elicited, results in cessation of inspiration by stimulating off-switch neurons in the medulla. This reflex is inactive during quiet breathing and plays a role in ventilatory control only at tidal volumes greater than 1 L in adults. It may help minimize the work of breathing by inhibiting large tidal volumes and preventing alveolar overdistention. Its importance in humans other than newborns is unclear.

A second described Hering-Breuer reflex is the **Hering-Breuer deflation reflex**. It is associated with an increase in ventilatory rate due to abrupt lung deflation. The mechanism for this reflex is unknown, but decreased stretch receptor activity and stimulation of other receptors such as J receptors have been implicated. The Hering-Breuer deflation reflex is thought to contribute to the increased ventilation in individuals with a pneumothorax and the periodic deep breaths (sighs) that occur normally; it may be important in preventing atelectasis (lung collapse), particularly in individuals who are being mechanically ventilated.

Stimulation of nasal or facial receptors with cold water initiates the **diving reflex**. When this reflex is elicited, apnea, or cessation of breathing, and bradycardia occur. This reflex protects individuals from aspirating in the initial stages of drowning. Activation of receptors in the nose is also responsible for the **sneeze reflex**.

Receptors are also present in the epipharynx and pharynx. Mechanical stimulation of these receptors produces the aspiration or **sniff reflex**. This is a strong, short-duration inspiratory effort that brings up material from the epipharynx to the pharynx where it can be swallowed or expectorated. These receptors are important in swallowing by inhibiting respiration and causing laryngeal closure.

The larynx contains both superficial and deep receptors. Activation of the superficial receptors results in apnea, cough, and expiratory movements that protect the lower respiratory tract from aspirating foreign materials. The deep receptors are located in the skeletal muscles of the larynx. Negative pressure in the upper airway causes reflex constriction of the dilator muscles.

In the tracheobronchial tree, there are three major types of receptors. Inhaled dust, noxious gases, and cigarette smoke stimulate **irritant receptors** in the trachea and large airways, which transmit information through myelinated, vagal afferent fibers. This results in an increase in airway resistance, reflex apnea, and cough. These receptors are also known as **rapidly adapting pulmonary stretch receptors** because their activity decreases rapidly during a sustained stimulus.

Slowly adapting pulmonary stretch receptors respond to mechanical stimulation and are activated by lung inflation. They also transmit information through myelinated, vagal afferent fibers. The increased lung volume in people with COPD stimulates these pulmonary stretch receptors and delays the onset of the next inspiratory effort. This allows the long, slow expiratory effort in these individuals that is essential to minimize dynamic, expiratory airway compression.

Specialized receptors exist in the lung parenchyma that respond to chemical or mechanical stimulation in the lung interstitium. These receptors are called **juxta-alveolar receptors or J receptors**. They transmit their afferent input through unmyelinated, vagal C-fibers. They may be responsible for the sensation of dyspnea (shortness of breath) and the altered ventilatory patterns (rapid, shallow) seen in

TABLE 10.2   Tracheobronchial Receptor Properties

Receptor Type	End Organ Location	Stimuli	Reflexes
Myelinated Vagal Fibers			
Slowly adapting receptor	Among airway smooth muscle cells	Lung inflation	Hering-Breuer inflation reflex Hering-Breuer deflation reflex Inspiratory time-shortening Bronchodilation Tachycardia
Rapidly adapting receptor (irritant receptor)	Among airway epithelial cells	Lung hyperinflation Exogenous and endogenous agents Histamine Prostaglandins	Hering-Breuer deflation reflex Cough Mucus secretion Bronchoconstriction
Unmyelinated Vagal Fibers			
C-fiber ending (J receptors)	Pulmonary interstitial space Close to pulmonary circulation Close to bronchial circulation	Large hyperinflation Exogenous and endogenous agents Capsaicin Phenyl diguanide Histamine Bradykinin Serotonin Prostaglandins	Apnea, followed by rapid shallow breathing Bronchoconstriction Bradycardia Hypotension Mucus secretion

individuals with interstitial lung edema and in some inflammatory lung states.

There are also **somatic receptors** in the intercostal muscles, rib joints, accessory muscles of respiration, and tendons that respond to changes in the length/tension of the respiratory muscles. Although they do not directly control respiration, they do provide information about lung volume and play a role in terminating inspiration. Somatic receptors are especially important in individuals with increased airway resistance and decreased pulmonary compliance because they can augment muscle force within the same breath. They also help minimize the chest wall distortion during inspiration in the newborn who has a very compliant rib cage.

NONPULMONARY REFLEXES

The ventilatory pattern is also under voluntary control. Purposeful hyperventilation can result in a decrease in $Paco_2$ and an increase in pH. The alkalosis that accompanies this hyperventilation can cause **carpopedal spasm**, contraction of the muscles of the hand and foot. An increase in arterial blood pressure stimulates aortic and carotid sinus baroreceptors and can cause reflex hypoventilation or apnea. Pain and temperature receptors can also affect ventilation.

RESPONSE TO CARBON DIOXIDE

Ventilation is regulated by the levels of CO_2, O_2, and pH in the arterial blood. Of these, the arterial Pco_2 is the most important. Both the rate and depth of breathing are controlled to maintain the $Paco_2$ close to 40 mm Hg. Even during periods of activity, rest, and sleep, the arterial Pco_2 is held at 40 ± 2 to 3 mm Hg. The importance of arterial CO_2 in ventilation can be demonstrated by having an individual breathe a low concentration of oxygen to which CO_2 is added to maintain a constant level of CO_2. Hypoxemia is sensed by the peripheral chemoreceptors, which increase their rate of firing in response to the decrease in Pao_2. This stimulation in ventilation, however, does not occur until the Pao_2 has dropped below 60 mm Hg. Below 60 mm Hg, there is marked stimulation of ventilation. However, if arterial $Paco_2$ is increased only a small amount (~5 mm Hg), ventilation is increased even in the presence of an increased level of Pao_2 (Fig. 10.9). Only voluntary hyperventilation and the hyperpnea of exercise can surpass the minute ventilation observed with increasing hypercapnia.

The relationship between $Paco_2$ and ventilation is best shown in a classic experiment that was first performed many years ago. In this experiment, the alveolar Po_2 is maintained at a constant level and the subject rebreathes from a bag so

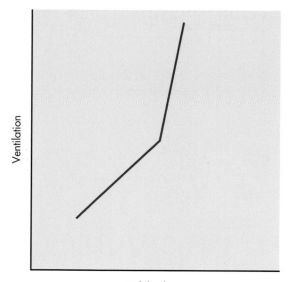

Fig. 10.9 Relationship between overall ventilation and tidal volume is depicted in awake state when ventilation is increased in response to respiratory stimuli such as hypercapnia. (Redrawn from Broaddus VC, Mason RJ, Ernst JD, King TE Jr, Lazarus SC, Murray JF, et al., eds. *Murray & Nadel's Textbook of Respiratory Medicine*, 6th ed. Philadelphia: W.B. Saunders; 2016.)

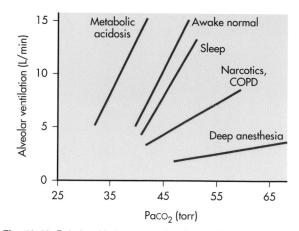

Fig. 10.10 Relationship between alveolar ventilation and changing P_{CO_2}. Responses to sleep and wakefulness, narcotic ingestion, chronic obstructive pulmonary disease (COPD), deep anesthesia, and metabolic acidosis. Both the slopes and the positions of the response curves are changed, indicating differences in ventilatory responses and response thresholds. (Redrawn from Levitzky MG. *Pulmonary Physiology*, 8th ed. New York: McGraw-Hill, 2013.)

that the inspired P_{CO_2} gradually rises. Ventilation is then plotted against alveolar P_{CO_2}, as shown in Fig. 10.10. The central and peripheral chemoreceptors detect the change in Pa_{CO_2} and transmit this information to the medullary respiratory centers. The respiratory control center then regulates minute ventilation to control arterial P_{CO_2} within the normal range. Ventilation increases as P_{CO_2} increases. In the presence of a normal Pa_{O_2}, the ventilation increases by about 3 L/min for each millimeter rise in Pa_{CO_2}. In the presence of a low Pa_{O_2}, there is greater ventilation for any given Pa_{CO_2} and the increase in ventilation with increasing Pa_{CO_2} is greater (steeper slope). The relationship between minute ventilation and the inspired CO_2 concentration is used as a test of CO_2 sensitivity. The slope of the response between minute ventilation and inspired CO_2 is termed the **ventilatory response to CO_2**. It is important to recognize that this relationship is amplified by low oxygen levels. This is because separate mechanisms are responsible for sensing P_{O_2} and P_{CO_2} in the peripheral chemoreceptors. Thus the presence of both hypercapnia and hypoxemia (sometimes called **asphyxia** when hypoxia is present) has an additive effect on chemoreceptor output and the resulting ventilatory stimulation (Fig. 10.11).

The ventilatory response to CO_2 is reduced by sleep, hyperventilation, increasing age, and genetic, racial, and personality factors. Trained athletes and divers, in general, have a lower CO_2 response. Drugs that depress the respiratory center such as morphine, barbiturates, and anesthetic agents decrease the ventilatory response to both CO_2 and O_2. In these instances, there is an inadequate stimulus to drive the motor neurons that innervate the muscles of respiration. Hypoventilation results, and arterial P_{CO_2} increases.

The ventilatory response to CO_2 is also reduced if the work of breathing is increased. This is primarily because the neural output of the respiratory center, which is (almost) normal, is not as effective in producing ventilation because of the mechanical limitation to ventilation. In addition, in individuals with COPD, there is evidence that the sensitivity of the respiratory control center is reduced. Metabolic acidosis shifts the CO_2 response to the left, demonstrating an increase in ventilation during metabolic acidosis for any particular Pa_{CO_2}.

RESPONSE TO HYPOXIA

The ventilatory response to hypoxia arises solely from stimulation of peripheral chemoreceptors and, most especially, stimulation of the carotid body. If an individual rebreathes air from a bag in which the P_{CO_2} is held constant at 40 mm Hg, there is little change in ventilation until the arterial P_{O_2} falls below 50 to 60 mm Hg. As one might anticipate, the response to arterial P_{O_2} is potentiated at higher arterial

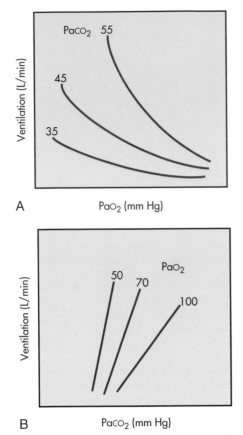

Fig. 10.11 The effects of hypoxia **(A)** and hypercapnia **(B)** on ventilation as the other respiratory gas partial pressure is varied. **A,** At a given Pa_{CO_2}, ventilation increases more and more as Pa_{O_2} decreases. When Pa_{CO_2} is allowed to decrease (the normal condition) during hypoxia, there is a little stimulation of breathing until P_{O_2} falls below 60 mm Hg. The hypoxic response is mediated through the carotid body chemoreceptors. **B,** The sensitivity of the ventilatory response to CO_2 is enhanced by hypoxia. (From Koeppen BM, Stanton BM, eds. *Berne and Levy's Physiology,* 7th ed. Philadelphia: Elsevier; 2018.)

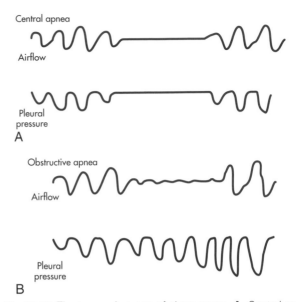

Fig. 10.12 The two main types of sleep apnea. **A,** Central apnea is characterized by the absence of an attempt to breathe, as demonstrated by no pleural pressure oscillations. **B,** In obstructive sleep apnea, the pleural pressure oscillations increase as CO_2 rises. This indicates that airflow resistance is very high, owing to upper airway obstruction. (From Koeppen BM, Stanton BM, eds. *Berne and Levy's Physiology*, 7th ed. Philadelphia: Elsevier; 2018.)

P_{CO_2} levels. The response to hypoxia is the response to P_{O_2}, not to O_2 content. This is why neither anemia nor carbon monoxide poisoning stimulates ventilation.

ABNORMALITIES IN CONTROL OF BREATHING

Changes in ventilatory pattern can occur for both primary and secondary reasons. During sleep, the carbon dioxide response curve shifts to the right (increased set point), and the slope of the response decreases slightly. As a result, during slow-wave sleep, arterial P_{CO_2} rises as much as 5

to 6 torr. Approximately one-third of normal individuals have brief episodes of apnea or hyperventilation during sleep that have no significant effect on arterial P_{O_2} and P_{CO_2}. These apneas usually last less than 10 seconds and occur during the lighter stages of slow-wave and rapid eye movement (REM) sleep. In a small number of individuals, the duration of apnea is abnormally prolonged, resulting in changes in arterial P_{O_2} and P_{CO_2}. These individuals have **sleep-disordered breathing.**

There are two major categories of sleep-disordered breathing—**obstructive sleep apnea (OSA)** and **central sleep apnea.** OSA (Fig. 10.12) is the most common of the sleep apnea abnormalities and occurs when the upper airway (usually the hypopharynx) closes during inspiration. Although the process is similar to what happens during snoring, it has more severe effects, obstructing the airway and causing cessation of airflow.

The histories of individuals with OSA are similar. A spouse usually reports that the individual snores. The snoring becomes louder and louder and then suddenly stops while the individual continues to make vigorous respiratory efforts. The individual is then aroused, goes back to sleep, and begins the same process repetitively throughout the night.

The upper airway is the source of the airway obstruction and the obstruction is due to failure of the pharyngeal muscles to contract properly as a result of excessive fat around the pharynx or airway blockage by the tongue. The arousal occurs when the arterial hypoxemia and hypercarbia stimulate both peripheral and central chemoreceptors. Respiration is restored briefly before the next apneic event occurs. Individuals with OSA can have hundreds of these events each night. As a consequence, they are sleep-deprived even though they do not awaken fully with each episode.

Other complications of OSA include polycythemia, right-sided cardiac failure (**cor pulmonale**), and increased risk for aortic dissection and pulmonary hypertension secondary to the recurrent hypoxic events. The most common cause of OSA is obesity. Other causes include excessive compliance of the hypopharynx, upper airway edema, and structural abnormalities of the upper airway. Treatment includes weight loss, oral appliances to pull the tongue forward, and continuous positive airway pressure (CPAP), which keeps the upper airway distended during inspiration.

Central sleep apnea occurs when there is a decrease in ventilatory drive to the respiratory motor neurons. The individual with central sleep apnea makes no respiratory efforts for abnormally long periods (1–2 minutes). Although the mechanism for this disorder is not clear in all individuals, a depressed response to CO_2 during sleep may be involved.

Central alveolar hypoventilation (CAH) is a rare disease in which voluntary breathing is intact but abnormalities in automaticity exist. It is also called **Ondine's curse**, named after a mythological tale in which the suitor of Neptune's daughter (Ondine) was cursed to lose automatic control over all bodily functions during sleep.

While awake, individuals with CAH have sufficient voluntary control over ventilation to maintain normal blood gas values, but during sleep or during times when ventilation is dependent on automatic ventilatory control (e.g., the individual is distracted by reading, watching TV, or playing a game), marked hypoventilation or apnea may occur. For these individuals, mechanical ventilation or, more recently, bilateral diaphragmatic pacing (similar to a cardiac pacemaker) can be lifesaving.

Another problem potentially related to abnormal ventilatory control is **sudden infant death syndrome** (SIDS). SIDS is the most common cause of death in infants in the first year of life outside of the perinatal period. Although the cause of SIDS is not known, abnormalities in ventilatory control and particularly in CO_2 responsiveness have been implicated. Placing infants on their back to sleep (reducing the potential for CO_2 rebreathing) has

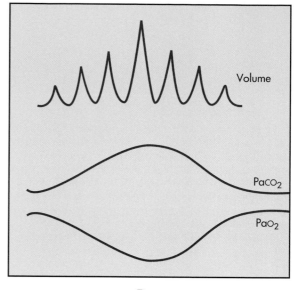

Fig. 10.13 In Cheyne-Stokes breathing, tidal volume and consequently arterial blood gases wax and wane. Generally, Cheyne-Stokes breathing is a sign of vasomotor instability, particularly low cardiac output. (From Koeppen BM, Stanton BM, eds. *Berne and Levy's Physiology*, 7th ed. Philadelphia: Elsevier; 2018.)

dramatically decreased (but not eliminated) the death rate from this syndrome.

Cheyne-Stokes ventilation, another abnormality in ventilatory control, is characterized by a varying tidal volume and ventilatory frequency (Fig. 10.13). After a period of apnea, tidal volume and respiratory frequency increase progressively over several breaths and then progressively decrease until apnea occurs. This irregular breathing pattern is seen in some individuals with central nervous system diseases including head trauma and increases in intracranial pressure. It is also present occasionally in normal individuals during sleep at high altitude. The mechanism for Cheyne-Stokes respiration is unknown. In some individuals it appears to be due to slow blood flow in the brain associated with periods of overshooting and undershooting ventilatory efforts in response to changes in P_{CO_2}.

Apneustic breathing, another abnormal breathing pattern (Fig. 10.14), is characterized by sustained periods of inspiration separated by brief periods of exhalation. The mechanism for this ventilatory pattern appears to be the loss of inspiratory-inhibitory activities that results in the augmented inspiratory drive. The pattern is sometimes seen in individuals with central nervous system injury.

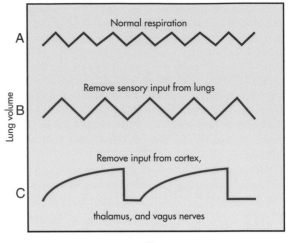

Fig. 10.14 Some patterns of breathing. **A,** Normal breathing at about 15 breaths/min in humans. **B,** The effect of removing sensory input from various lung receptors (mainly stretch) is to lengthen each breathing cycle and to increase tidal volume so that alveolar ventilation is not significantly affected. **C,** When input from the cerebral cortex and thalamus is also eliminated, together with vagal blockade, the result is prolonged inspiratory activity broken after several seconds by brief expirations (apneusis). (From Koeppen BM, Stanton BM, eds. *Berne and Levy's Physiology*, 7th ed. Philadelphia: Elsevier; 2018.)

CLINICAL BOX

In 1968, the summer Olympic games were held in Mexico City, Mexico. Mexico City is 7240 feet above sea level or a half mile higher than Denver, Colorado. Imagine that you are an athlete who lives in Boston and flies to Mexico City for the competition. The barometric pressure in Boston is ~760 mm Hg, whereas the barometric pressure in Mexico City is 585 mm Hg. At sea level, your Po_2 in arterial blood = ~95 torr. (Using the alveolar air equation in Chapter 5, Pao_2 = [760 – 47 mm Hg] × 0.21 – 40/0.8 = 100 torr. Assuming an $AaDo_2$ of 5 torr, your Pao_2 = 100 – 5 = 95 torr.) In the cerebrospinal fluid (CSF), your pH would be ~7.33, your Pco_2 would be 44 torr ($Paco_2$ = CO_2 produced by metabolism of the brain cells), and your CSF HCO_3^- would be approximately 22 mEq/L.

When you arrive in Mexico City, there is an abrupt decrease in inspired O_2 (Pio_2 = [585 – 47] × 0.21 = 113 torr) and a decrease in alveolar O_2 (Pao_2 = 113 torr – 40 torr/ 0.8 = 63 torr). If your $AaDo_2$ remained at 5, your Pao_2 would decrease to 58 torr. This decrease in arterial O_2 will result in stimulation of peripheral chemoreceptors and an increase in alveolar ventilation. The increase in ventilation will produce a decrease in $Paco_2$ and an increase in arterial pH. The net result of the increase in ventilation and decrease in $Paco_2$ is to minimize the hypoxemia by increasing your Pao_2. (For example, assume that the $Paco_2$ decreases to 31 torr; then Pao_2 = [585 – 47 torr] × 0.21 – 31 torr/0.8 = 74 torr, an increase in Pao_2 of 16 torr.) The decrease in arterial Pco_2 also produces a decrease in CSF Pco_2. Because

the bicarbonate concentration is unchanged, there is an increase in CSF pH. This increase attenuates the rate of discharge of central chemoreceptors and decreases their contribution to ventilatory drive.

Over the next 12 to 36 hours, the bicarbonate concentration in the CSF decreases as ion pumps or other mechanisms in the blood–brain barrier are activated. The result is that the CSF pH returns toward normal. Central chemoreceptor discharge increases and minute ventilation is further increased. At the same time that the bicarbonate concentration in the CSF is decreasing, there is a gradual excretion of bicarbonate ions from plasma by the kidney. This results in a gradual return of the arterial pH toward normal. Peripheral chemoreceptor stimulation increases further as arterial pH becomes normal (peripheral chemoreceptors are inhibited by elevated arterial pH).

The final result is that within 36 hours of arriving at high altitude, there is a significant increase in minute ventilation that is greater than the immediate effect of the hypoxemia on ventilation. This further increase is due to both central and peripheral chemoreceptor stimulation. Thus by the end of the weekend, both arterial and CSF pH are approaching normal, minute ventilation is increased, arterial Po_2 is decreased (but less than when you arrived), and arterial Pco_2 is decreased.

You now return home. When you land in Boston, your Pio_2 returns to normal and the hypoxic stimulus to ventilation is removed. Arterial Po_2 returns to normal and the peripheral chemoreceptor stimulation to ventilation decreases. This results in an increase in arterial CO_2 toward normal. CSF CO_2 also increases toward normal. This increase is associated with a decrease in CSF pH because the bicarbonate concentration in CSF is now reduced and ventilation is augmented.

Over the next 12 to 36 hours, ion pumps in the blood–brain barrier move HCO_3^- ions back into the CSF, with a gradual return of the CSF pH toward normal. Similarly, the pH in the blood decreases as the arterial P_{CO_2} rises because the arterial bicarbonate concentration is also decreased. This stimulates peripheral chemoreceptors, and minute ventilation remains augmented. Over the next 12 to 36 hours, renal mechanisms increase the blood HCO_3^- concentrations, the arterial pH returns to normal, and minute ventilation returns to normal.

SUMMARY

1. Respiratory control is both automatic and voluntary.
2. Ventilatory control is composed of sensors (central chemoreceptors, peripheral chemoreceptors, and pulmonary mechanoreceptors), controllers (the respiratory control center), and effectors (respiratory muscles).
3. The arterial P_{CO_2} is the major factor influencing ventilation.
4. The respiratory control center is composed of the dorsal respiratory group and the ventral respiratory group. Rhythmic breathing depends on a continuous (tonic) inspiratory drive from the dorsal respiratory group and on intermittent (phasic) expiratory inputs from the cerebrum, thalamus, cranial nerves, and ascending spinal cord sensory tracts.
5. The peripheral and central chemoreceptors respond to changes in P_{CO_2} and pH. The peripheral chemoreceptors (carotid and aortic bodies) are the only chemoreceptors that respond to changes in P_{O_2}.
6. The blood–brain barrier is relatively impermeable to H^+ and HCO_3^- but CO_2 readily diffuses across it. Acute and chronic hypercarbia affect breathing differently because of slow adjustments in cerebrospinal fluid $[H^+]$ and $[HCO_3^-]$, which alter CO_2 sensitivity.
7. Hypoxia enhances CO_2 responsiveness. The ventilatory response to hypoxia alone arises solely from stimulation of peripheral chemoreceptors, and in particular the carotid body, and occurs in response to decreases in P_{O_2} and not to changes in O_2 content.
8. The pneumotaxic center regulates tidal volume and respiratory rate and is important in fine-tuning respiratory rhythm.
9. Pulmonary stretch receptors respond to mechanical stimulation and are activated by lung inflation.
10. Irritant receptors protect the lower respiratory tract from particles, chemical vapors, and physical factors, primarily by inducing cough.
11. C-fiber juxta-alveolar or J receptors in the terminal respiratory units are stimulated by distortion of the alveolar walls (lung congestion or edema).
12. The two most important clinical abnormalities of breathing are obstructive sleep apnea and central sleep apnea.

KEYWORDS AND CONCEPTS

Aortic body
Apneustic breathing
Apneustic center
Blood–brain barrier
Carotid body
Central alveolar hypoventilation
Central chemoreceptors
Central sleep apnea
Cerebrospinal fluid
Cheyne-Stokes respiration
CO_2 ventilatory response curve
Diving reflex
Dorsal respiratory group

Henderson-Hasselbach equation
Hering-Breuer inspiratory inhibitory reflex
Hering-Breuer lung deflation reflex
Integrator
Irritant receptor
Juxta-alveolar receptor (J receptor)
Obstructive sleep apnea (OSA)
Peripheral chemoreceptors
Pneumotaxic center
Pulmonary mechanoreceptors
Pulmonary stretch receptors (rapidly adapting)
Pulmonary stretch receptors (slowly adapting)
Respiratory control center

Sneeze reflex
Sniff reflex
Somatic receptors
Sudden infant death syndrome

Ventilatory control
Ventilatory pattern generator
Ventral respiratory group

SELF-STUDY PROBLEMS

1. Underwater swimmers sometimes hyperventilate before they go under water for long periods of time. What then is the impetus for respiration, and why is this potentially dangerous?

2. Explain the acute and chronic ventilatory responses to altitude. What regulatory processes take place as a consequence of the change in arterial pH that develops during the first day of exposure to altitude?

3. How does an increase in Pa_{CO_2} influence the sensitivity of carotid bodies to Pa_{O_2}?

4. What is the mechanism of respiratory failure in individuals who have ingested an overdose of sleeping pills?

ADDITIONAL READINGS

Coleridge HM, Coleridge JC. Pulmonary reflexes: neural mechanisms of pulmonary defense. *Annu Rev Physiol*. 1994;56:69–91.

Corne S, Webster K, Younes M. Hypoxic respiratory response during acute stable hypocapnia. *Am J Resp Crit Care Med*. 2003;167:1193–1199.

de Castro D, Lipski J, Kanjhan R. Electrophysiological study of dorsal respiratory neurons in the medulla oblongata of the rat. *Brain Res*. 1994;639:49–56.

Funk GD, Feldman JL. Generation of respiratory rhythm and pattern in mammals: insights from developmental studies. *Curr Opin Neurobiol*. 1995;5:778–785.

Gonzalez C, Dinger B, Fidone SJ. Mechanisms of carotid body chemoreception. In: Dempsey JA, Pack AI, eds. *Regulation of Breathing*. New York: Marcel Dekker; 1995.

Jammes Y, Speck DF. Respiratory control by diaphragmatic and respiratory muscle afferents. In: Dempsey JA, Pack AI, eds. *Regulation of Breathing*. New York: Marcel Dekker; 1995.

Lee LY, Kou YR, Frazier DT, et al. Stimulation of vagal pulmonary C-fibers by a single breath of cigarette smoke in dogs. *J Appl Physiol*. 1989;66:2032–2038.

Robin ED, Whaley RD, Crump CH, Travis DM. Alveolar gas tensions, pulmonary ventilation and blood pH during physiologic sleep in normal subjects. *J Clin Invest*. 1958;37:98–989.

Sampol G, Romero O, Salas A, et al. Obstructive sleep apnea and thoracic aorta dissection. *Am J Resp Crit Care Med*. 2003;168:1528–1531.

Sant'Ambrogio G, Tsubone H, Sant'Ambrogio FB. Sensory information from the upper airway: Role in the control of breathing. *Respir Physiol*. 1995;102:1–16.

Voipio J, Ballanyi K. Interstitial P_{CO_2} and pH and their role as chemostimulants in the isolated respiratory network of neonatal rats. *J Physiol (Lond)*. 1997;499:527–542.

Younes M. Contributions of upper airway mechanics and control mechanisms to severity of obstructive apnea. *Am J Resp Crit Care Med*. 2003;168:645–658.

Nonrespiratory Functions of the Lung

OBJECTIVES

1. Describe patterns of particle deposition in the nose and airways and how they relate to lung defense and disease.
2. Describe the role of the nose in lung defense.
3. Describe the three major components of mucociliary transport and their interaction in the defense of the lung.
4. Explain how the lung functions as an organ of the mucosal immune system.
5. Explain the roles of phagocytic, dendritic, and natural killer cells in lung defense.
6. Describe the function of the lung in humoral immune mechanisms.
7. Outline the immune response to bacteria in the normal lung.
8. List four pulmonary diseases associated with abnormalities in mucociliary transport and innate and adaptive immunity.

In addition to its primary function of gas exchange, the lung also functions as a major defense organ to protect the body from the outside world. Just as the respiratory system has developed unique systems to effect gas exchange, it has also developed a unique series of defense systems to cope with environmental exposure and the constant insult of foreign agents.

The respiratory tract is continuously exposed to dust, pollen, ash, and other products of combustion; to microorganisms such as pathogenic viruses and bacteria; to particles or substances such as asbestos and silica; and to hazardous chemicals and toxic gases. In addition, liquids and food particles can be accidentally aspirated (inhaled) from the oropharynx or nasopharynx into the airways. The respiratory tract processes and disposes of these foreign substances using three categories of defense mechanisms: (1) mucociliary clearance that moves inhaled and trapped particles cephalad toward the mouth, (2) phagocytic and inflammatory cells that destroy inhaled material, and (3) a specialized mucosal immune system.

AEROSOL DEPOSITION IN THE LUNG

Aerosols are collections of particles that remain airborne for a substantial length of time. Large-particle aerosols tend to settle rapidly to the floor in a sealed room, whereas fine-particle aerosols remain airborne for longer periods of time. In the respiratory tract, the pattern of aerosol deposition is based on particle size (Fig. 11.1), distance traveled, mode and pattern of breathing, size and shape of the airways, particle density, and relative humidity.

There are three major mechanisms of particle deposition in the airways: impaction, sedimentation, and diffusion (Fig. 11.2). **Impaction** is due to the inertia of particles, causing them be moved toward an airway wall when there is a change in direction of the airstream. (This is similar to the sensation of being pushed against the outer wall of a car when going around a corner at high speed.) In general, particles larger than 5 μm in diameter are deposited by impaction in the nasal passages, where airflow is high and changes direction abruptly as a result of the upper airway anatomy. The anatomy of the nose is ideally suited for this function (see Fig. 1.1), with ribbons of tissue (**turbinates**) and nasal hairs (**vibrissae**) over which air is scrubbed. In more distal areas, where airflow is slower, smaller particles (0.2–2.0 μm in diameter) deposit on the surface or on mucus secondary to gravity. This gradual settling of particles based on their weight is called **sedimentation**. Particle deposition by sedimentation occurs extensively in the small airways, including the terminal and respiratory bronchioles, in large measure because these airways are so small that particles

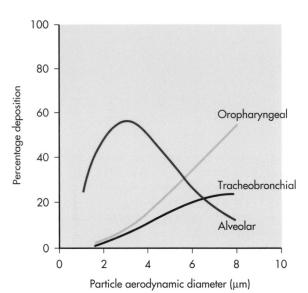

Fig. 11.1 Inhaled particles are trapped at different locations in the airways, according to their size. Particles with diameters greater than ~5 μm tend to impact into the nasopharynx, oropharynx, or large conducting airways. Smaller particles are more likely to become trapped in the distal airways or in the alveoli. (Redrawn from Clarke SW, Pavia D. Mucociliary clearance. In Crystal RG, West JB (eds.). *The Lung: Scientific Foundation.* New York: Raven Press; 1991.)

have a short distance to fall, and airflow is so slow. Random movement of particles (**Brownian motion**) as a result of their continuous bombardment by gas molecules is called **diffusion** and is the third mechanism of particle deposition. Particle deposition by diffusion occurs with particles less than 0.1 μm in diameter and mainly takes place in the smallest airways and alveoli. These particles are cleared by endocytosis by the alveolar macrophages, or they are carried away by lymphatics/lymphoid tissue or transported to the beginning of the mucociliary transport system.

INHALED TOXICANTS, AIR POLLUTION, AND DISEASE

Because the respiratory tract is one of the few organ systems in direct contact with the external environment, inhaled toxic materials can cause severe respiratory tract injury. The bronchioles and the alveoli are the most sensitive to inhaled toxicants in part because they are thin (one cell thick) and not coated by a layer of mucus. Protection of these airways from inhaled toxicants represents an important respiratory defense mechanism. A physiologic function of the nose and large airways is to scrub toxicants from the inhaled airstream, a process that limits penetration to the more distal bronchiolar and alveolar airways. The structure and function of the nose and bronchi are well suited for this purpose. This phenomenon occurs for both particulates and gases and vapors.

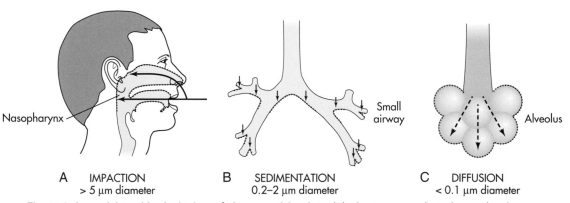

Fig. 11.2 Aerosol deposition in the lung. **A,** Large particles deposit in the nose, mouth, and posterior pharynx by impaction. **B,** Smaller particles deposit by gravity and sediment in smaller airways and at the bifurcations of larger airways. **C,** The smallest particles reach the alveoli and deposit on the alveolar surface by diffusion. (Adapted from West J. Pulmonary Physiology and Pathophysiology, 2nd ed. Philadelphia: Lippincott Williams & Wilkins; 2007.)

CLINICAL BOX

Particle size is the fundamental basis for the establishment of particulate air pollution standards. The U.S. National PM2.5 (particulate matter 2.5 μm) and PM10 standards are based on potential risks of particles smaller than 2.5 and 10 μm, respectively. In the nasal cavity, impaction is the primary mechanism of particle deposition for particles with diameters greater than 5 μm in diameter. Because of impaction, approximately 50% of inhaled 2.5-μm particles and greater than 90% of 10-μm particles deposit in the nose. Thus approximately one-half of inhaled 2.5-μm particles penetrate through the nose to the lower respiratory tract, whereas less than 5% of 10-μm particles so do. During mouth breathing the nose is bypassed, and there is a large increase in the delivery of inhaled particulates to the lower respiratory tract.

As noted earlier, particles of differing size deposit with differing efficiency within the various regions of the respiratory tract. Less well appreciated is that the nose also scrubs airborne vapors and gases. The same structural and physiologic properties that optimize the ability of the nose to heat and humidify the airstream, specifically narrow airspace, large surface area, and large blood flow, also serve to enhance the scrubbing of vapors and gases. Nasal scrubbing is most efficient for water-soluble, chemically reactive gases and vapors. An extreme example is sulfur dioxide, the ubiquitous air pollutant that is associated with acid rain and derived in large part from combustion of coal. More than 95% of inhaled sulfur dioxide is absorbed in the nose during nose breathing, and less than 5% penetrates to the lower airways. Clearly this serves to protect the lower airways from the harmful effects of such materials.

The protection offered by the nasal cavity is lost during mouth breathing during exercise. Moreover, there is a large increase in ventilation during exercise. These two factors lead to a profound increase in delivery of inhaled materials to the lower respiratory tract during exercise. Consider the pollutant sulfur dioxide. Switching to mouth breathing increases delivery to the lower respiratory tract 20-fold (100% penetration rather than 5% penetration); if accompanied by a 4-fold increase in ventilation, then the total delivered dose to the lower airways would increase 80-fold during exercise. For this reason, persons who exercise outdoors are considered to be at much greater risk from air-pollutant-induced lung injury and diminished lung function than sedentary individuals. This includes not only labor-intensive workers but also children playing outdoor sports and joggers who run in polluted cities.

Analogous to the nose, the bronchial airways also scrub inhaled toxicants from the airstream, a process that limits penetration to the distal bronchiolar and alveolar airways. Few, if any, inhaled particles greater than 10 μm penetrate to the alveoli. In contrast to 10-μm particles, 2.5-μm particles can penetrate to the alveoli; in fact, approximately 25% of inhaled 2.5-μm particles deposit in this region. Thus it can be appreciated that markedly differing alveolar health risks would be anticipated from PM2.5 versus PM10. Gases and vapors can also be absorbed efficiently within the bronchial airways. These airways are considered to be inert (e.g., dead space) with respect to oxygen or carbon dioxide, but this is not the case for soluble and reactive vapors and gases. Such materials are efficiently absorbed in the bronchial airways, resulting in very little penetration to the alveoli. An illustrative example is formaldehyde. This carcinogenic gas is near completely absorbed in the large airways; no inhaled formaldehyde penetrates to the alveoli. As a result, formaldehyde, although it causes large airway injury, does not pose a risk of causing alveolar injury. Diacetyl, the vapor associated with popcorn worker's lung disease, provides another example of this phenomenon (see Clinical Box: Popcorn Lung Disease).

CLINICAL BOX: POPCORN LUNG DISEASE

In the early 2000s an astute physician noted a cluster of individuals with bronchiolitis obliterans among employees in a single microwave popcorn factory. Some workers demonstrated such severe fibrosis of the bronchioles (associated with a forced expiratory volume in 1 second [FEV$_1$] <20% of predicted) that lung transplantation was required. Surveys of the workplace air were performed and revealed the presence of more than 60 hazardous chemicals. A chemical of particular interest, **diacetyl** (2,3-butane-dione), was present in high concentrations. Inhalation toxicity safety evaluation studies in rodents revealed that diacetyl caused nasal and large bronchial, but not bronchiolar, injury. Importantly, this testing was performed in sedentary nose-breathing rodents, a physiologic condition considerably different from exercise with mouth breathing such as that experienced by the workers in the popcorn industry. Subsequent studies revealed that the dose of diacetyl that is delivered to the bronchiolar airways of mouth-breathing exercising workers exceeded that in the sedentary rat by 30-fold or more. Moreover, introduction of diacetyl into the small airways of the rat caused small airway fibrotic disease similar to that observed in workers. It is now accepted that diacetyl causes small airway disease in humans. Diacetyl is the natural chemical that imparts the taste of butter. Diminished lung function has been observed not only in workers in the microwave popcorn industry but also in workers in other occupations that are exposed to butter flavorings, including coffee roasting and certain baking occupations. This exemplifies not only the difficulties in safety evaluation of inhaled materials but also the importance of understanding occupational exposure history in evaluating individuals with lung dysfunction.

Mucociliary Transport

The mucociliary transport system is another one of the lung's structural, primary defense mechanisms. It protects the conducting airways by trapping and removing bacteria, inhaled particles, and cellular debris from the lung. In general, the longer inhaled material remains in the airways, the greater the probability that lung damage will occur. Once particles in the terminal airways have entered the interstitium, clearance is even slower, and the likelihood of lung damage is even greater.

There are three major components of mucociliary transport: (1) the periciliary fluid, (2) the mucus layer, and (3) the cilia that beat in a lower layer of nonviscid, serous fluid (periciliary fluid) (Fig. 11.3). Effective clearance requires both ciliary activity and respiratory tract fluid (periciliary fluid and mucus). Inhaled material is trapped in the relatively tenacious and viscous mucus, whereas the watery periciliary fluid allows the cilia to move freely with only their tips contacting the mucus and propelling it toward the mouth.

Periciliary Fluid

The periciliary fluid layer is produced by the pseudostratified, columnar epithelium that lines the respiratory system and that is joined together by tight junctions (see Fig. 1.10). Airway epithelial cells are ciliated and line the entire respiratory tract to the level of the bronchioles, where they are replaced by a cuboidal, nonciliated epithelium. The only exceptions are parts of the pharynx and the anterior third of the nasal cavity. The respiratory epithelial cells are responsible for maintaining the level of the periciliary fluid, a layer of water 5 μm in depth, and

electrolytes in which the cilia and mucociliary transport system function. The depth of the periciliary fluid is maintained by the movement of ions across the epithelium. Active (i.e., dependent on energy, as in adenosine triphosphate) chloride secretion into the airway lumen occurs through chloride (Cl^-) channels in the apical membrane. These channels are regulated by intracellular cyclic adenosine monophosphate (cAMP) and calcium. Sodium (Na^+) is absorbed through sodium channels in the apical membrane (Fig. 11.4). Both chloride secretion and sodium absorption translocate water secondarily (osmotic equilibrium), and it is the balance between Cl^- secretion and Na^+ absorption that regulates the depth of the periciliary fluid. A sodium-potassium adenosine triphosphatase (ATPase; Na^+,K^+-ATPase) pump in the basolateral membrane maintains the sodium gradient, allowing for sodium absorption. An Na^+-Cl^- cotransporter in the basolateral membrane links sodium and chloride flux, leading to a buildup in chloride in the cell above its electrochemical equilibrium and to diffusion down a favorable gradient into the airway lumen. The sodium that accompanies chloride is then transported back across the basolateral membrane by the Na^+,K^+-ATPase pump.

Thus active secretion of Cl^- into the airway lumen produces fluid secretion, whereas active Na^+ absorption accounts for the ability to absorb fluid. It is the balance between chloride secretion and sodium absorption that regulates

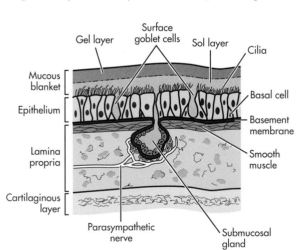

Fig. 11.3 Epithelial lining of the tracheobronchial tree. The cilia of the epithelial cell reside in the periciliary fluid layer with the mucus on top. Interspersed between the ciliated epithelial cells are surface secretory (goblet) cells and submucosal glands. (From Berne RM, Levy ML, Koeppen BM, Stanton BM (eds.). *Physiology*, 5th ed. St. Louis: Mosby; 2004.)

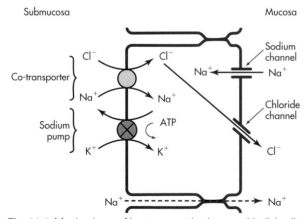

Fig. 11.4 Mechanisms of ion transport in airway epithelial cells. A cotransporter in the basolateral membrane links sodium and chloride flux, leading to a buildup in chloride above its electrochemical equilibrium. A sodium-potassium ATPase pump in the same membrane transports sodium out of the cell and thus maintains a sodium gradient inside the cell. A sodium channel and a chloride channel in the apical membrane provide for sodium influx into the cell and chloride efflux out of the cell. ATP, adenosine triphosphate. Osmotic equilibrium is maintained by the diffusion of water accompanying net solute flux. (From Berne RM, Levy ML, Koeppen BM, Stanton BM (eds.). *Physiology*, 5th ed. St. Louis: Mosby; 2004.)

the depth of the periciliary fluid at 5 to 6 μm (Table 11.1). This depth is important for the normal functioning of the cilia. If it is too deep, cilia splash around, and if it is not deep enough, ciliary function is markedly diminished.

Mucus Layer

The mucus or gel layer lies on top of the periciliary fluid layer and is propelled by the cilia. Airway mucus is a complex mixture of macromolecules including proteins, glycoproteins, electrolytes, and water. The mucus layer is 5 to 10 μm thick and exists as a discontinuous blanket (i.e., islands of mucus). Three cells produce the mucus layer: surface secretory cells, submucosal tracheobronchial glands, and Clara cells. These cells control both the quantity and composition of macromolecules in the mucus.

Mucus is composed of glycoproteins and consists of groups of oligosaccharides that are attached to a protein backbone like the bones of a fish to the vertebral column (Fig. 11.5). The oligosaccharides are bound to the amino acids by "O" glycosidic bonds (i.e., oxygen links the carbohydrate to the protein), and unlinked proteins form disulfide or peptide bonds. The result is a high-molecular-weight glycoprotein with low viscosity and high elasticity. It is this elasticity that prevents mucus from backsliding during clearance. Mucus is 95% to 97% water.

Surface secretory cells (also called **goblet cells**) line the respiratory epithelium and are present in approximately every five to six ciliated cells (see Fig. 1.10). They decrease in number between the 5th and 12th lung divisions and disappear completely beyond the 12th tracheobronchial

TABLE 11.1 Agents that Stimulate Chloride Secretion in Airway Epithelia

Agent	Surface*	cAMP
β-Adrenergic agonist	Submucosal	↑
Prostaglandin E_2	Submucosal	↑
Prostaglandin F_2	Submucosal	—
Vasoactive intestinal peptide	Submucosal	↑
Adenosine	Mucosal	↑
Leukotrienes LTC_4 and LTD_4	Mucosal and submucosal	↑?
Substance P	Mucosal and submucosal	?
Bradykinin	Mucosal and submucosal	↑?

*Surface is the side of the epithelium on which the agents act. ↑, increase; ?, uncertainty; —, no measurable change. cAMP, cyclic adenosine monophosphate.
From Welsh MJ. Production and control of airway secretions. In Fishman AP, ed. *Pulmonary Diseases and Disorders*, 2nd ed. New York: McGraw-Hill; 1988.

division. They secrete neutral and acidic glycoproteins rich in sialic acid. In response to a chemical signal, goblet cells discharge their stored material by the process of exocytosis, in which membrane-bound storage granules fuse with the plasma membrane and subsequently open to the airway lumen and release their contents. In the presence of cigarette smoke or in individuals with chronic bronchitis, surface secretory cells increase in size and number and extend further down the respiratory tract toward the alveolus. Their output also increases, and there is a change in the chemical composition of their secretions.

Submucosal tracheobronchial glands are present normally wherever there is cartilage; they empty into the airway lumen through a ciliated duct. In patients with chronic bronchitis, these glands are increased in number and size and can extend to the bronchioles. The glands' secretory component consists of mucous cells near the distal end of the tubule, which is lined by "nonspecified" cells, and of serous cells at the most distal end of the tubule (Table 11.2). Mucous cells contain large, often confluent, electron-lucent granules; serous cells contain small, discrete electron-dense secretory granules. The mucous cells of the submucosal tracheobronchial glands secrete acid glycoproteins, whereas the serous cells secrete neutral glycoproteins and contain lysozyme, lactoferrin, and antileukoprotease. In disease, the chemical composition of the glycoproteins does not change, but there is an increase in the volume of the secretions and a change in the ratio of neutral glycoproteins to acidic glycoproteins that modifies the physical properties of the mucus. This change in viscosity and elasticity affects the subsequent clearance of the mucus. Gland secretion is under parasympathetic, adrenergic, and peptidergic (vasoactive intestinal peptide) neural control. Local inflammatory mediators such as histamine and arachidonic acid metabolites stimulate mucus production.

Clara cells are located in the bronchioles and contain granules. Although their exact function is not known, they secrete a nonmucinous material containing carbohydrate and protein. They also appear to play a role in bronchial regeneration after injury.

Healthy individuals produce approximately 100 mL of mucus each day. Although some people even today refer to the "mucous blanket" in the airways, the mucus layer is actually "spotty" and varies in thickness between 2 and 5 μm. Most of the volume of the mucus is absorbed by the ciliated, columnar, epithelial lining cells, with only 10 mL reaching the glottis per day. This mucus is propelled to the back of the throat, where it is swallowed.

Cilia

Cilia are the microscopic hairlike scrubbers of the respiratory system. It is estimated that there are approximately 200 to 250 cilia per cell (Fig. 11.6).

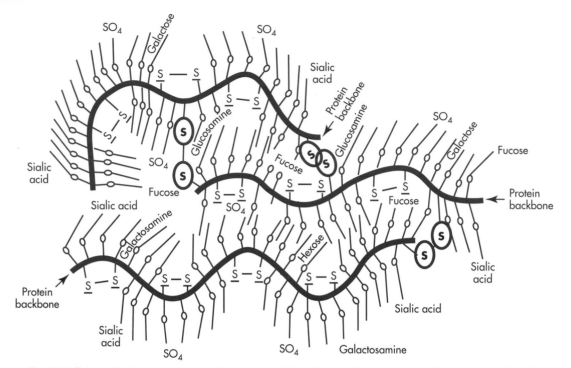

Fig. 11.5 Schematic drawing of mucus. Note the protein backbone with glycoprotein side chains and the "O" glycosidic and disulfide bonds. (From Berne RM, Levy ML, Koeppen BM, Stanton BM (eds.). *Physiology*, 5th ed. St. Louis: Mosby; 2004.)

TABLE 11.2	**Properties of Submucosal Gland Cells**	
	Serous Cells	**Mucous Cells**
Granules	Small, electron-dense	Large, electron-lucent
Glycoproteins	Neutral Lysozyme, lactoferrin	Acidic
Hormone Receptors	α > β-Adrenergic Muscarinic	β > α-Adrenergic Muscarinic
Degranulation	α-Adrenergic Cholinergic Substance P	β-Adrenergic Cholinergic

From Welsh MJ. Production and control of airway secretions. In Fishman AP, ed. *Pulmonary Diseases and Disorders*, 2nd ed. New York: McGraw-Hill; 1988.

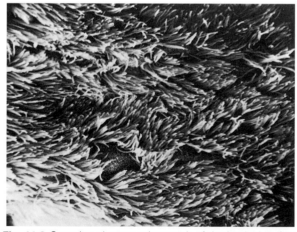

Fig. 11.6 Scanning electron micrograph of the luminal surface of a bronchiole from a normal man; many cilia are evident surrounding a nonciliated cell (~2000). (Reprinted by permission from Ebert RV, Terracio MJ. The bronchiolar epithelium in cigarette smokers. Observations with the scanning electron microscope. *Am Rev Resp Dis*. 1975;111:4-11.)

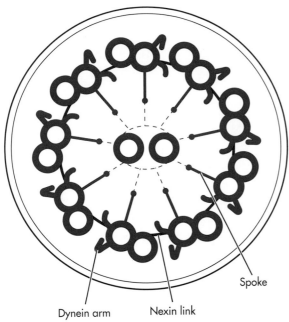

Dynein arm   Nexin link   Spoke

Fig. 11.7 Schematic cross-sectional diagram of cilium showing its main structural components. (From Palmbald J, Mossberg B, Afzelius BA. Ultrastructural, cellular, and clinical features of the immotile-cilia syndrome. *Ann Rev Med.* 1984;35:481-492. Reprinted with permission from Annual Reviews Inc.)

They are 2 to 5 μm in length and have a structure that has been preserved through evolution from protozoa. Cilia are composed of nine microtubular doublets that surround two central microtubules and are held together by dynein arms, nexin links, and spokes (Fig. 11.7). This structure is ideally suited for their function. The central microtubule doublet contains an ATPase enzyme that is likely responsible for the contractile beat of the cilium. Coordinated ciliary beating can be detected by the 13th week of gestation.

Cilia beat with a coordinated oscillation in a characteristic biphasic, wavelike rhythm called metachronism (Fig. 11.8). They beat 900 to 1200 strokes/min with a "power forward" stroke and a slow return or recovery stroke. During their power forward stroke, the tips of the cilia extend upward into the viscous layer, dragging it and entrapped particles. On the reverse beat, the cilia release the mucus and are contained completely in the sol layer. Cilia in the nasopharynx beat in the direction that will propel mucus into the pharynx, whereas cilia in the trachea propel mucus upward toward the pharynx, where it is swallowed. Ciliary beating is powered by ATP. The bending of the cilia occurs by the sliding

of dynein arms interlinking each microtubule pair. This causes a bending to one side. Cilia beat in a coordinated fashion; this coordination occurs by cell-to-cell ion flow, resulting in electrical and metabolic coordination. The mechanism by which cilia and the adjoining cells communicate is unknown. Ciliary function is inhibited or impaired by cigarette smoke, hypoxia, and infection.

Cough, stimulated by irritant receptors that are activated by inhaled or aspirated foreign material, is also an important protective mechanism. Coughing achieves rapid airflow acceleration and extremely high flow rates and, when coupled with dynamic airway compression, is effective in squeezing and clearing material and mucus from the airways (see Fig. 3.11).

When functioning normally, the mucociliary transport system is highly effective. Deposited particles can be removed in a matter of minutes to hours. In the trachea and mainstem bronchi, the rate of particle clearance is 5 to 20 mm/min, whereas it is slower in the bronchioles (0.5–1.0 mm/min).

Phagocytic and Inflammatory Cells

Pulmonary alveolar macrophages and **dendritic cells** (DCs) are mononuclear phagocytic cells that scavenge particles and bacteria in the airways and in the alveoli. DCs and alveolar macrophages are differentiated cells of the myeloid lineage and are the first nonepithelial cells to contact and respond to foreign substances. They are important components of the innate immune system.

Although B and T lymphocytes are the predominant cells involved in mounting an immune response, DCs are a major cell type for antigen presentation to T cells and are required for a maximum response. The major functions of DCs are to capture, process, and present antigen to T cells as well as to either activate or suppress the T-cell response (Table 11.3).

DCs are commonly found from the trachea to the alveoli in the parenchyma of the lung and are usually associated with the epithelium (Fig. 11.9). The upper airways are more densely populated with DCs than the smaller airways in the more peripheral regions of the lung. The anatomic location of these cells correlates well with particle deposition in the airways.

Alveolar macrophages are large, foamy, highly active phagocytic cells derived from myeloid progenitor cells in the bone marrow. Alveolar macrophages have a mean life span of 1 to 5 weeks and are derived from blood monocytes, usually as the result of secondary division by other alveolar macrophages. In inflammatory states such as

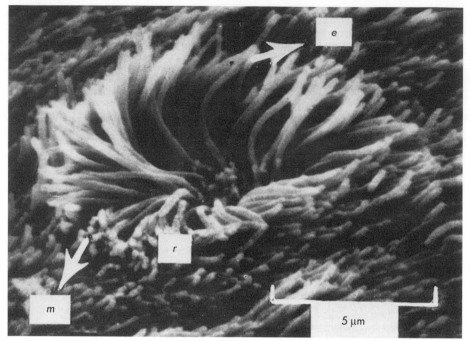

Fig. 11.8 Scanning electron micrograph of a metachronal wave on rabbit tracheal epithelium. Cilia that move to the left close to the cell surface in their recovery stroke (r) swing over toward the right in the more erect effective stroke (e). The metachronal wave moves in the direction indicated by arrow (m). (Micrograph by MJ Sanderson.) (From Sanderson MJ, Sleigh MS. Ciliary activity of cultured rabbit tracheal epithelium: beat pattern and metachrony. *J Cell Sci.* 1981;47:331-347.)

TABLE 11.3   **Functions of the Dendritic Cell**
Capture and process antigen
Migrate to lymphoid tissues
Present antigen to lymphocytes via major histocompatibility complex
Activate lymphocytes and enhance stimulatory response
Express lymphocyte costimulatory molecules
Secrete cytokines
Induce tolerance

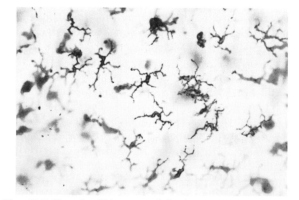

Fig. 11.9 The dendritic network in the conducting airways. The long, delicate processes of the dendritic cells can be seen throughout the conducting airways. (Reproduced with permission of the © ERS 2018: *European Respiratory Journal* Oct 2001;18(4):692-704.)

tuberculosis, blood monocytes can, however, migrate into the lung and differentiate into new alveolar macrophages. Alveolar macrophages are found mostly in the alveolus adjacent to the epithelium and less frequently in the terminal airways and interstitial space (Fig. 11.10).

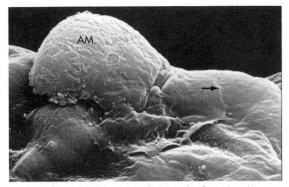

Fig. 11.10 Scanning electron micrograph of an alveolar macrophage (AM) sitting on an epithelial cell in the lung. Arrow points to the advancing edge of the cell. (From Weibel, 1980. Reproduced with permission.)

They migrate freely throughout the alveolar spaces and serve as a first line of defense in the lower air spaces. They readily and rapidly (usually within 24 hours) phagocytize foreign particles and substances, as well as cellular debris from dead cells. Once a particle is engulfed, the major mechanisms for killing are typical of phagocytic cells and include oxygen radicals, enzymatic activity, and halogen derivatives within lysosomes. Alveolar macrophages kill foreign material rapidly and without mounting an inflammatory response, which enhances lung defense and contributes to the overall defense system. Rapid phagocytosis inhibits binding of these substances to the alveolar surface and prevents possible invasion into the interstitial spaces and tissue damage.

Polymorphonuclear leukocytes (PMNs) are important cells in lung defense against established bacterial infection of the lower respiratory tract. Although rarely found in normal small airways and alveoli, PMNs are a prominent, histologic feature of a bacterial pneumonia. These cells are recruited to the lung by chemotactic factors released by alveolar macrophages and by products of complement activation. Movement into the lung from the pulmonary vasculature is orchestrated by many factors that mediate the process of adhesion, including integrins on the PMN surface and adhesion molecules on the vascular endothelial cells. PMNs phagocytose and kill invading bacteria by generating products of oxidative metabolism toxic to microbes.

Surface enzymes and factors in serum and airway secretions assist in destroying or detoxifying particles and include **lysozymes** found primarily in PMNs and known to have bactericidal properties; **interferon** (IFN), a potent antiviral compound produced by macrophages and lymphocytes; **complement,** an important cofactor in antigen-antibody reactions; and the **bacteriostatic lactoferrin,** produced by PMNs and glandular mucosal cells. Antiproteases found in normal lungs are especially important in inactivating the elastase enzymes released by macrophages and PMNs during phagocytosis. The most important of the antiproteases is α1-antitrypsin. Individuals with α1-antitrypsin deficiency lack the ability to synthesize this enzyme and are predisposed to the development of emphysema in their 30s and 40s. Some individuals who smoke produce increased levels of these proteases beyond the capacity of the antiprotease systems, resulting in pulmonary inflammation that leads to degradation of the alveolar septal walls and emphysema.

The transition between the conducting airways and the mucociliary transport system and the terminal respiratory units where alveolar mechanisms are important is the Achilles' heel in what is otherwise a highly effective defense system, because the risk of particle retention at this location is high. In the occupational lung disease called pneumoconiosis (the "black lung" disease of coal miners) or silicosis (the lung disease caused by inhalation of silica during quarrying, mining, or sandblasting), particle sedimentation occurs in the region of the terminal and respiratory bronchioles. The relatively slow rate of particle clearance in this area provides an opportunity for particles to invoke toxic reactions (in the case of silica) or to leave the airway space and enter the interstitial spaces and invoke less intense fibrotic responses. The terminal respiratory unit is the most common location of airway damage in all types of occupational lung disease. It is also likely that deposition of atmospheric particles such as tobacco smoke in this area causes some of the earliest changes in chronic bronchitis.

CLINICAL BOX: SILICOSIS AND ASBESTOSIS

Silica dust and asbestos are mineral crystals that cannot be dissolved by the macrophage after phagocytosis. The sharp crystals puncture lysosomal membranes, resulting in intracellular lysosomal enzyme release and cell death. Chemotactic factors released from the dying macrophage cause fibroblast migration and collagen synthesis in the region. Migration of additional macrophages into the region to ingest the dead macrophages occurs, and these macrophages are also killed by the nondissolved, sharp mineral

Continued

CLINICAL BOX: SILICOSIS AND ASBESTOSIS—cont'd

crystals. Their death stimulates additional fibroblast migration and additional collagen synthesis (see the accompanying figure). The end result is that the alveolar macrophage now has localized and concentrated silica or asbestos particles in a region of the lung in association with the development of pulmonary fibrosis, a disease associated with reduced lung compliance, impaired gas exchange, and increased work of breathing.

The fate of the alveolar macrophage is varied. It can be taken up into the mucociliary clearance system, it can die within the alveolus and be phagocytized by other alveolar macrophages, or it can migrate into lymphoid tissue or the lung interstitium.

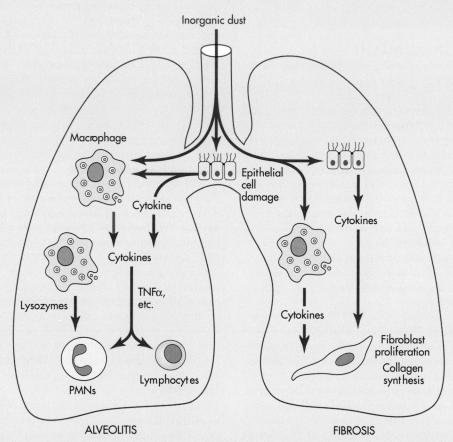

The pathophysiology of alveolitis and fibrosis in pneumoconiosis. In the inflammatory process (left side), inhaled dust is ingested by alveolar macrophages that are damaged and activated to release cytotoxic O, lysosomal enzymes, and inflammatory cytokines (TNF-α, IL-1). These in turn recruit inflammatory cells (lymphocytes, neutrophils, and PMNs) into the alveoli. Epithelial cells are also damaged, and they release additional inflammatory cytokines. Alveolar macrophages, lymphocytes, and neutrophils are the cells mainly responsible for the development of alveolitis. In the process of fibrosis (right side) following the inflammatory process, reparation, and fibrosis develop. Growth factors (e.g., TNF, IL-1) stimulate the recruitment and proliferation of type II pneumocytes and fibroblasts and induce overproduction of fibronectin and collagen. IL-1, interleukin-1; TNF, tumor necrosis factor.

(Adapted from Fujimura N. Pathology and pathophysiology of pneumoconiosis. *Curr Opin Pulm Med.* 2000;6:140-144.)

THE LUNG AS A SECONDARY LYMPHOID ORGAN

The lymphatic system and lymphoid tissues in the lung include organized lymphoid structures such as lymph nodes, lymph nodules, and lymph aggregates, in addition to a diffuse submucosal network of scattered lymphocytes and dendritic cells. These lymphoid structures are found throughout the respiratory tract in different anatomic locations. Because there is regional variation in inhaled particle deposition, each lymphoid tissue plays an important and unique role in the overall defense of the lung.

Regional Lymph Nodes of the Lung

The lymph nodes draining the lung are part of the mediastinal network, which drains the head and neck, the lungs, and the esophagus. The peribronchial and hilar lymph nodes are the prominent nodes in the local lung region; less prominent are the intrapulmonary nodes in the pleura and interlobar septal areas. Lymph nodes in these areas have the encapsulated organization typical of lymph nodes in other areas of the body, including the cortex, paracortex, and medulla. When activated, a germinal center is apparent in B cells and plasma cells in the cortical follicles and medullary cords, and in T cells in the paracortical areas between the follicles.

In addition to being the site of antigen presentation via lymph drainage, regional lymph nodes are the sites to receive cancer cells. Thus these mediastinal nodes have significant diagnostic importance for lung cancer.

Mucosal-Associated Lymphoid Tissue (MALT)

The lymphoid tissue of the mucosal areas in the gastrointestinal, respiratory, and urinary systems consist of loosely organized aggregates of cells known as **MALT**. In contrast to lymph nodes, these tissues are not encapsulated and are composed mainly of aggregates or clusters of lymphocytes residing in submucosal regions. In addition to aggregates of cells, MALT contains a substantial number of solitary B and T lymphocytes. The B cells found in MALT can selectively differentiate into IgA-secreting plasma cells when stimulated by antigen. MALT in the lung is called **BALT (bronchus-associated lymphoid tissue)** and provides a first line of defense for this highly exposed mucosal surface. In the upper airways of the respiratory tract, BALT is present in adenoids and tonsils.

BALT predominates throughout the conducting airways, with aggregates of lymph nodules or solitary lymph nodules found sporadically. The epithelium associated with areas of BALT is specialized and is called lymphoepithelium. It is composed of a mix of epithelial cells and lymphocytes. Lymphoepithelium lacks ciliated epithelial

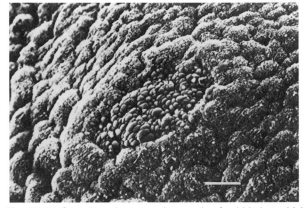

Fig. 11.11 Scanning electron micrograph of rabbit bronchial epithelium showing island of lymphoepithelium surrounded by ciliated epithelium. Bar = 1 mm. (Reprinted by permission from Bienenstock J, Johnston N. A morphologic study of rabbit bronchial lymphoid aggregates and lymphoepithelium. *Laboratory Invest.* 1976;35:343-348.)

cells, which results in a break in the mucociliary clearance system. This enhances fluid and particulate flow into the BALT area (Fig. 11.11). These epithelial cells secrete cytokines (e.g., interleukin-6, which favors induction of IgA synthesis); express adhesion molecules essential for antigen-presenting cell (APC) contact with T cells; and have also been shown to have APC capabilities. BALT is observed in humans but only in the presence of pathologic conditions such as upper respiratory tract infections. There are no organized lymphoid structures in the alveolar spaces.

HUMORAL IMMUNE MECHANISMS

IgA and IgG

Humoral immunity in the respiratory system consists of two major immunoglobulins: IgA and IgG. IgA, and a particular form of IgA known as **secretory IgA**, is especially important in the nasopharynx and upper airways. Secretory IgA is composed of two IgA molecules (a dimer) joined by a polypeptide that contains an extra glycoprotein called the secretory component. Secretory IgA is synthesized locally in submucosal areas by plasma cells and secreted in a dimer form linked by a J-chain. The antibody-dimer migrates to the submucosal surface of epithelial cells where it binds to a surface protein receptor called poly Ig (Fig. 11.12). The poly Ig receptor aids in the pinocytosis of the dimer into the epithelial cell and its eventual secretion into the airway lumen. During exocytosis of the IgA complex, the poly Ig is enzymatically cleaved, leaving a portion of it (the secretory

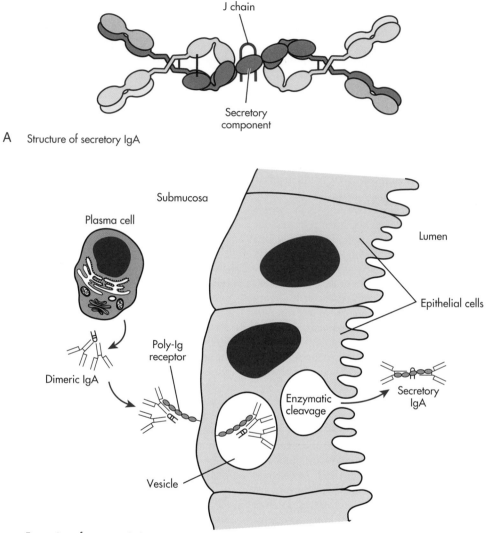

A   Structure of secretory IgA

B   Formation of secretory IgA

Fig. 11.12 Structure and formation of secretory immunoglobin A (IgA). **A,** Secretory IgA consists of at least two IgA molecules that are covalently linked via a J chain and covalently associated with the secretory component. The secretory component contains five Ig-like domains and is linked to dimeric IgA (thick black line) between its fifth domain and one of the IgA heavy chains. **B,** Secretory IgA is formed during transport through mucous membrane epithelial cells. Dimeric IgA binds to a poly Ig receptor on the basolateral membrane of an epithelial cell and is internalized by receptor-mediated endocytosis. After transport of the receptor-IgA complex to the luminal surface, the poly Ig receptor is enzymatically cleaved, releasing the secretory component bound to the dimeric IgA. (From Koeppen BM, Stanton BM, eds. *Berne and Levy's Physiology*, 7th ed. Philadelphia: Elsevier; 2018.)

component) still associated with the complex. The secretory piece stays attached to the IgA complex in the airway and aids in its protection from proteolytic cleavage in the lumen. Secretory IgA binds to antigens including viruses and bacteria and prevents their attachment to epithelial cells. The IgA also agglutinates microorganisms, which makes them more easily cleared by mucociliary transport.

Unlike IgA, IgG is abundant in the lower respiratory tract. Synthesized locally, IgG neutralizes viruses, is an opsonin (a macromolecular coat around bacteria) for macrophage handling of bacteria, agglutinates particles, activates complement, and in the presence of complement causes lysis of Gram-negative bacteria.

NORMAL ADAPTIVE IMMUNE RESPONSE AND THE RESPONSE TO BACTERIA

The adaptive immune system in the respiratory tract is summoned only after the insulting agent has avoided the unique defense systems established in the respiratory tract. Once triggered, however, it is similar to the response in any other systemic organ.

Under normal circumstances, bacteria such as *Streptococcus pneumoniae* that commonly come into contact with the upper respiratory system (i.e., bronchus to nasopharynx) are expelled by the mucociliary clearance system or are handled by BALT via an IgA response. However, if the bacteria elude these first-line defenses, an inflammatory response develops (e.g., bacterial pneumonia), which is followed by a classic adaptive immune response with T-cell activation and antibody synthesis (Fig. 11.13). These responses take 1 to 2 weeks to develop fully before a resolution of the pneumonia occurs. A typical inflammatory response to a bacterial or viral pneumonia is initially dominated by polymorphonuclear leukocytes and if it persists, a more mononuclear cell infiltrate. As with other organ systems, a transient population of bloodborne phagocytic cells (polymorphonuclear leukocytes and macrophages) resides in local vessels and is on the ready to emigrate into sites of injury. The first inflammatory cells to respond to the injury via chemotactic mechanisms, usually within 4 to 12 hours, are the polymorphonuclear leukocytes, and if the injury persists, they are followed by macrophages within 24 to 72 hours.

Under circumstances in which the bacteria or other inciting agent persists and is hard to phagocytize, a granulomatous response occurs. The lung's reaction to *Mycobacterium tuberculosis* is a classic example of a granulomatous response; that is, a rim of mononuclear cells (lymphocytes and macrophages) forms around the agent in an attempt to wall it off and prevent it from infiltrating into other tissues. This is a T-cell response dominated by CD4+ T cells and T-helper (Tн-1) cytokines such as IFN-γ. A granulomatous response is associated with diseases such as silicosis, sarcoidosis, and the hypersensitivity lung diseases (e.g., farmer's lung). Whereas the sequela of many acute bacterial and viral pneumonias is resolution to normal tissue, a common sequela of the chronic granulomatous type of response is scar formation (e.g., pulmonary fibrosis). Extensive injury and cell death (necrosis) occur during the granulomatous response; as a result, the body lays down collagen to form scar tissue, which in essence "sews" up the hole left by the necrotic tissue. Scar formation for the most part is nonreversible. It replaces normal functioning tissue and therefore imparts a dysfunctional state in affected areas. Thus if 10% of the lung scars, technically speaking it may lose 10% of its functional capacity, not taking into account compensatory mechanisms.

ALTERED PULMONARY DEFENSE

Today's urban industrial environment coupled with occupations in which airborne particles are inhaled can produce a significant burden even on a normal mucociliary transport system. Chronic lung injury often develops after many years of exposure to these foreign materials. Excessive mucus production stresses the mucociliary transport system and stimulates the cough reflex that helps remove these secretions.

LUNG DISEASES ASSOCIATED WITH ABNORMALITIES OF LUNG DEFENSE

Numerous diseases involving the lung have their origin in abnormalities of lung defense. **Cystic fibrosis** is an autosomal recessive disease characterized by thick, tenacious, dehydrated airway secretions. In this disease, the airway epithelium demonstrates decreased permeability to Cl^- because of failure of the chloride ion channel in the apical cell membrane to open even under stimulation by cAMP. The result is a thick mucus with a water content lower than normal. In addition, in cystic fibrosis there is proliferation of goblet cells and hypertrophy of submucosal glands secondary to irritation and/or abnormalities in surface liquid.

Bronchial secretions in normal individuals owe their viscoelastic properties to the size, length, coiling, and cross-linking of the mucus glycoproteins, resulting in flexible elastic fibers. Normal secretions have low viscosity and long relaxation times (highly elastic). In **asthma**—a disease associated with bronchospasm, airway inflammation, and airway edema—mucus viscosity instead of elasticity becomes the major physical property, and a glycoprotein

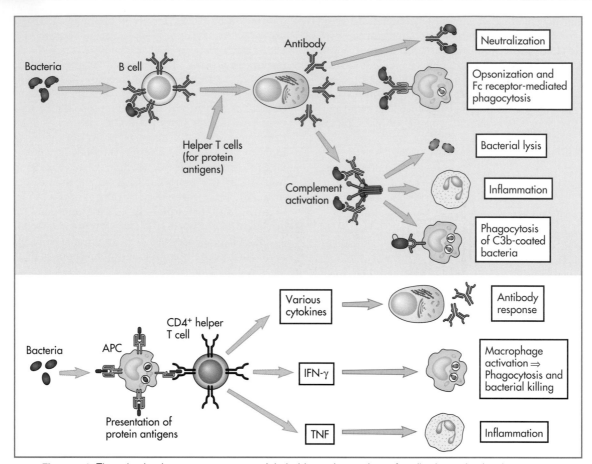

Fig. 11.13 The adaptive immune response to inhaled bacteria consists of antibody production (upper panel) and T-cell activation (lower panel). Antibodies neutralize and eliminate bacteria by several mechanisms, whereas T-cell responses stimulate B-cell antibody responses, macrophage activation, and inflammation. APC, antigen-presenting cell; IFN-γ, interferon-γ; TNF, tumor necrosis factor. (Modified from Abbas AK, Lichtman AH. *Cellular and Molecular Immunology*, 8th ed. Philadelphia: Elsevier; 2015.)

gel is formed. Secretions from individuals with asthma have the highest viscosity of mucus in any disease; on occasion, entire mucus casts of a lobe have been expectorated.

Many processes that result in abnormal ciliary beating are associated with abnormal clearance. Ciliary beating is decreased by hypoxia, repeated exposure to the gas phases of tobacco smoke, very dry air, inflammation, and pollution, particularly of ozone.

Cilia are also destroyed by infection. **Immotile cilia syndrome** is associated with abnormal ciliary microstructure throughout the body and consequently cilia that do not beat. The triad of situs inversus associated with bronchiectasis and sinusitis associated with immotile cilia is known as **Kartagener's syndrome**.

DISEASES ASSOCIATED WITH ABNORMALITIES IN INNATE AND ADAPTIVE IMMUNITY

By far the most common pathologic conditions associated with mucosal tissues are allergic diseases (e.g., allergic asthma, allergic rhinitis, and food and skin allergies). In an allergic response, an antibody synthesis switchover response occurs and IgE, instead of IgA, becomes the predominant antibody synthesized to the allergen. Sensitized T cells and the cytokine IL-4 are required for this to occur. The IgE binds to the surface of tissue mast cells and, upon antigen stimulation, leads to the degranulation of mast cells (Fig. 11.14). The released granules

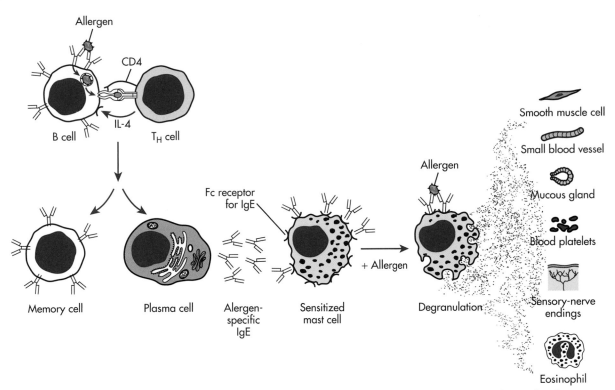

Fig. 11.14 The general mechanism underlying an allergic reaction. Exposure to an allergen activates B cells to form IgE-secreting plasma cells. The secreted IgE molecules bind to IgE-specific Fc receptors on mast cells and blood basophils. Upon a second exposure to the allergen, the bound IgE is cross-linked, triggering the release of pharmacologically active mediators (red) from mast cells and basophils. The mediators cause smooth-muscle contraction, increased vascular permeability, and vasodilation. IgE, immunoglobin E. (From Berne RM, Levy ML, Koeppen BM, Stanton BM, eds. *Physiology*, 5th ed. St. Louis: Mosby; 2004.)

contain many factors, including eosinophil chemotactic factor and leukotrienes with bronchoconstrictor activity. Symptoms of wheezing, cough, and shortness of breath occur within minutes, and locally there is intense eosinophilia and airway edema. Resolution of the inflammatory response can occur spontaneously or in response to therapy (antiinflammatory drugs). Low-grade inflammation may, however, persist and can result in permanent changes in airway structure referred to as **airway remodeling**.

CLINICAL BOX: PERSONALIZED MEDICINE

As our understanding of various lung diseases has increased, so have therapeutic options. In the past asthma was treated with bronchodilators; when the role of inflammation was recognized, treatment with antiinflammatory drugs became first line. More recently, however, monoclonal antibodies against IgE, and against specific inflammatory markers such as IL-4 and IL-5, have been developed. These monoclonal antibodies offer opportunities for targeted therapies tailored to the needs of individuals, especially individuals with difficult-to-control or severe asthma.

Similarly markers have been identified on the surface of non–squamous cell lung cancers (not related to smoking), and drugs to selectively target these cancer cells have recently been developed. This is especially noteworthy because chemotherapeutic agents have for the most part been unsuccessful in treating these cancers.

Continued

CLINICAL BOX: PERSONALIZED MEDICINE—cont'd

An interesting group of difficult-to-diagnose lung diseases, first described in the 1930s, are caused by nonpathologic organisms and dusts. These diseases are known as **hypersensitivity lung diseases** and are associated with an altered immune response to the inciting agent. Only a small percentage of exposed individuals contract the disease, which is caused by the immune response to the agent, and not by the agent itself. It is not a typical allergic response, because the symptoms usually occur 4 to 6 hours after exposure, in contrast to the immediate type of response to allergens; however, some individuals can also have an allergic response. Also, the lesion is not dominated by eosinophils but consists of a polymorphonuclear cell response or a granulomatous-type response followed by pulmonary fibrosis.

Pulmonary complications are common in chronic systemic diseases with possible autoimmune etiologies, including rheumatoid arthritis, systemic lupus erythematosus, and inflammatory bowel diseases (e.g., Crohn's disease, ulcerative colitis). It is not clear why this association exists, but it may be due to a dysregulation of immune responses that initiates a local pulmonary type of autoimmune disease. **Goodpasture's syndrome** is the classic autoimmune response in the lung. It is a pulmonary hemorrhagic disease due to an autoimmune IgG antibody response to type IV collagen in the basement membrane of the lung. Cell injury and death occur through complement activation via an antibody–antigen complex. It is also associated with an intense glomerulonephritis where the disease is thought to have been initiated. The type IV collagen antigen in the kidney basement membrane cross-reacts with the lung basement membrane.

The most common inherited immunoglobulin deficiency is selective **IgA deficiency**, with a prevalence of 1 in 800 births. Although the deficiency is not associated with any specific disease, individuals with the deficiency have a high rate of chronic lung disease, illustrating the importance of this antibody in host defense in the respiratory tract.

SUMMARY

1. The three major components of lung defense against inhaled particles and other inhaled materials are mucociliary transport in the larger airways, phagocytic and inflammatory cells, and a specialized mucosal immune system.

2. The bronchioles and the alveoli are the most sensitive to inhaled toxicants.

3. Sedimented particles (0.2–2.0 μm in diameter) deposit in small airways at the junction of the end of the mucociliary transport system and the terminal respiratory units where alveolar mechanisms are important. This is the Achilles' heel of the respiratory system and plays a significant role in many respiratory diseases.

4. The three components of mucociliary transport are periciliary fluid, mucus, and the cilia.

5. The depth of the periciliary fluid layer is maintained by the balance between chloride secretion and sodium absorption and is essential to normal ciliary beating.

6. Mucus is a complex macromolecule composed of glycoproteins, proteins, electrolytes, and water. The viscoelastic properties of mucus are due to the size,

length, coiling, and cross-linking of the mucus glycoproteins. Normal mucus has low viscosity and high elasticity.

7. Three cell types produce mucus: surface secretory cells, tracheobronchial glands, and Clara cells.

8. Pulmonary alveolar macrophages and dendritic cells are mononuclear phagocytic cells that scavenge particles and bacteria in the airways and alveoli. Polymorphonuclear leukocytes are important in lung defense against established bacterial infection.

9. BALT (bronchus-associated lymphoid tissue) is part of the mucosa-associated lymphoid tissue (MALT) system and is mainly composed of aggregates of lymph nodules throughout the conducting airways.

10. Lymphocytes and their products (B lymphocytes and humoral immunity; T lymphocytes and cell-mediated immunity) are the important components of adaptive immunity.

11. IgA is the predominant antibody produced by plasma cells in BALT; IgG is the predominant antibody in the lower respiratory tract.

12. Allergic diseases are characterized by a switchover response (IgE instead of IgA).

KEYWORDS AND CONCEPTS

Aerosol
Airway remodeling
Alveolar macrophages
Asthma
Bronchus-associated lymphoid tissue (BALT)
Cilia
Clara cells
Cystic fibrosis
Dendritic cells
Diacetyl
Diffusion
Goblet cells (surface secretory cells)
Goodpasture's syndrome
Granulomatous response
Hypersensitivity lung disease
IgA deficiency

Immotile cilia syndrome
Impaction
Kartagener's syndrome
Mucociliary transport
Mucosa-associated lymphoid tissue (MALT)
Mucus
Particulate matter 2.5 μm (PM2.5)
Particulate matter 10 μm (PM10)
Periciliary fluid
Polymorphonuclear leukocytes (neutrophils)
Popcorn lung disease
Secretory component
Secretory IgA
Sedimentation
Silica dust
Tracheobronchial glands

SELF-STUDY PROBLEMS

1. Describe the pathology of the lung in individuals with chronic bronchitis secondary to smoking.
2. What would be the effect on the periciliary fluid layer and mucociliary transport of a drug that blocks sodium absorption and increases intracellular levels of cAMP?
3. Describe the synthesis, structure, and transport mechanisms of IgA.
4. Describe the function of dendritic cells in the lung.
5. How does macrophage phagocytosis of asbestos differ from the usual macrophage processing of microorganisms?
6. Explain how mucosa-associated lymphoid tissues differ from the systemic immune system and lymph nodes.

ADDITIONAL READINGS

1. Arora S, Dev K, Agarwal B, Das P, Syed MA. Macrophages: their role, activation and polarization in pulmonary diseases. *Immunobiology*. 2017. https://doi.org/10.1016/j.imbio.2017.11.001, pii: S0171-2985(17)30207-3.
2. Cook PC, MacDonald AS. Dendritic cells in lung immunopathology. *Semin Immunopathol*. 2016;38(4):449–460.
3. Cosio MG, Bazzan E, Rigobello C, et al. *Ann Am Thoracic Soc*. 2016;13(suppl 4):S305–S310.
4. Daniele RP. Immunoglobulin secretion in the airways. *Annu Rev Physiol*. 1990;52:177.
5. Dickey BF, Knowles MR, Boucher RC. Mucociliary clearnace. In: Grippi MS, Elias JA, Fishman JA, Pack AI, Senior RM, Kotloff R, eds. *Fishman's Pulmonary Diseases and Disorders*. 5th ed. McGraw Hill; 2015.
6. Kubo M. Innate and adaptive type immunity in lung allergic inflammation. *Immunol Rev*. 2017;278(1):162–172. https://doi.org/10.1111/imr.12557.
7. Oberdorster G. Lung clearance of inhaled insoluble and soluble particles. *J Aerosol Med*. 1988;1:289–330.
8. Kerr A. The structure and function of human IgA. *Biochem J*. 1990;271:285.
9. Martonen TB. Deposition patterns of cigarette smoke in human airways. *Am Ind Hyg Assoc*. 1992;53:6–18.
10. Mirra V, Werner C, Santamaria F. Primary ciliary dyskinesia: an update on clinical aspects, genetics, diagnosis, and future treatment strategies. *Front Pediatr*. 2017;5:135. https://doi.org/10.3389/fped.2017.00135.
11. Quon BS, Rowe SM. New and emerging targeted therapies for cystic fibrosis. *BMJ*. 2016;352. https://doi.org/10.1136/bmj.i859.
12. Sheehan JK, Thornton DJ, Somerville M, et al. The structure and heterogeneity of respiratory mucus glycoproteins. *Am Rev Respir Dis*. 1991;144:S4–S9.
13. Sommerhoff CP, Finkbeiner WE. Human tracheobronchial submucosal gland cells in culture. *Am J Respir Cell Mol Biol*. 1990;2:41–50.
14. Verdugo P. Goblet cell secretion and mucogenesis. *Annu Rev Physiol*. 1990;52:157–176.

The Lung Under Special Circumstances

The lung can adapt to a number of special environments and special circumstances, some of which are described here.

EXERCISE

The ability to exercise depends on the capacity of the cardiac and respiratory systems to increase oxygen delivery to the tissues and to remove carbon dioxide from the body (Fig. 12.1). During exercise, energy metabolism is increased through muscle contraction and the conversion of glucose to chemical energy during moderate exercise and the generation of lactic acid during strenuous exercise. Also involved in exercise is the central nervous system (CNS), which delivers coordinated signals to the musculoskeletal system, and the autonomic nervous system, which redistributes blood flow among various organs to meet the demands of exercise.

Both tidal volume and respiratory rate increase with exercise, resulting in an increase in minute ventilation (Fig. 12.2). The increase in minute ventilation with exercise is linearly related to both CO_2 production and O_2 consumption at low to moderate levels (Fig. 12.3). With maximal exercise, a fit young man can achieve an oxygen consumption of 4 L/min with a minute volume of 120 L/min, almost 15 times resting levels, and a cardiac output that increases only 4 to 6 times above resting level. As a result, in normal individuals, the cardiovascular system and not the respiratory system is the rate-limiting factor in exercise.

Work of breathing is also increased during exercise secondary to increases in both lung and chest wall elastic recoil and increases in airway resistance. Larger tidal volumes result in higher lung volumes, and both the lung and the chest wall become less compliant at these higher lung volumes, resulting in increased work to overcome the lung and chest wall elastic recoil. In addition, the airway resistance component of work of breathing increases with the higher flow rates generated during exercise (Table 12.1). These normal changes in work of breathing are exaggerated in individuals with abnormalities in pulmonary mechanics due to airway obstruction or to changes in lung compliance or in oxygenation and can result in exercise limitation.

LUNG VOLUME CHANGES WITH EXERCISE

With exercise, the increase in tidal volume occurs mainly through the inspiratory reserve capacity. Total lung capacity decreases slightly as the central blood volume increases (secondary to increased venous return). Residual volume (RV) and functional residual capacity (FRC) are unchanged or increase slightly. Anatomic dead space increases slightly as a result of airway distention at higher lung volumes. This is associated with a decrease in alveolar dead space as cardiac output increases with exercise. The net effect is no change in physiologic dead space. The ratio of dead space volume to tidal volume (V_{DS}/V_T), however, decreases as V_T increases.

Pulmonary Blood Flow During Exercise

Cardiac output increases linearly with oxygen consumption during exercise (Fig. 12.4). The increase in cardiac output is secondary to primarily an increase in heart rate

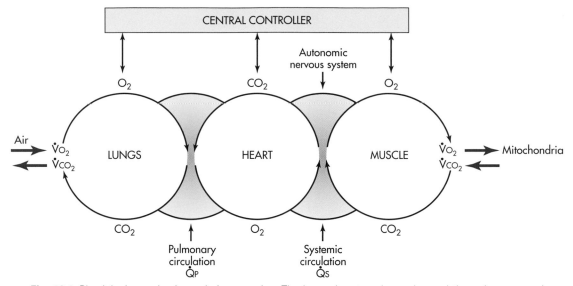

Fig. 12.1 Physiologic mechanisms during exercise. The lungs, heart, and muscles and the pulmonary and systemic circulations are interrelated and regulated by the central controller and the autonomic nervous system and result in processes commensurate with oxygen consumption ($\dot{V}_{O_2}$) and carbon dioxide production ($\dot{V}_{CO_2}$). (Modified and redrawn from Murray J. *The Normal Lung*, 2nd ed. Philadelphia: W.B. Saunders; 1986.)

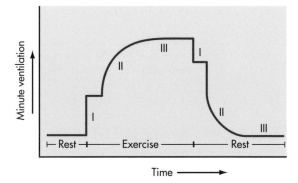

Fig. 12.2 Ventilation before, during, and after exercise. In phase I there is an abrupt increase in ventilation during the transition between rest and exercise. Phase II occurs after approximately 15 s and involves a gradual (exponential) rise in ventilation to reach a new steady state (phase III). Phase III is reached approximately 4 minutes after the onset of exercise. At the end of exercise, there is an abrupt decrease in ventilation (I) followed by a gradual return (II) to the former resting ventilation (III). (Modified from Berne RM, Levy ML, Koeppen BM, Stanton BM. *Physiology*, 5th ed. St. Louis: Mosby; 2004.)

and increased venous return due to deeper inspiratory efforts. Mean pulmonary artery and mean left atrial pressures increase out of proportion to changes in pulmonary blood flow. As a result, there is a decrease in pulmonary vascular resistance. Recruitment of pulmonary blood vessels occurs, especially in upper regions of the lung, and this is associated with a decrease in the regional inhomogeneity observed at rest.

Exercise results in a more uniform ventilation-perfusion ratio ($\dot{V}/\dot{Q}$) throughout the lung, with regional ratios close to 1.0 (Fig. 12.5). Increased pulmonary blood flow during exercise increases the diffusion capacity as oxygen uptake increases. The surface area for diffusion increases as pulmonary blood flow to the upper lung regions increases. Increased velocity of blood flow occurs, and this maintains the partial pressure gradient for diffusion. At maximum levels of exercise associated with high blood velocities, diffusion limitation of gas transfer can occur even in healthy individuals.

Exercise is most remarkable for the lack of significant changes in blood gas values. Except at maximal levels, in general, arterial P_{CO_2} (Pa_{CO_2}) decreases slightly and arterial P_{O_2} (Pa_{O_2}) increases slightly during exercise. Arterial pH remains normal at moderate exercise. During heavy exercise, arterial pH begins to fall as lactic acid is liberated during anaerobic metabolism. This decrease in arterial pH stimulates ventilation out of proportion to the level of exercise intensity and results in a fall in Pa_{CO_2}. The level of exercise at which a sustained metabolic acidosis begins is called the **anaerobic threshold** (Fig. 12.6). This level is different in fit compared with unfit individuals. The AaD_{O_2} also increases during exercise as a result of a number of factors, including

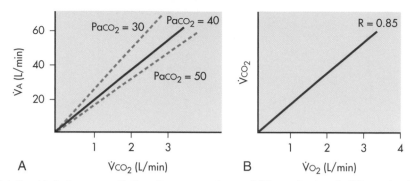

Fig. 12.3 Relationship between ventilation, O_2 consumption, and CO_2 production. **A,** CO_2 production increases linearly with increased minute ventilation ($\dot{V}A$) during exercise to maintain the $Paco_2$ at 40 mm Hg. Levels of ventilation at a moderate level of exercise $CO_2 = 2$ L/min) change with different levels of $Paco_2$. **B,** CO_2 production and O_2 consumption are linearly related. (Modified and redrawn from Leff A, Schumacker P. *Respiratory Physiology: Basics and Applications*. Philadelphia: W.B. Saunders; 1993.)

TABLE 12.1 **Response of the Respiratory System to Exercise**		
Variable	**Moderate Exercise**	**Severe Exercise**
Mechanics of Breathing		
Elastic work of breathing	↑	↑↑
Resistance work of breathing	↑	↑↑
Alveolar Ventilation		
Tidal volume	↑↑	↑↑
Frequency	↑	↑↑
Anatomic dead space	↑	↑
Alveolar dead space (if present)	↓	↓
V_D/V_T	↓	↓↓
Pulmonary Blood Flow	↑	↑↑
Perfusion of upper lung	↑	↑↑
Pulmonary vascular resistance	↓	↓↓
Linear velocity of blood flow	↑	↑↑
Ventilation–Perfusion Matching	↑	↑
Diffusion through the alveolar–capillary barrier	↑	↑↑
Surface area	↑	↑↑
Perfusion limitation	↓	↓↓
Partial pressure gradients	↑	↑↑
Oxygen Unloading at the Tissues	↑	↑↑
Carbon Dioxide Loading at the Tissues	↑	↑↑
PAo_2	↔	↑
Pao_2	↔	↑, ↔, or ↓
$Paco_2$	↔	↓
pH	↔	↓
O_2 extraction ratio	↑	↑↑

↑, increase; ↓, decrease; ↔, no change; ↑↑, greater increase than ↑; ↓↓, greater decrease than ↓.

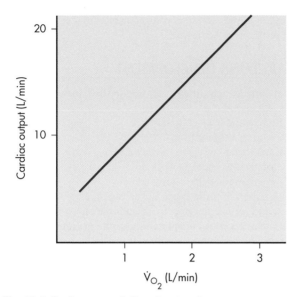

Fig. 12.4 Cardiac output is linearly related to oxygen consumption. (Modified and redrawn from Wilmot R, (ed.). *Chernick and Kendig's Disorders of the Respiratory Tract in Children*, 8th ed. Philadelphia: Elsevier; 2012.)

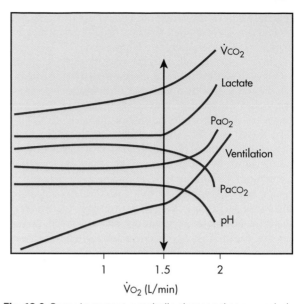

Fig. 12.6 Some important metabolic changes that occur during exercise. The anaerobic threshold (arrow) is marked by a sudden change in the measured variables, which is due mainly to the developing lactic acidosis as anaerobic glycolysis takes over more and more of the muscle energy supply, which is caused by the relative failure of the body to supply sufficient oxygen to the muscles at the rate demanded by the level of exercise. (Modified from Koeppen BM, Stanton BM. *Berne and Levy's Physiology*, 7th ed. Philadelphia: Elsevier; 2018.)

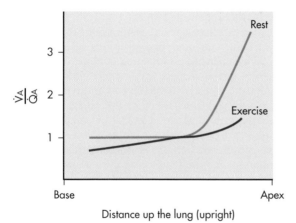

Fig. 12.5 Regional ventilation/perfusion ratios ($\dot{V}_A/\dot{Q}_A$) in the lung at rest and during exercise. During exercise the $\dot{V}_A/\dot{Q}_A$ is more homogeneous than at rest. (Modified and redrawn from Levitzky MG. *Pulmonary Physiology*, 8th ed. New York: McGraw-Hill; 2013.)

diffusion limitation of gas transfer, decreased mixed venous Po_2 ($P\bar{v}_{O_2}$), increased alveolar Po_2 (P_{AO_2}), and shifts in the oxyhemoglobin dissociation curve resulting in increased O_2 unloading at the level of the muscle.

With activity, CO_2 production increases, and as a result, ventilation must increase. At low levels of exercise (CO_2 production of 1 L/min), there are only small differences in the alveolar ventilation needed to maintain the $Paco_2$ over a wide range of values (see Fig. 12.3). As CO_2 production increases with increasing exercise, greater increases in alveolar ventilation are required to maintain the $Paco_2$ within this range of values. Although this is not difficult for the individual with normal pulmonary mechanics, CO_2 elimination can be a significant problem for individuals with altered pulmonary mechanics.

The actual cause of the increased ventilation during exercise remains largely unknown. No single mediator or mechanism has been identified to explain why ventilation remains so closely matched to carbon dioxide production. Hypoxic or hypercarbic mechanisms do not play a role because neither occurs during most exercise. Mechanisms believed to contribute include neural inputs from the motor cortex to the medullary respiratory control center, afferents from muscle and joint mechanoreceptors, and unknown mediators released from working muscles.

EXERCISE TESTING

Exercise testing provides a quantitative assessment of an individual's exercise capacity. A variety of simple and sophisticated tests can be performed to assess exercise capacity. Many of the simpler tests can be performed in the office; more sophisticated tests are usually performed in a hospital's pulmonary function laboratory.

The simplest of all exercise tests is exercise oximetry. Oxygen saturation by pulse oximetry is measured at rest; the individual then exercises until becoming short of breath, and the oxygen saturation is recorded. Two types of tests are commonly done: walking and stair climbing.

In the 6- and 12-minute walk test, the individual is instructed to walk back and forth over a 100-ft distance, and the number of laps is counted. The distance walked over a 6- or 12-minute time period is recorded, and the average rate of walking in miles per hour is calculated. This test is particularly useful for titrating oxygen therapy to ensure adequate oxygenation and enhanced exercise capacity. This test is also used in assessing the severity and response to therapy in individuals with pulmonary artery hypertension.

In the stair-climbing test, the number of steps climbed is counted until the individual's symptoms become limiting. On average, the ability to climb 83 steps is equivalent to a maximal oxygen consumption of 20 mL/kg/min. This value is associated with fewer complications after thoracotomy; thus this is a useful test for individuals with chronic obstructive pulmonary disease (COPD) who are undergoing thoracic surgical procedures.

Formal cardiorespiratory exercise testing requires sophisticated equipment and experienced physiologic direction and medical supervision. Such testing is useful in distinguishing between cardiac and pulmonary causes of dyspnea, determining whether symptoms are the result of deconditioning, conducting disability evaluations, assessing work/job capacity, and identifying the malingering patient.

TRAINING EFFECTS

Training increases the ability to perform exercise. Most of the training effect occurs in skeletal muscles and in the cardiovascular system. Maximum oxygen uptake increases with exercise in large part because of an increase in maximal cardiac output. Training lowers the resting heart rate and increases the resting stroke volume without affecting the maximum heart rate. Physical training increases the oxidative capacity of skeletal muscle, improves the strength and endurance of respiratory muscles, induces mitochondrial proliferation, and increases the concentration of oxidative enzymes and the synthesis of glycogen and triglyceride. This results in increased aerobic energy production capacity and lower blood lactate levels in trained subjects. The lower lactate levels in turn result in decreases in ventilation during submaximal exercise. Physical training, however,

does not appear to affect resting or maximal ventilation or the response to lactic acid.

FETAL LUNG DEVELOPMENT

Fetal lung development can be divided into five stages (Fig. 12.7):
1. Embryonic (day 26 to day 52)
2. Pseudoglandular (day 52 to week 16)
3. Canalicular (week 16 to week 28)
4. Saccular (week 28 to week 36)
5. Alveolar (week 36 to term).

In the embryonic stage, the cells of the conducting airways and alveoli develop from endodermally derived epithelium as a ventral outpouching of the primitive gut. The primary bronchi then elongate into the mesenchyme and divide into two main bronchi and undergo dichotomous branching to form the conducting airways. About 23 to 27 generations of conducting airways are formed, each lined by a columnar epithelium (Fig. 12.8). At the same time, the mesenchyme differentiates around the airways into cartilage, smooth muscle, and connective tissue. By the end of the pseudoglandular stage (16 weeks' gestation), all of the conducting airways, including the terminal respiratory bronchioles, are fully developed.

In the canalicular stage, respiratory bronchioles with terminal air sacs—the first primitive alveoli—develop. There is also marked proliferation of blood vessels in close proximity to the air sacs with a marked decrease in the amount of connective tissue. Type I and type II epithelial cells appear, and lamellar bodies, the storage place for surfactant, become apparent. Toward the end of the canalicular stage, gas exchange becomes possible as the capillaries rapidly proliferate and the epithelial surface thins. This is important for the fetus because ex utero life becomes possible.

During the saccular stage, there is a marked increase in lung growth; the lung grows to fill the thoracic cavity, and increasing numbers of gas exchanging units develop. Acinar development is complete and is the major site of gas exchange, as there are relatively few true alveoli at birth. Alveolar development occurs rapidly after birth, with marked growth in the first 2 years of life.

FETAL RESPIRATION DEVELOPMENT

Respiratory movements have been observed in utero, but regular, automatic respiration begins at birth. The fetus is well suited to its environment in which the lung is not the gas exchange unit. In utero, the placenta is the organ of gas exchange for the fetus. Its microvilli interdigitate with the maternal uterine circulation and O_2 transport and CO_2

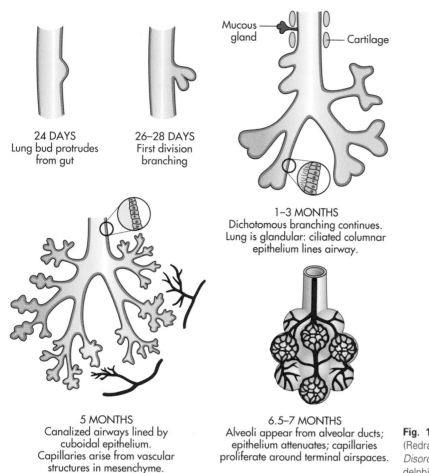

24 DAYS
Lung bud protrudes from gut

26–28 DAYS
First division branching

Mucous gland

Cartilage

1–3 MONTHS
Dichotomous branching continues. Lung is glandular: ciliated columnar epithelium lines airway.

5 MONTHS
Canalized airways lined by cuboidal epithelium. Capillaries arise from vascular structures in mesenchyme.

6.5–7 MONTHS
Alveoli appear from alveolar ducts; epithelium attenuates; capillaries proliferate around terminal airspaces.

Fig. 12.7 Stages of lung fetal development. (Redrawn from Avery ME. *The Lung and Its Disorders in the Newborn Infant*, 3rd ed. Philadelphia: W.B. Saunders; 1974.)

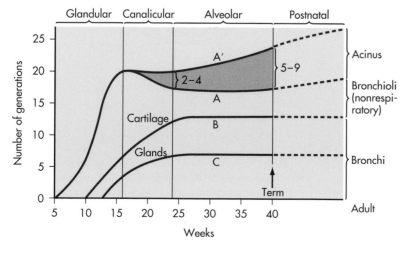

Fig. 12.8 Development of the tracheobronchial tree in utero. Line A represents the number of bronchial generations; line A′ represents the number of respiratory bronchioles and alveolar ducts; line B is the extension of cartilage along the bronchial tree; and line C is the extension of mucous glands. (Redrawn from Bucher U, Reid L. Development of the intrasegmental bronchial tree: the pattern of branching and development of cartilage at various stages of intrauterine life. *Thorax.* 1961;16:207-218.)

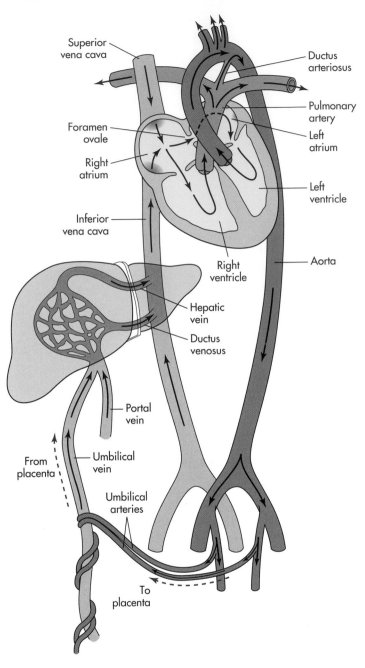

Fig. 12.9 Fetal circulation. In utero, blood is diverted away from the lungs through the foramen ovale and the ductus arteriosus. (Redrawn from Leff A, Schumacker P. *Respiratory Physiology: Basics and Applications*. Philadelphia: W.B. Saunders; 1993.)

removal from the fetus occur by passive diffusion across the maternal circulation. Blood travels through the umbilical artery to the placenta and returns to the fetus through the umbilical vein (Fig. 12.9). Maternal and fetal circulations are separate and the blood of the fetus and mother do not mix, although micro RNA of fetal origin has been detected in the maternal circulation. Compared with adult arterial partial pressures, the Po_2 being delivered to the fetus is low because the uterus extracts its oxygen before delivery to the fetus (Fig. 12.10). Thus the Po_2 in the umbilical vein is only

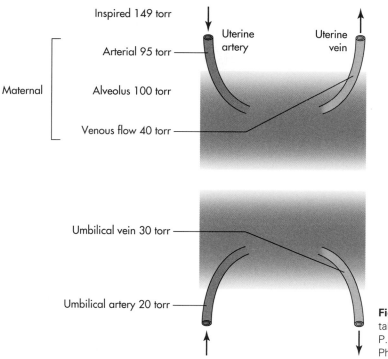

Inspired 149 torr

Maternal
- Arterial 95 torr
- Alveolus 100 torr
- Venous flow 40 torr

Uterine artery

Uterine vein

Umbilical vein 30 torr

Umbilical artery 20 torr

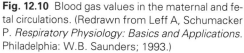

Fig. 12.10 Blood gas values in the maternal and fetal circulations. (Redrawn from Leff A, Schumacker P. *Respiratory Physiology: Basics and Applications.* Philadelphia: W.B. Saunders; 1993.)

30 torr and in the umbilical artery is only 20 torr. The fetus, however, is able to thrive in this environment because of the presence of fetal hemoglobin, which has a substantially greater affinity for oxygen than does adult hemoglobin. Fetal hemoglobin is discussed in Chapter 8.

The fetal lung has no respiratory function in utero, and in fact, very little blood actually circulates through the fetal lung. Venous return from the fetus bypasses the lung, instead passing through a **patent foramen ovale**, an opening in the atrial septum of the fetal heart. The foramen ovale remains open because of the high pulmonary vascular resistance in the fetal lung (due to pulmonary hypoxic vasoconstriction), which results in increased pressure in the right atrium. Most of the venous blood that reaches the right ventricle is diverted into the systemic circulation through a **patent ductus arteriosus**, a connection between the pulmonary artery and the aorta. Again, it is the high pulmonary vascular resistance in the lung that produces a pressure gradient favoring blood flow from the pulmonary artery to the aorta.

Birth marks the end of the placenta and the beginning of respiration. With the first breath, there is an increase in oxygen in the lungs. This results in a rapid and marked decrease (to one-fifth of the systemic circulation) in pulmonary vascular resistance and an increase in blood flow

through the lung. The foramen ovale now closes, and over the first several days of life, the ductus arteriosus also closes, favored by the change in pressure gradients secondary to further decreases in pulmonary vascular resistance and the increased oxygen content in the systemic circulation which closes the ductus arteriosus (unlike other vascular tissue). In some individuals, especially in premature infants, the ductus arteriosus does not close, and surgical closure is required.

POSTNATAL DEVELOPMENT

In the first several months of life, many changes occur in the respiratory system. Newborn infants show a strong preference for nasal breathing ("obligate nose breathers"). This adaptation allows newborn infants to breathe and swallow at the same time, a feat lost in the first year of life. It also results in high airway resistance that can be made worse by nasal congestion. Pulmonary vascular resistance falls and the relatively thick-walled smooth muscle of the pulmonary arterial system thins to adult levels. Airways grow in length and diameter but do not change in number. Alveoli increase in number from approximately 50 million at birth to 300 million in adulthood. Although it is unclear at what age alveolarization

TABLE 12.2   Physiologic Responses to High-Altitude Compared With Sea-Level Control Values

	Immediate	Early Adaptive (72 Hours)	Late Adaptive (2–6 Weeks)
Spontaneous Ventilation			
Minute ventilation	↑	↑	↑
Respiratory rate	Variable	Variable	Variable
Tidal volume	↑	↑	↑
Arterial P_{O_2}	↓	↓	↓
Arterial P_{CO_2}	↓	↓	↓
Arterial pH	↑	↑ ↔	↑ ↔
Arterial HCO_3^-	↔	↓	↓
Evaluation of Lung Function			
Vital capacity	↔	↔	↔
Maximum airflow rates	↑	↑	↑
Functional residual capacity	↔	↔	↔
Ventilatory response to inhaled CO_2	↔	↑	↑
Ventilatory response to hypoxia	↔	↔	↔
Pulmonary vascular resistance	↑	↑	↑
Oxygen Transport			
Hemoglobin	↔	↑	↑
Erythropoietin	↑	↔	↔
P_{10}	↓	↑	↑
2,3-DPG	↔	↑	↑
Cardiac output	↑	↔	↔ ↓
Central Nervous System			
Headaches, nausea, insomnia	↑	↔	↔
Perception, judgmenet	↓	↔	↔
Spinal fluid pH	↑	↔	↔
Spinal fluid HCO_3^-	↔	↓	↓

2,3-DPG, 2,3-diphosphoglycerate; ↑, increased; ↓, decreased; ↔, no change.
Source: Adapted with permission from Guenter CA, Weich MH, Hogg JC: *Clinical Aspects of Respiratory Physiology*. Philadelphia, Lippincott. 1976. p 3–37.

is completed, it is known that it occurs early, perhaps by 2 to 3 years of age and certainly no later than 8 years of age. After completion of alveolarization, alveolar surface area increases in relation to increasing O_2 requirements because alveoli become more complex in shape as they grow.

HIGH ALTITUDE AND ACCLIMATIZATION

At high altitude, ambient air still contains 21% oxygen, but the barometric pressure is lower and the inspired P_{O_2} and alveolar P_{O_2} are decreased. Alveolar and thus arterial P_{CO_2} are also lower because the decreased P_{O_2} stimulates peripheral chemoreceptors. The result of hyperventilation is an increase in arterial P_{O_2} (recall the alveolar air equation) (Table 12.2).

Individuals who ascend from sea level to high altitude (unacclimatized) can experience sudden decreases in arterial oxygen and the rapid onset of signs and symptoms of hypoxia with altered CNS function. These same symptoms are seen in people on airplanes when there is a sudden loss of cabin pressure. Some individuals who ascend quickly to moderate altitudes develop a syndrome called **acute mountain sickness**. Symptoms include headache, sleeplessness, nausea, vision and hearing diminution, weakness, breathlessness, and dyspnea on exertion. The symptoms are secondary to hypoxia and hypocapnia and require immediate descent. In most individuals, symptoms disappear 1 to 3 days after descent.

Another problem in some individuals who go to high altitude is **high-altitude pulmonary edema.** Symptoms include severe dyspnea, orthopnea, cough, and copious crackles, sometimes to the point of coughing up pink, frothy fluid. High-altitude pulmonary edema is a life-threatening illness. Individuals with this problem should be advised against returning to high altitude, as the problem is likely to recur. A similar problem, known as **high-altitude cerebral edema,** associated with the CNS symptoms of confusion, ataxia, hallucinations, and loss of consciousness, can also occur and requires immediate descent.

Some individuals who reside in high-altitude areas develop a syndrome known as **chronic mountain sickness,** characterized by cyanosis, fatigue, marked polycythemia, and profound hypoxemia. These individuals need to descend to lower altitudes.

Long-term acclimatization to high altitude, however, occurs in most individuals and begins within hours of ascent to high altitude. Hyperventilation is one of the most important features of acclimatization. Renal compensation for the respiratory alkalosis begins within hours, characterized by bicarbonate excretion and hydrogen ion conservation. Hypoxia stimulates erythropoiesis, increasing the hematocrit and oxygen-carrying capacity. As a result, oxygen content (not Pao_2) increases. Although the polycythemia (increased hematocrit) increases oxygen content, it also increases blood viscosity, which increases ventricular workload. Oxygen release at the tissues is enhanced through increased production of 2,3-diphosphoglycerate secondary to respiratory alkalosis and a rightward shift of the oxyhemoglobin dissociation curve.

Hypoxic stimulation of the peripheral chemoreceptors continues at high altitude, but the ventilatory response curve to CO_2 shifts to the left. Thus at any level of arterial CO_2, the ventilatory response is greater after several days at high altitude. Coincident with this shift, cerebrospinal fluid pH returns to normal and CNS symptoms abate.

Cardiac output, heart rate, and systemic blood pressure increase with ascent to high altitude. After a month or so, these changes return to baseline as a result of a decrease in sympathetic activity. However, pulmonary hypoxic vasoconstriction and pulmonary hypertension persist, leading to right ventricular hypertrophy and cor pulmonale.

Persons born at high altitude have a diminished ventilatory response to hypoxia, whereas those who are born at sea level and subsequently move to high altitude have a normal ventilatory response to hypoxia even after residing at high altitude for a long time. Thus it appears that the ventilatory response to hypoxia is determined at a young age.

CLINICAL BOX

Carbon dioxide and black carbon are the leading greenhouse gases implicated in global warming, and increased levels have resulted in changing weather patterns, including hotter seasonal temperatures in the summer and increased ground-level ozone and outdoor air pollutants such as fine particulate matter (PM). They also drive more extreme weather events. These changes increase the volume of allergenic materials. One result of climate change is **thunderstorm asthma.** The rainwater from thunderstorms hydrates and ruptures pollen grains, releasing inhalable aeroallergens that normally would be too large for respiration. When these thunderstorms occur during a high pollen season such as spring and summer, asthma epidemics can occur. In Australia, eight people with asthma died and 10,000 required hospital treatment after a severe thunderstorm released high levels of rye grass pollen. Hurricanes have been similarly implicated, as have wildfires, which can also result in dissemination of PM matter.

SUMMARY

1. With moderate levels of exercise, the increase in minute ventilation is linearly related to both CO_2 production and O_2 consumption.
2. In normal individuals, the cardiovascular system, and not the respiratory system, is the rate-limiting factor in exercise.
3. Cardiac output increases linearly with oxygen consumption during exercise.
4. In general, arterial blood gases change little during exercise.
5. The anaerobic threshold occurs when a sustained metabolic acidosis develops during exercise. Training shifts the location of the anaerobic threshold to the right but does not change the maximum heart rate that is achievable.
6. Fetal lung development is divided into five stages: embryonic, pseudoglandular, canalicular, saccular, and alveolar.
7. Airways are fully formed by the 16th week of gestation. Alveoli at birth are relatively few in number and increase dramatically in the first 2 to 3 years of life.
8. Primitive alveoli develop during the latter stages of the canalicular phase of growth and mark the earliest stage of gas exchange and possible extrauterine life.

9. The fetal lung has no respiratory function in utero. Pulmonary hypoxic vasoconstriction is responsible for the maintenance of the patency of the foramen ovale and the ductus arteriosus.

10. High altitude is associated with a decrease in barometric pressure and decreases in Pao_2 and $Paco_2$.

11. Various syndromes are associated with high altitude, including acute and chronic mountain sickness, high-altitude pulmonary edema, and high-altitude cerebral edema.

12. Hyperventilation is a major feature of acclimatization and results in renal, CNS, and hematologic compensatory mechanisms. Hypoxia stimulates red blood cell production, resulting in polycythemia and an increase in oxygen-carrying capacity.

KEYWORDS AND CONCEPTS

6- and 12-minute walk test
Acclimatization
Acute mountain sickness
Anaerobic threshold
Canalicular stage
Chronic mountain sickness
Climate change
Embryonic stage
Global warming
High-altitude cerebral edema

High-altitude pulmonary edema
Oximetry
Patent ductus arteriosus
Patent foramen oval
Pseudoglandular stage
Saccular stage
Stair-climbing test
Thunderstorm asthma
Training

SELF-STUDY PROBLEMS

1. What factors limit maximal exercise?
2. What happens to minute ventilation before and after the anaerobic threshold? Why?
3. What is the effect of training on maximum heart rate and cardiac output, respiratory muscle strength, and endurance and ventilation?
4. In congenital diaphragmatic hernia (CDH), the diaphragm fails to close between the thoracic and abdominal cavity. This normally occurs by the 16th week of gestation. As a result, abdominal cavity contents fill the space and prevent normal lung development. What components of the respiratory tract (airways, blood vessels, interstitium, and alveoli) will be involved in individuals with CDH?
5. Describe fetal circulation and the circulatory changes that occur at birth.
6. What are the effects of high altitude on arterial oxygenation, lung fluid balance, and the central nervous system?

ADDITIONAL READINGS

Adamson IY. Development of lung structure. In: Crystal RG, West JB, Barnes PJ, eds. *The Lung: Scientific Foundation*. New York: Raven Press; 1997.

Bangsbo J. Quantification of anaerobic energy production during intense exercise. *Med Sci Sports Exerc*. 1998;30:47–52.

Bhaqi S, Srivastava S, Singh SB. High-altitude pulmonary edema: a review. *J Occup Health*. 2015;52(4):235–243.

Cibella F, Cuttitta G, Romano S, et al. Respiratory energetics during exercise at high altitude. *J Appl Physiol*. 1999;86:1785–1792.

D'Amato G, Holgate ST, Pawankar R, et al. Meteorological conditions, climate change, new emerging factors and asthma and related allergic disorders. A statement of the world allergy organization. *World Allergy Organ J*. 2015;8(1):25. https://doi.org/10.1186/s40413-015-0073-0.

Harding R, Hooper SB. Regulation of lung expansion and lung growth before birth J. *Appl Physiol*. 1996;81:209–224.

Kotecha S. Lung growth: implications for the newborn infant. *Arch Dis Child Fetal Neonatal Ed*. 2000;82:F69–F74.

Shoene RB. Limits of human lung function at high altitude. *J Exp Biol*. 2001;204:3121–3127.

*West J, Hackett P, Maret K, et al. Pulmonary gas exchange on the summit of Mt Everest. *J Appl Physiol*. 1983;55:678–687.

---

*A classic.

Answers to Self-Study Problems

CHAPTER 1

1. The alveolar–capillary unit has a large surface area for gas exchange. In addition, there is a short distance between the alveolus and the red blood cell, and the unit as a whole takes the entire cardiac output. These features make it ideal to function as the gas-exchanging unit.

2. Type II cells cover almost the entire alveolar surface (93%) with their broad, thin extensions. They do not divide and are especially susceptible to injury. Type II cells are cuboidal and located in the corners of alveoli. They are more numerous than type I cells. The hallmark of type I cells are the osmiophilic lamellar inclusion bodies that contain surfactant. Upon injury, type II cells multiply and eventually become type I cells.

3. The pulmonary circulation is a low-pressure, high-compliance system. At rest, many of the vessels are either compressed or not open. Increases in pulmonary flow either universally, as would occur during exercise, or locally, as would occur if one of the main pulmonary arteries were occluded, are associated with maintenance of low pressure, as compressed or occluded vessels open and open vessels distend. Thus transient occlusion of the left main pulmonary artery would double the blood flow through the right pulmonary artery, but this increase in flow would produce only a small change in the pressure in the right pulmonary artery and would certainly not double it.

4. The barrier between gas in the alveolus and the red blood cell consists of the type I alveolar epithelial cell, the capillary endothelial cell, and their respective basement membranes. The distance of the barrier is approximately 1 to 2 μm.

5. The principal function of the lung is gas exchange. The anatomic features that make the lung ideally suited for this function include the large surface area for gas exchange, with millions of alveoli and capillaries; the close proximity between gas in the alveolus and the red blood cell; the dual circulation of the lung, resulting in the entire cardiac output going through the lung; the

structure of the type I cell, with its thin, elongated cytoplasm that reduces the distance between alveolar gas and the pulmonary capillary; and the highly distensible, low-pressure pulmonary circulation that allows for accommodation over a wide range of cardiac outputs without a significant change in pressure.

CHAPTER 2

1. Factors that determine total lung capacity (TLC) include lung elastic recoil and the properties of the muscles of the chest wall. TLC occurs when the forces of inspiration decrease because of chest wall muscle lengthening and are insufficient to overcome the lung's elastic recoil.

2. Residual volume occurs when the forces exerted by expiratory muscle shortening decrease and are insufficient to overcome the outward recoil of the chest wall.

3. Acute hypersensitivity pneumonitis is associated with an increased number of cells and material in the alveoli and interstitium and is an example of a restrictive lung disease. Thus lung volumes will be reduced. Specifically, TLC and, to a lesser extent, functional residual capacity (FRC) and residual volume (RV) are decreased, resulting in an increase in the RV/TLC ratio.

4. Surfactant increases lung compliance overall. In addition, surfactant stabilizes individual alveoli by increasing surface tension at high alveolar volumes and decreasing surface tension as lung volume decreases.

CHAPTER 3

1. Increasing lung volume increases the length and diameter of the airways. As a result, resistance to airflow decreases with increases in lung volume, but the relationship is curvilinear. At lung volumes greater than FRC, there is little effect on total airway resistance. Below FRC, resistance increases rapidly and approaches infinity at RV.

2. The cross-sectional area of a conducting airway is determined by the forces of contraction (i.e., the elastic forces

in the airways and the tension of the smooth muscle surrounding the airways) and the forces of dilation or outward traction (i.e., a positive transpulmonary pressure or the interdependence of alveoli and terminal bronchioles).

3. A reduction in elastic recoil pressure, which is present in individuals with emphysema, will result in a decrease in the driving pressure for expiratory gas flow and in premature airway closure in association with movement of the equal pressure point closer to the alveoli.

4. Airway resistance is determined by flow rate (the more laminar the airflow, the lower the resistance), and airflow velocity becomes very low as the effective cross-sectional area increases. Furthermore, the airways exist in parallel, and as a result the many small airways contribute little to the resistance.

CHAPTER 4

1. A–D.
   A. The test appears to be performed in a satisfactory way with a rapid rise to peak flow and a gradual, smooth decline to residual volume. Compared with the normal curve (dotted line), peak flow and expiratory flow rates are decreased. Forced vital capacity (FVC) is normal, with a decreased forced expiratory volume after 1 second (FEV_1); this would result in a decrease in the FEV_1/FVC ratio. These changes are consistent with obstructive pulmonary disease (OPD); the magnitude is approximately 50%, and thus this is moderate OPD.

   B. The test demonstrates a rapid rise and a smooth decline to the baseline compatible with acceptable quality. The FVC and FEV_1 are reduced, with a normal FEV_1/FVC ratio. Expiratory flow rates are normal. These changes are consistent with restrictive pulmonary disease; the magnitude is reduced 25% to 50%; thus this is mild-to-moderate restrictive lung disease.

   C. The test demonstrates a rapid rise to peak flow, a saw-toothed decline, and an abrupt drop in flow to the baseline. The effort as demonstrated by the initial rise is good, but the subject either coughed (sawtooth) or periodically closed the glottis when exhaling. In addition, the subject did not exhale to residual volume (abrupt drop in flow). Thus this flow volume curve is uninterpretable.

   D. There is a rapid rise to peak flow followed by a gradual, smooth decline to zero flow or baseline. This is an acceptable test. The FVC and FEV_1 are normal and have a normal ratio. Expiratory flow rates at high lung volume (i.e., early in the maneuver or close to TLC) are normal; flow rates at low lung volume (i.e., late in the maneuver or close to RV) are reduced. This is an example of mild obstructive pulmonary disease (OPD) involving the small airways. It is what you might find in an asymptomatic 20 pack-per-year cigarette smoker.

2. Early in chronic OPD, the spirogram and flow volume curve are normal, but evidence of air trapping (i.e., an elevated RV/TLC ratio) may be present. As the disease progresses, there is further air trapping in association with decreased expiratory flow rates, particularly involving the small airways (see Answer 1D). With further progression, peak flow and airway resistance (Raw) are affected and FEV_1 becomes decreased. When the FVC begins to decrease, the individual has moderate-to-severe obstructive pulmonary disease; when the FVC is below 50% of predicted, the individual has severe obstructive pulmonary disease. Emphysema and chronic bronchitis can both produce pulmonary function abnormalities as already described. The two diseases can be distinguished by the diffusion capacity for carbon monoxide (DLco). The DLco is normal in chronic bronchitis, whereas it is decreased in emphysema.

3. In individuals with restrictive pulmonary disease, both the FVC and the FEV_1 are decreased but proportionately. This occurs in association with normal (and even supernormal) expiratory flow rates (see Answer 1B) and with decreases in TLC, and less so in RV (resulting in an elevated RV/TLC ratio due to a decrease in TLC). Compliance is also reduced in many (but not all) restrictive lung diseases. As the disease progresses, there is further reduction in these pulmonary function measurements with eventual decreases in expiratory flow rates.

4. A normal DLco requires a normal surface area for gas diffusion. This is the major requirement. However, decreased perfusion secondary to emboli or decreased cardiac output or decreased capillary blood volume such as in anemia also contributes to an abnormal DLco.

CHAPTER 5

1. As tidal volume (V_T) increases, there is a decrease in dead space ventilation (V_{DS}) for the same minute ventilation (V_E):

   V_T = 500 mL If V_{DS} is 150mL then
   V_E = V_T − V_{DS} = 350 mL
   When V_T is 600 mL for the same V_E
   V_{DS} = 600 mL − 350 mL = 250 mL

2. Using Fowler's method, the dead space is equal to the volume of the anatomic dead space that contains 100% oxygen and 0% nitrogen plus ½ of the rising nitrogen volume, or

$$V_{DS} = 130 + 1/2 \ (170 - 130) = 150 \ ml \ .$$

3. At Pike's Peak, the partial pressure of inspired air is

$$PI_{O_2 dry} = (445 \ mm \ Hg) \times 0.21 = 93 \ mm \ Hg \ .$$

The air in the conducting airways is

$$PIO_2 = (445 \ mm \ Hg - 47 \ mm \ Hg) \times 0.21$$
$$= 83.6 \ mm \ Hg \ .$$

4. From the alveolar air equation, it can be seen that an increase in Pa_{CO_2} will result in a decrease in alveolar P_{O_2}. This has significant implications in the face of a decrease in the oxygen in inspired air (PI_{O_2}). One of the ways that we can increase alveolar P_{O_2} is by changing alveolar P_{CO_2}. At high altitudes we hyperventilate and decrease alveolar CO_2; this results in an increase in alveolar P_{O_2}.

5. If alveolar ventilation is constant but CO_2 production increases, there will be an increase in alveolar (arterial) CO_2. As a result, using the alveolar air equation, alveolar P_{O_2} will decrease. This is most commonly seen in individuals who are being mechanically ventilated under significant sedation or in patients who are paralyzed, who are on mechanical ventilators, and who develop fever. These individuals will develop an increase in P_{CO_2} in association with a decrease in P_{O_2} as a result of the increase in CO_2 production that is due to the fever.

6. In the upright position, the pleural pressure gradient is most negative at the apex and decreases (becomes less negative) in the dependent regions of the lung. As a result, alveoli at the apex of the lung are bigger, and because of where they are located on the pressure volume curve of the lung, they are less compliant. Thus with tidal volume breathing, most of the ventilation goes to the alveoli at the base or dependent region. The vertical pressure gradient is maintained when you are standing on your head, but it is now reversed. Namely, the apex of the lung is the dependent portion; its surrounding pleural pressure is less negative; as a result, the alveoli in the apex are now smaller than alveoli at the base of the lung and are positioned at the steeper portion of the pressure volume curve; thus these now dependent alveoli receive a greater portion of the tidal volume.

CHAPTER 6

1. The relationship between total pulmonary vascular resistance and lung volume in the entire lung is described by a U-shaped curve. Total pulmonary vascular resistance (PVR) is lowest near FRC and increases at both high and low lung volumes. The pulmonary vascular resistance in alveolar vessels increases with increasing lung volume and distention of the air-filled alveoli. Pulmonary vascular resistance in extraalveolar vessels decreases with increasing lung volume due to stretching and an increase in vessel diameter caused by radial traction.

2. Pulmonary blood flow is dramatically affected by gravity. In the absence of gravity, pulmonary blood flow throughout the lung would be equal.

3. A decrease in pulmonary artery pressure, if sufficient, would result in the appearance of Zone I regions in the uppermost areas of the lung. A decrease in pulmonary venous pressure could also convert Zone II regions into Zone III regions.

4. Exposure to high altitude results in a decrease in alveolar oxygen tension. This can cause hypoxic vasoconstriction throughout the lung, resulting in an increase in pulmonary arterial pressures due to an increase in pulmonary vascular resistance.

5. Oxygen is a potent vasodilator. During cardiac catheterization, oxygen is administered to determine whether the pulmonary vasculature is responsive to oxygen. Responsiveness to oxygen is measured by a decrease in pulmonary artery pressure with oxygen administration.

CHAPTER 7

1. An anatomic shunt does not respond to breathing 100% oxygen, whereas a physiologic shunt will have a blunted response (the extent of which is dependent on the degree of the physiologic shunt). In contrast, low $\dot{V}/\dot{Q}$ will respond to increasing the ambient oxygen concentration. Hypoventilation with hypoxemia will have a normal AaD_{O_2}.

2. At the level of a single alveolus, the Pa_{O_2} is equal to the alveolar ventilation divided by the capillary flow.

3. With $\dot{V}/\dot{Q}$ inequality, blood from normally ventilated alveoli mixes with blood from lung regions with low ventilation. Because the relationship between oxygen content and partial pressure is sigmoidal, ventilation of normally ventilated alveoli cannot significantly increase the oxygen content in the blood leaving them. This same relationship for CO_2 is more linear; thus excessive ventilation of some alveoli can effectively compensate for underventilation of other alveoli with regard to CO_2

exchange. This difference results in a low arterial P_{O_2} with a normal P_{CO_2} in many lung diseases until the process is very advanced and compensation can no longer occur for CO_2.

CHAPTER 8

1. The oxyhemoglobin dissociation curve is shifted to the right (increased P_{50}, decreased O_2 affinity) with increases in temperature, P_{CO_2}, and levels of 2,3-diphosphoglycerate (2,3-DPG) and decreases in pH. The curve is shifted to the left (decreased P_{50}, increased O_2 affinity) with decreases in temperature, P_{CO_2}, and 2,3-DPG and increases in pH.
2. The shifts in the oxyhemoglobin dissociation curve aid in the uptake of O_2 and unloading of CO_2 in the lung and in the uptake of O_2 and unloading of CO_2 by the tissues.
3. Yes. Oxygen content and oxygen saturation do not measure the same thing. For example, oxygen content is low in anemia, but the saturation is normal. Other causes include poor circulation and poisoning of the mitochondrial transport systems (e.g., CO poisoning).
4. O_2 is primarily transported in two forms: dissolved and chemically bound to hemoglobin. CO_2 is transported in three forms: physically dissolved, as carbamino compounds, and as bicarbonate ions.
5. When hemoglobin is fully saturated, supplemental oxygen will not appreciably affect the Hgb O_2 content. When hemoglobin is not fully saturated, such as in individuals with a P_{aO_2} less than 60 mm Hg, supplemental oxygen will markedly increase oxygen saturation and thus increase Hgb O_2 content.
6. Tissue hypoxia occurs when the cells or tissues in the body do not receive adequate oxygen to carry out their metabolic functions, and as a result, tissues switch from oxidative metabolism to anaerobic metabolism. There are four mechanisms of tissue hypoxia: hypoxic hypoxia due to lung disease, anemic hypoxia secondary to inadequate numbers of red blood cells, circulatory hypoxia when there is a marked decrease in cardiac output, and histologic hypoxia due to mitochondrial function poisons.
7. A gas leaving the capillary that has reached equilibrium with alveolar gas is perfusion-limited, whereas a gas leaving the capillary that has not reached equilibrium with alveolar gas is diffusion-limited. The major factors determining whether a gas is perfusion- or diffusion-limited are its solubility in the membrane, its solubility in the blood, and its ability to bind chemically to hemoglobin. Under normal conditions, both O_2 and CO_2 are perfusion-limited; however, they can become diffusion-limited, with very rapid red cell transit in the pulmonary circulation.

CHAPTER 9

1–5. Correct matches are in boldface type.
- a–3. Using the alveolar air equation, the AaD_{O_2} is $[0.21 \times (760 - 47) - 40/0.8] - 110 = -10$ mm Hg; thus this is an impossible gas value on room air. Looked at another way, the sum of the P_{aO_2} and P_{aCO_2} on room air at sea level should not be greater than 130 mm Hg.
- b–4. The pH is less than 7.4, suggesting that there is an acidosis. For the elevated P_{aCO_2} to account for the change in pH of 0.06 units, the increase must be chronic ($0.03 \times 20/10$ mm Hg = 0.06 units). Using the alveolar air equation, the AaD_{O_2} is $[0.21 \times (760 - 47) - 60/0.8] - 60 = 15$ mm Hg; this is a normal alveolar-arterial difference demonstrating normal lung parenchyma. Therefore this individual has chronic hypoventilation with normal lung parenchyma.
- c–1. The pH is less than 7.4, suggesting that there is an acidosis. In this case the P_{aCO_2} is also low—a compensation for the acidosis. Therefore this must be a metabolic acidosis. What would you predict the base excess to be in this individual? The answer is −10 (0.15 change in pH is associated with a 10 mEq/L change in base excess.) Using the alveolar air equation, the $AaD_{O_2} = [(0.21 \times 760 - 47) - 25/0.8] - 110 = 9$ mm Hg, which is normal, demonstrating no pulmonary parenchymal disease. Thus this individual has a metabolic acidosis (with respiratory compensation).
- d–5. This individual has an abnormal AaD_{O_2}. ($AaD_{O_2} = P_{AO_2} - P_{aO_2} = [0.21 \times (760 - 47) - 30/0.8] - 50$ mm Hg = 62 mm Hg). The hyperventilation (low P_{aCO_2}) appears acute in nature (pH increases 0.08 units for a 10 mm Hg decrease in P_{aCO_2}). Why is this individual hyperventilating? In the presence of hypoxia, hyperventilation will increase the P_{aO_2}. The P_{aO_2} in this individual would be approximately 10 mm Hg lower if this individual did not hyperventilate (if the partial pressure of one gas increases, the other must decrease). The actual amount can be calculated again using the alveolar air equation: $0.21 \times (760 - 47) - 40/0.8 = 100$; in the presence of an $AaD_{O_2} = 62$ mm Hg, the P_{aO_2} is $100 - 62 = 38$ mm Hg. Thus by hyperventilating and decreasing the P_{aCO_2} by 10 mm Hg, this individual achieved a 12 mm Hg increase in P_{aO_2}.
- e–2. This individual has an elevated pH and a mildly elevated P_{aCO_2}. Because it is unusual

to overcompensate, the underlying process is most likely a metabolic alkalosis with respiratory compensation. Is there evidence of underlying lung disease in this arterial blood gas? Using the alveolar air equation, the $AaDo_2 = [0.21 \times (760 - 47) - 45/0.8] - 80 = 14$ mm Hg. This is within the normal range, so this individual does not have pulmonary parenchymal disease. What would the HCO_3^- be in this individual? (Answer: >24 mEq/L)

6. The correct answer is a. The pH is less than 7.35, and therefore the infant has an acidosis. The base excess of -12 mEq/L is indicative of a metabolic acidosis probably secondary to dehydration. This acidosis should be associated with a 0.15 unit decrease in pH. The pH, however, is decreased only 0.08 units. This is because there is a 15 mm Hg decrease in $Paco_2$, a compensatory respiratory alkalosis (expected pH increase of between 0.12 units with a 15 mm decrease in $Paco_2$ if acute and 0.045 units if chronic). In addition, there is mild hypoxemia ($Pao_2 = 0.21 \times (760 - 47) - 25/0.8 = 119$; $AaDo_2 = 119 - 66 = 53$. The hypoxemia in this case is due to the bronchiolitis.

7. The correct answer is d. The pH is less than 7.35, and therefore this individual has an acidosis. Because of his underlying lung disease, you suspect that the increase in $Paco_2$ is at least partially chronic. An increase of 27 mm Hg, if chronic, should be associated with a decrease in pH of ~0.08 units. Thus all of the change in pH is due to chronic respiratory disease. Despite oxygen therapy, this individual remains hypoxemic.

CHAPTER 10

1. Hyperventilation will reduce the arterial $Paco_2$ and will cause an increase in cerebrospinal fluid (CSF) and arterial pH and a reduction in respiratory drive. When an individual is swimming, O_2 will be consumed (CO_2 will begin to rise), but the major stimulus to breathe—a fall in Pao_2—will not occur until the Pao_2 is reduced to 50 to 60 torr. The swimmer is thus at risk for hypoxemia before the hypercarbic stimulus to breathe is activated.

2. The decrease in Pio_2 with altitude results in a decrease in Pao_2 and Pao_2, according to the alveolar air equation. The reduced Pao_2 stimulates the carotid bodies, and ventilation increases in response to this hypoxic stimulus. This results in a decrease in $Paco_2$ and a respiratory alkalosis. CO_2 also diffuses freely out of the CSF, whereas H^+ and HCO_3^- diffuse very slowly. This results in a marked increase in CSF pH and a decrease in the respiratory stimulus to the central respiratory center.

The increased arterial pH may be brought back to normal by renal compensation that occurs over 24 to 48 hours. At the same time, through ion transport in the brain, the CSF pH approaches the pH of arterial blood, and the central respiratory center is again stimulated by a near normal $[H^+]$, so that the hypoxic stimulus on the carotid bodies becomes fully effective.

3. The sensitivity of the carotid bodies to low Pao_2 is elevated when $Paco_2$ is elevated.

4. Barbiturates and other centrally active anesthetics are known to depress the respiratory center. Central respiratory depression occurs as a result of overdosage of these drugs and results in life-threatening hypercapnia and hypoxia.

CHAPTER 11

1. Smoking can result in emphysema, chronic bronchitis, and lung cancer. In individuals with chronic bronchitis, the lung pathology consists of goblet cell hyperplasia and hypertrophy with extension of the goblet cells into smaller airways beyond the 12th tracheobronchial division, where they normally disappear. In addition, there is mucus gland hypertrophy, with a change in mucus viscosity and elasticity. The airway lumen contains increased mucus, including mucous plugs. Cilia are affected by the smoke, with decreased activity. The combination of decreased ciliary activity and increased and abnormal mucus production results in decreased mucociliary transport. Carbon from the smoke is deposited at bifurcations in small airways due to impaction and sedimentation of particles in the smoke.

2. A drug that inhibits sodium absorption from the airway lumen (such as amiloride) would result in an increase in periciliary fluid. Increased cyclic adenosine monophosphate (cAMP) levels in the airway epithelial cell would open chloride channels and result in increased chloride and secondary water in the airway lumen. Both of these would increase the depth of the periciliary fluid and could result in cilia splashing around in the fluid and a decrease in mucociliary transport effectiveness. This is an example of too much of a good thing. Fortunately, most drugs either inhibit sodium absorption or increase chloride secretion but do not do both.

3. Plasma cells in the submucosa of the lung in response to interleukin (IL)-6 synthesize and secrete immunoglobulin (Ig)A in a dimer form linked by a J-chain. The dimer migrates to the submucosal surface of epithelial cells where it binds to the protein receptor poly Ig, which aids in its pinocytosis and secretion into the airway lumen. During exocytosis of the IgA complex, the poly Ig is enzymatically cleaved, leaving a portion, the

secretory piece, still associated with the complex. The secretory piece stays attached to the dimer and aids in its protection from proteolytic cleavage in the lumen.

4. Dendritic cells (DCs) are derived from the myeloid lineage of monocytes and macrophages and are a major cell type for antigen presentation to T cells. DCs have been found in the periphery of many tissues and function most likely as sentinels, not only to capture antigens but also to bring and process them to lymphocytes in the various lymphoid tissues. There are two known sources of DCs, the first being developmentally from CD 34$^+$ progenitor cells in the bone marrow. The other source is the differentiation of blood monocytes in response to the cytokines such as granulocyte macrophage-colony stimulating factor (GM-CSF) GM-CSF and IL-4. DCs are commonly found throughout the respiratory tract in the parenchyma of the lung, from the trachea to the alveolus, and are usually associated with the epithelium. The upper airways are more densely populated with DCs than the smaller airways in the more peripheral regions of the lung. The anatomic location of these cells correlates well with particle deposition in the airways. Immature DCs capture and process antigen, and mature DCs have a more immunoregulatory role.

5. Macrophages phagocytize particles and digest them to amino acids in lysosomes. After ingesting an organism or particle, macrophages undergo a burst of metabolic activity and kill the organism or dissolve the particle. Ingestion is rapid and is not associated with an inflammatory response. The alveolar macrophage, however, is unable to dissolve asbestos; the sharp crystal punctures lysosomes that release their product intracellularly. The macrophage dies and, in the process of dying, releases chemotactic factors that cause fibroblast migration and collagen synthesis, which attracts other macrophages into the area. These macrophages ingest the asbestos, and the process recurs. As a result, the alveolar macrophage localizes asbestos in the airways, and this process results in pulmonary fibrosis.

6. The lymphoid tissues of the mucosal areas (MALT) somewhat resemble actual lymph nodes with a similar repertoire of immune cells. In contrast to lymph nodes, however, these tissues are not encapsulated and are composed mainly of aggregates or clusters of lymphocytes residing in submucosal regions. In addition to aggregates of cells, MALT contains a substantial number of solitary B and T lymphocytes, which are scattered regularly throughout the tissue within the connective tissue of the lamina propria (lamina propria lymphocytes) and the epithelial layer (intraepithelial lymphocytes). The B cells found in MALT have a selectivity for differentiation into IgA-secreting plasma cells when stimulated by antigen.

CHAPTER 12

1. In healthy individuals, maximal exercise is cardiac-limited—specifically, limited by the heart rate and stroke volume. These factors determine the amount of oxygen delivery to the muscles during maximal activity. In normal, healthy individuals, exercise is never pulmonary-limited.

2. At the beginning of exercise, both tidal volume and respiratory rate increase, resulting in an increase in minute ventilation. This increase is linearly related to both CO_2 production and O_2 consumption. At high to maximal levels of exercise, arterial pH begins to fall as lactic acid is liberated during anaerobic metabolism. The fall in pH stimulates ventilation out of proportion to the level of exercise intensity, and this results in a fall in arterial P_{CO_2}.

3. Maximum heart rate does not change with training. Rather, training lowers the resting heart rate and increases the resting stroke volume. Training increases the oxidative capacity of skeletal muscles and improves strength and endurance of respiratory muscles. As a result, there is increased aerobic capacity with greater exercise, as well as lower lactic acid levels, which results in a decrease in ventilation during submaximal exercise (compared with the untrained individual).

4. By the 16th week of gestation, all conducting airways, terminal bronchioles, and the primitive acini have formed. Neither rudimentary alveoli nor intraacinar capillaries have formed. Thus congenital diaphragmatic hernia (CDH) affects the development of the alveolar–capillary barrier and airway growth, but the number of airway divisions is not affected.

5. Before birth, blood flow in the fetus bypasses the lung and is diverted by the foramen ovale and the ductus arteriosus. The circulation is distributed to the developing organs through the systemic circulation, returns to the right side of the heart, passes through the foramen ovale into the left side, and returns to the systemic circulation. Any blood that enters the right ventricle leaves the heart and is diverted across the ductus arteriosus into the descending aorta. After birth, with the first breath, pulmonary vascular resistance decreases, the pressure in the left side of the heart becomes greater than the pressure in the right, and thus the foramen ovale, which is flap-like, closes. As the pressure in the right side of the heart decreases, oxygenated blood in the aorta passes through the ductus arteriosus and causes it to close, establishing the adult circulation.

6. High altitude results in hypoxemia with hyperventilation. High-altitude pulmonary edema and high-altitude cerebral edema can occur in susceptible individuals.

Multiple-Choice Examination

1. If a patient's total lung capacity is 5.0 L with a tidal volume of 0.5 L, an inspiratory reserve volume of 3.0 L, and an expiratory reserve volume of 1.0 L, then the residual volume is:
   a. 0.5 L
   b. 1.0 L
   c. 1.5 L
   d. 2.0 L
   e. 2.5 L
2. The minute ventilation of an individual with a tidal volume of 500 mL and a respiratory rate of 12 breaths per minute is:
   a. 42 mL
   b. 500 mL
   c. 42 L/min
   d. 5 L/min
   e. 6 L/min
3–9. Match the arterial blood gas values (a to g) with the most likely condition (3 to 9). A condition can be used more than once.

	Pao_2 mm Hg	$Paco_2$ mm Hg	Cao_2 Vol %	Sao_2%
a.	100	40	20	97
b.	100	40	10	98
c.	100	40	10	50
d.	120	20	20	99
e.	650	40	22	100
f.	60	60	17	85
g.	45	48	20	80

3. A person with normal lungs breathing 100% oxygen
4. Anemia
5. Hypoventilation
6. Carbon monoxide poisoning
7. Severe chronic bronchitis
8. Normal
9. Hyperventilation
10. Flow resistance across a set of airways is lowest under the following conditions:
    a. Airway radius is large, airways are in series, gas is of low viscosity
    b. Airway radius is large, airways are in parallel, gas is of high viscosity
    c. Airway radius is small, airways are in series, gas is of low viscosity
    d. Airway radius is small, airways are in parallel, gas is of high viscosity
    e. Airway radius is large, airways are in parallel, gas is of low viscosity
11. The airways most responsible for the resistance of the respiratory system during nasal breathing are:
    a. The nose to the larynx
    b. The trachea to segmental bronchi
    c. The subsegmental airways
    d. The terminal bronchioles
    e. The alveoli and alveolar ducts
12. Which of the following factors does not contribute to lung resistance?
    a. Lung volume
    b. Number and length of conducting airways
    c. Airway smooth muscle tone
    d. Elastic recoil
    e. Static lung compliance
13. Expiratory flow limitation occurs when:
    a. Pleural (intrathoracic) pressure exceeds elastic recoil pressure
    b. The pressure outside an airway is greater than the pressure inside the airway
    c. Dynamic lung compliance is greater than static lung compliance
    d. Lung volume is increased
    e. Expiratory flow rates are high
14. A person's respiratory rate at rest is determined by:
    a. The compliance and resistance of their respiratory system
    b. The minimal oxygen cost of breathing

c. The metabolic demands of the body

d. The work of breathing

e. All of the above

15. Which of the following statements about the measurement of lung volumes is correct?

a. FRC by helium dilution technique is the same as FRC measured by body plethysmography in individuals with obstructive and restrictive pulmonary disease.

b. TLC is determined by inspiratory muscle strength and lung elastic recoil.

c. The FVC is greater than the SVC in individuals with obstructive pulmonary disease.

d. The functional residual capacity is increased in individuals with muscle weakness.

e. One of the hallmarks of obstructive lung disease is an RV/TLC ratio less than 25%.

16. Which of the following pulmonary function test results best describes an individual with moderate chronic bronchitis?

a. Normal vital capacity, normal FEV_1, normal FEV_1/FVC, reduced expiratory flow rates, decreased D_{LCO}

b. Normal vital capacity, reduced FEV_1, decreased FEV_1/FVC, reduced expiratory flow rates, decreased D_{LCO}

c. Normal vital capacity, normal FEV_1, normal FEV_1/FVC, reduced expiratory flow rates, normal D_{LCO}

d. Normal vital capacity, reduced FEV_1, decreased FEV_1/FVC, reduced expiratory flow rates, normal D_{LCO}

e. Reduced vital capacity, reduced FEV_1, normal FEV_1/FVC, reduced expiratory flow rates, normal D_{LCO}

17. A 55-year-old woman, a former smoker, complains of shortness of breath. She has an FVC of 2.4 L and an SVC of 2.9 L. These findings suggest:

a. Restrictive lung disease

b. Obstructive lung disease

c. Muscle weakness

d. Anemia

e. Upper airway obstruction

18. Pulmonary function tests (spirometry and lung volumes) might be indicated in all of the following except:

a. Smokers older than 20 years of age

b. Evaluation of the severity of pulmonary hypertension

c. Assessment of the risk of lung resection

d. Congestive heart failure

e. Children with asthma

19. Factors affecting normal values for pulmonary function tests include all except:

a. Age

b. Sex

c. Ethnicity

d. Barometric pressure

e. Height

20. Which of the following statements about the effort-independent part of the expiratory flow volume curve is correct?

a. It occurs in the first 20% of the expiratory maneuver.

b. It depends on expiratory muscle force.

c. It is a measure of small airway function.

d. Abnormalities are indicative of severe airway obstruction.

e. Abnormalities occur early in restrictive lung disease.

21. The D_{LCO} is frequently abnormal in all except which of the following conditions?

a. Lung resection

b. Chemotherapy-induced pulmonary toxicity

c. Pulmonary hypertension

d. Multiple pulmonary emboli

e. Idiopathic pulmonary fibrosis

22. A 40-year-old mountain climber has the following blood gas values at sea level (760 mm Hg): Pa_{O_2} = 96 torr, Pa_{CO_2} = 40 torr, pH = 7.40, and F_{IO_2} = 0.21. He climbs to the top of Pike's Peak (barometric pressure, 445 mm Hg). What is his PA_{O_2} at the top of Pike's Peak (assume that his Pa_{CO_2} and R are unchanged)?

a. 25 mm Hg

b. 34 mm Hg

c. 44 mm Hg

d. 55 mm Hg

e. 60 mm Hg

23. An increase in dead space ventilation without a change in tidal volume will result in:

a. An increase in alveolar P_{CO_2} without significant change in alveolar P_{O_2}

b. An increase in alveolar P_{CO_2} with a decrease in alveolar P_{O_2}

c. A decrease in alveolar P_{CO_2} without significant change in alveolar P_{O_2}

d. A decrease in alveolar P_{CO_2} without significant change in alveolar P_{O_2}

e. No change in alveolar P_{CO_2} or alveolar P_{O_2}

24. The inspired oxygen tension at the level of the trachea when an individual is at the summit of Mt. Everest (barometric pressure, 250 torr) is:

a. 25 mm Hg

b. 43 mm Hg

c. 62 mm Hg

d. 75 mm Hg

e. 100 mm Hg

25. Anatomic dead space is determined by:

a. The size and number of the airways

b. The number of alveoli that are ventilated but not perfused

c. The mechanical properties of the chest and chest muscles

d. The characteristics of inspired gas

e. Physiologic dead space

26. If the alveolar ventilation is 4 L/min and the CO_2 production is 200 mL/min, what is the P_{ACO_2} (assume barometric pressure is 760 torr)?
    a. 31 torr
    b. 36 torr
    c. 38 torr
    d. 50 torr
    e. 55 torr

27. How many milliliters of O_2 does 100 mL of blood contain at a P_{aO_2} of 40 mm Hg?
    a. 4 mL
    b. 6 mL
    c. 8 mL
    d. 10 mL
    e. 12 mL

28. A patient has a hemoglobin level of 10 g/100 mL of blood. What is his O_2-carrying capacity?
    a. 10 mL O_2/100 mL blood
    b. 13 mL O_2/100 mL blood
    c. 15 mL O_2/100 mL blood
    d. 20 mL O_2/100 mL blood
    e. 25 mL O_2/100 mL blood

29. If the arterial–venous difference is 5 mL O_2/100 mL blood in the preceding question, what is the O_2 content of the venous blood?
    a. 5 mL O_2/100 mL blood
    b. 8 mL O_2/100 mL blood
    c. 10 mL O_2/100 mL blood
    d. 15 mL O_2/100 mL blood
    e. 18 mL O_2/100 mL blood

30. A sample of blood has a P_{O_2} of 100 mm Hg and is 98% saturated. The hemoglobin is 15 g/100 mL. The O_2 content of this blood is:
    a. 10 mL/100 mL blood
    b. 15 mL/100 mL blood
    c. 20 mL/100 mL blood
    d. 23 mL/100 mL blood
    e. 25 mL/100 mL blood

31. Investigators are studying a recently discovered gas. This gas has a high solubility in the alveolar–capillary membrane and a low solubility in the plasma. It does not appear to bind chemically to blood. Which of the following statements is true about this gas?
    a. The amount of gas absorbed into the blood is inversely proportional to the partial pressure gradient across the alveolar–capillary membrane.
    b. Diffusion across the capillary–tissue interface will be greater than diffusion across the alveolar–capillary interface.
    c. Diffusion will be directly related to the thickness of the membrane.

d. The higher the molecular weight, the greater the diffusion.
    e. Diffusion will be perfusion-limited.

32. Which of the following factors is associated with enhanced O_2 release to the tissues?
    a. Decreased temperature
    b. Increased P_{CO_2}
    c. Decreased 2,3-DPG
    d. Increased pH
    e. Tissue bicarbonate levels

33. What of the following statements about the Bohr effect is correct?
    a. It is primarily due to the effect of CO_2 on pH and on hemoglobin.
    b. It shifts the oxyhemoglobin dissociation curve to the left in the tissues.
    c. It enhances CO_2 uptake from the tissues and CO_2 unloading in the lung.
    d. It increases the levels of 2,3-DPG in red blood cells.
    e. It is related to chloride exchange processes in the red blood cell.

34–37. Match the blood gas values in a to e with the acid–base disorders shown in 34 to 37.

	pH	HCO_3^-	P_{aCO_2}
a.	7.23	10	25
b.	7.34	26	50
c.	7.37	28	50
d.	7.46	30	44
e.	7.66	22	20

34. Metabolic acidosis with respiratory compensation
35. Respiratory acidosis with renal compensation
36. Metabolic alkalosis with respiratory compensation
37. Respiratory alkalosis with renal compensation

38. A 65-year-old retired man has been homebound for 5 years because of shortness of breath. He has increased sputum production after a cold and complains of dyspnea so severe that it interferes with his smoking cigarettes. His chest is hyperinflated, with distant breath sounds and loud rhonchi on auscultation. Of the three possible sets of arterial blood gas values shown (A, B, C), which best fits the patient's condition and history?

	A	B	C
pH	7.30	7.18	7.45
P_{aO_2}	45	28	65
P_{aCO_2}	70	70	70
HCO_3^-	35	24	50
B_E	+10	0	+20

39. Which of the following would increase the ventilatory response to CO_2?
    a. Barbiturates
    b. Hypoxia
    c. Sleep
    d. Chronic obstructive pulmonary disease
    e. Anesthesia

40. Breath-holding for 90 seconds will:
    a. Increase P_{CO_2}
    b. Decrease P_{O_2}
    c. Stimulate central chemoreceptors
    d. Stimulate peripheral chemoreceptors
    e. Result in all of the above

41. Which of the following statements is not true about peripheral chemoreceptors?
    a. They respond to decreases in P_{O_2} and O_2 content.
    b. They respond to changes in arterial pH.
    c. They respond to increases in P_{CO_2}.
    d. They account for ~40% of the ventilatory response to CO_2.
    e. They are rich in dopamine.

42. Which of the following responses would be expected in a normal individual after 1 week of residence at an altitude of 12,500 ft?
    a. Increased alveolar ventilation (relative to sea level)
    b. Normal Pa_{CO_2}
    c. Normal pulmonary artery pressure
    d. Normal Pa_{O_2}
    e. Normal plasma bicarbonate

43. An 80-year-old man in congestive heart failure has a respiratory rate of 26 breaths/min, arterial pH of 7.08, P_{O_2} of 60 torr, and P_{CO_2} of 31 torr. He is treated with diuretics, oxygen, and digitalis and is given bicarbonate intravenously. The following day his respiratory rate remains elevated, and he has an arterial pH of 7.49, P_{O_2} of 102 torr on 28% O_2, and P_{CO_2} of 31 torr. The best explanation for his current respiratory alkalosis is:
    a. Excessive bicarbonate administration
    b. Cerebrospinal fluid central acidosis
    c. Compensatory metabolic acidosis
    d. Peripheral chemoreceptor stimulation
    e. Hypoxia-induced hyperventilation

44. An individual with pneumonia is receiving 30% supplemental O_2 by a facemask. Arterial blood gas values are pH = 7.40, Pa_{CO_2} = 44 mm Hg, and a Pa_{O_2} = 70 mm Hg (assume that the individual is at sea level and his respiratory quotient is 0.8). What is his AaD_{O_2}?
    a. 15 mm Hg
    b. 35 mm Hg
    c. 55 mm Hg
    d. 89 mm Hg
    e. 94 mm Hg

45. Moderate levels of exercise result in:
    a. An increase in total lung capacity
    b. An increase in pulmonary vascular resistance
    c. A decrease in the diffusion capacity for carbon monoxide
    d. A lack of significant changes in arterial blood gases
    e. A decrease in CO_2 production

46. The effects of training on the ability to perform exercise can be described as:
    a. A lowering of the resting heart rate
    b. An increase in the maximum heart rate
    c. No change in resting stroke volume
    d. Decreases in glycogen synthesis
    e. Increases in blood lactate levels

47. The first time that extrauterine life can exist is:
    a. When the airways are fully developed.
    b. When acinar development is complete
    c. At the end of the canalicular stage
    d. At the end of the saccular stage
    e. At birth

48. The most important change in the pulmonary circulation at birth is:
    a. The decrease in pulmonary vascular resistance
    b. Stimulation of respiration by progesterone
    c. Delivery of the placenta
    d. Pulmonary vasoconstriction
    e. All of the above

49. Ascent to high altitude is associated with:
    a. Hyperventilation
    b. A decrease in inspired oxygen
    c. A respiratory alkalosis
    d. A rightward shift of the oxyhemoglobin dissociation curve
    e. All of the above

50. The respiratory control center is located in the:
    a. Cerebral cortex
    b. Pons
    c. Medulla oblongata
    d. Cerebellum
    e. Spinal motor tract

51. The carotid body responds to:
    a. Hypoxia
    b. Hypercarbia
    c. Change in pH
    d. All of the above
    e. None of the above

52. The response to increases in P_{CO_2} is characterized by:
    a. A curvilinear increase in minute ventilation
    b. A linear increase in alveolar ventilation
    c. Decreased carotid sinus nerve firing
    d. Inhibition by low levels of O_2
    e. Inhibition by low pH

53. Central chemoreceptors respond to:
    a. Low Po_2
    b. Changes in blood bicarbonate levels
    c. Changes in H^+ ion concentrations
    d. Changes in molecular CO_2
    e. All of the above
54. The Hering–Breuer reflex is stimulated by:
    a. Spinal motor neurons
    b. Nasal or facial receptors
    c. Increases in lung volume
    d. Irritant receptors
    e. J receptors
55. Which of the following statements about obstructive sleep apnea (OSA) is true?
    a. OSA is most commonly caused by obesity.
    b. OSA is associated with a decrease in ventilatory drive to the respiratory motor neurons.
    c. OSA is associated with an absence of ventilatory effort.
    d. OSA is associated with lower respiratory tract obstruction.
    e. OSA is never associated with hypoxia.
56. Which of the following statements about mucus in chronic bronchitis is not true?
    a. Submucosal glands increase in number and size with chronic bronchitis.
    b. Surface secretory cells increase in number and size with chronic bronchitis.
    c. The chemical composition of surface secretory cells changes with chronic bronchitis.
    d. The chemical composition of submucosal glands changes with chronic bronchitis.
    e. Particulate smoke deposition occurs in respiratory bronchioles in chronic bronchitis.
57. Particle retention in the lung most often occurs:
    a. At the transition between the conducting airways and the terminal respiratory units
    b. At bifurcations in large airways
    c. At bifurcations in small airways
    d. In the nose
    e. In the trachea
58. Important defense systems in the respiratory system include:
    a. Mucociliary transport
    b. Innate immunity
    c. Adaptive immunity
    d. Migratory phagocytic and inflammatory cells
    e. All of the above
59. Alveolar macrophages:
    a. Are derived from blood monocytes
    b. Live 1 to 5 weeks in the respiratory tract
    c. Both dissolve and engulf foreign materials
    d. Are characterized by all of the above
    e. Are characterized by none of the above
60. Surfactants:
    a. Decrease surface tension at all lung volumes
    b. Increase surface tension at low lung volumes and decrease surface tension at high lung volumes
    c. Are resistant to hypoxia and sheer stress
    d. Are produced by type I epithelial cells
    e. Are characterized by all of the above

ANSWERS TO MULTIPLE-CHOICE EXAMINATION

1. a	13. b	25. a	37. e	49. e
2. e	14. e	26. b	38. a	50. c
3. e	15. b	27. e	39. b	51. d
4. b	16. d	28. b	40. e	52. b
5. f	17. b	29. b	41. a	53. d
6. b	18. b	30. c	42. a	54. c
7. g	19. d	31. e	43. b	55. a
8. a	20. c	32. b	44. d	56. d
9. d	21. c	33. a	45. d	57. a
10. e	22. b	34. a	46. a	58. e
11. a	23. b	35. c	47. c	59. d
12. e	24. b	36. d	48. a	60. a

C APPENDIX

Abbreviations, Gas Laws

ABBREVIATIONS

1.1 Pressures

P_B, barometric (ambient) pressure
P_{H_2O}, water vapor pressure

1.2 Respiratory Gases

P_A, partial pressure of a gas in alveolar air; for example, P_{AO_2}, partial pressure of oxygen in the alveolus
Pa, partial pressure of a gas in arterial blood; for example, P_{aO_2}, partial pressure of oxygen in arterial blood
P_V, partial pressure of a gas in mixed venous blood; for example, P_{vO_2}, partial pressure of oxygen in mixed venous blood

1.3 Volumes

TV or V_T, Tidal volume
FRC, Functional residual capacity
RV, Residual volume
VC, Vital capacity
FVC, Forced vital capacity
TLC, Total lung capacity
V_D, Anatomic dead space volume
V_D/V_T, Ratio of dead space volume to tidal volume

1.4 Blood Flow

Q_T, cardiac output

1.5 Ventilation

MV, Minute ventilation
$\dot{V}O_2$, Oxygen consumption
$\dot{V}CO_2$, Carbon dioxide consumption
$\dot{V}A$, Alveolar ventilation
$\dot{V}/\dot{Q}$ Ventilation perfusion ratio

1.6 Concentration

Ca_{O_2}, oxygen content (C) of arterial oxygen

1.7 Fraction (F)

F_{AO_2}, fraction of oxygen in alveolar gas

1.8 Hemoglobin

Hgb, hemoglobin concentration
$HgbO_2$, oxyhemoglobin
SO_2, oxygen saturation

THE GAS LAWS

The behavior of gases is described by the **ideal gas equation**, which relates volume, pressure, and temperature:

$$PV = nRT,$$

where P is pressure, V is volume, T is temperature, n is the number of moles of gas molecules, and R is the gas constant, which is fixed at 0.0821.

When nR is constant, the equation can be used to determine changes in pressure, volume, and temperature under different conditions. That is,

$$\frac{P_1 \times V_1}{T_1} = \frac{P_2 \times V_2}{T_2}$$

Boyle's law characterizes the relationship between temperature and volume. That is, if temperature (T_1 and T_2 in the preceding equation) remains constant, pressure will vary inversely to volume:

$$P_1 \times V_1 = P_2 \times V_2$$

Boyle's law is used to calculate lung volumes (Chapter 2).

Charles's law characterizes the relationship between volume and temperature in the presence of a constant pressure. That is, if pressure (P_1, P_2) remains constant, volume and temperature will vary directly:

$$\frac{P_1}{T_1} = \frac{P_2}{T_2}$$

2.1 Gases

Air is composed of a mixture of gases that exert a pressure. Each individual gas exerts its own pressure, known as its **partial pressure**. This pressure is generated by the collision of gas molecules along the wall of the container. The partial pressure of the individual gases is the product of the total gas pressure and the proportion of total gas composition made up by the specific gas of interest (see Chapter 5). For example, at sea level, the total ambient pressure, also known as the **barometric pressure,** is 760 mm Hg. (The basic pressure unit in respiratory physiology is millimeters of mercury—mm Hg.) Air is composed of approximately 21% oxygen. Thus, at sea level the partial pressure of oxygen is 0.21 × 760 mm Hg = 160 mm Hg. Small pressure differences are often expressed in cm H_2O where there is 1.36 cm H_2O for every 1 mm Hg of pressure.

Dalton's law states that the total pressure of a gas mixture is equal to the sum of the partial pressure of the gases in a gas mixture. That is, each individual gas in a gas mixture acts independently and exerts its own partial pressure, and the sum of all of the partial pressures is equal to the total pressure. Because the total pressure is fixed, as the pressure exerted by one specific gas increases, the pressure exerted by another must decrease. When water vapor is added or when carbon dioxide is added in the alveolus, the partial pressure of oxygen decreases.

2.2 Vapor Pressure

At the interface of a liquid and an open space, the rate of escape of molecules from the liquid phase equals the rate at which gas molecules return to the liquid phase. The vapor pressure of a gas is defined as the partial pressure exerted by gas molecules when they are in equilibrium between the gas and liquid phase. For the respiratory system, water is the major liquid, and the vapor pressure of water is solely dependent on temperature. Water vapor pressure increases with increasing temperature; at body temperature, this water vapor pressure is 47 mm Hg. The amount of moisture in the air is defined by its relative humidity, which is defined as the ratio of the measured partial presssure of water in the air to the vpaor pressure of water (determined solely on the basis of the temperature of the air). The air that we breathe is usually less than body temperature and rarely fully saturated. Inspired air, however, by the time it reaches the trachea, has been warmed to body temperature and is fully saturated. If the total pressure is 760 mm Hg and water vapor pressure (P_{H_2O}) is 47 mm Hg, the remaining 713 mm Hg is equal to the sum of all the remaining gases in the inspired air (Dalton's law). Thus, in the trachea, the partial pressure of O_2 in the ambient air is now .21 × (760 − 47) = 150 mm Hg, or an approximately 10 mm decrease in the partial pressure of oxygen in the inspired air that enters the nose and mouth.

2.3 Measuring Gas Volumes

Gas volumes can be measured and reported under three conditions. When gas is exhaled into a spirometer or bag, it is reported at ambient temperature and pressure, saturated (ATPS). Gas volumes measured in the lung are reported at body temperature and pressure, saturated (BTPS), while oxygen consumption and carbon dioxide production are reported at standard temperature and pressure, dry (STPD). When reporting gas volumes, it is important to make sure that different volumes have been measured until the same conditions. For example, in going from ATPS to BTPS, there is an increase of volume of approximately 10%.

2.4 Gas Solubility

In the respiratory system, we must also consider the partial pressure of a gas in a liquid phase—namely, the blood. When a liquid is in contact with a gas mixture, the partial pressure of the particular gas in the liquid is the same as its partial pressure in the gas mixture, assuming that full equilibration has occurred. Therefore the partial pressure of the gas acts as the "driving force" for the gas to be carried in the liquid phase.

Henry's law states that the amount of a gas absorbed by a liquid such as blood, to which it is not chemically combined, is directly proportional to the positive pressure of the gas to which the liquid is exposed and the solubility of the gas in the liquid. For example, if a gas is very soluble in the liquid, more of that particular gas will be carried in a given pressure compared to a less soluble gas. In addition, and most important for the respiratory system, if the liquid is able to bind or carry more of the gas, more of the gas will be transported at a particular partial pressure.

The interaction of hemoglobin in the red blood cells and oxygen allows more oxygen to be transported at any partial pressure and is the major transport system in the body for oxygen (see Chapter 8).

The transport and delivery of O_2 from the lungs into the blood and from the blood into the tissue (and vice versa for CO_2) are dependent on the gas diffusion laws and is described by **Fick's law** (see Fig. 8.2).

The diffusion constant for a gas is directly proportional to the solubility of the gas and inversely proportional to the square root of the molecular weight of the gas.

$$D = \frac{\text{solubility}}{\sqrt{\text{molecular weight}}}$$

Solubility is defined as the volume of gas in milliliters that must be dissolved in 100 mL of the barrier liquid to raise the partial pressure by 1 torr.

2.5 Airflow in Airways

Air or liquid flows through a tube or a set of tubes when there is a pressure difference from one end of the tube to the other (analogous to **Ohm's law** for the flow of electricity: the voltage [V] across a circuit is equal to the current [I] × the resistance [R]. V = IR). The same is true in the airways, in which air flows when a pressure difference exists from one point in the airways to another. The speed or average velocity (in cm/sec) of flow is equal to the overall flow rate (in mL/sec) divided by the cross-sectional area of the tube (cm²).

Analogous to electric resistance, resistances in series are added directly:

$$R_{tot} = R_1 + R_2 + R_3 \ldots$$

Resistances in parallel are added as reciprocals:

$$1/R_{tot} - 1/R_1 + 1/R_2 + 1/R_3 \ldots$$

There are two major patterns of gas flow—laminar and turbulent (Fig. Appendix C-1). Gas flow patterns in between laminar and turbulent also occur and are called transitional, or disturbed. The pattern of gas flow depends on the velocity and the characteristics of the airway. Laminar flow occurs when the stream of gas in a cylindrical tube is parallel to the walls of the tube. Laminar flow occurs at low flow rates. At high flow rates, there is disorganization of the flow stream with flow occurring both parallel and perpendicular to the overall flow axis and turbulence occurs.

In laminar flow, the gas traveling in the center of the tube moves most rapidly, whereas the gas in direct contact with the wall of the tube remains stationary. In laminar flow, pressure (P) and flow ($\dot{V}$) are proportional (i.e., P = k × $\dot{V}$). This telescope arrangement of multiple cylinders within the tube results in the cylinder closest to the vessel wall having the slowest velocity (due to frictional forces) and the center cylinder, where K is a constant,

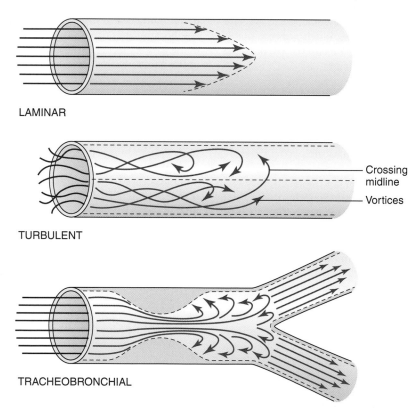

LAMINAR

TURBULENT

— Crossing
  midline
— Vortices

TRACHEOBRONCHIAL

Figure Appendix C-1 Types of airflow. In laminar flow, air moves in the same direction parallel to the walls of the airways. The fluid in the center moves twice as fast as the fluid toward the edges, whereas the fluid at the wall does not move. In turbulent flow, air moves irregularly in axial, radial, and circumferential directions and vortices are common. Gas density is important but viscosity is not. Turbulent flow requires higher pressures than does laminar flow. Flow changes from laminar to turbulent when the Reynolds number exceeds 2000. Turbulent flow occurs in the large airways (tracheobronchial) and wherever there are irregularities in the airways (e.g., bifurcations, mucus).

having the highest velocity. This changing velocity across the diameter of the tube is known as the velocity profile and occurs because fluid velocity decreases with the square of the radial distance away from the center of the tube. Thus, laminar flow has a parabolic velocity profile. In fact, when laminar flow is fully developed, the gas in the center of the tube moves exactly twice as fast as the average velocity.

In turbulent flow, gas movement occurs both parallel and perpendicular to the axis of the tube and differs from laminar flow in two important ways. First, pressure is no longer proportional to the flow rate but to the flow rate squared (i.e., $P = k \times \dot{V}^2$). Second, the viscosity of the gas becomes unimportant, but an increase in gas density increases the pressure drop for a given flow. Gas along the wall still remains stationary, but there is less variation in gas velocity as a function of position in the tube. Overall, gas velocity is blunted because energy is consumed in the process of generating the eddies and chaotic movement. A higher driving pressure is needed to support a given flow under turbulent conditions compared with laminar flow conditions. There is a linear relationship between pressure and flow under laminar conditions and a nonlinear relationship under turbulent conditions (Fig. Appendix C-2).

Whether flow through a tube is laminar or turbulent depends on the **Reynolds number** (Re). Re is a dimensionless value that expresses the ratio of two dimensionally equivalent terms (kinematic/viscosity):

$$Re = \frac{2 \, rvd}{n}$$

where r is the radius, v is the average velocity, d is the density, and n is the viscosity.

In straight tubes, turbulence occurs when the Reynolds number is greater than 2000. From this relationship it can be seen that turbulence is most likely to occur when the average velocity of gas flow is high and the radius is large. In contrast, a low-density gas such as helium is less likely to cause turbulent flow at any given flow rate. Airflow in the trachea during tidal volume (Vτ) breathing is turbulent because the trachea has a large diameter (3 cm in the adult) and gas flow at the mouth during quiet breathing is approximately 1 L/sec, which results in an average velocity of 150 cm/sec. Thus, the Reynolds number for the trachea during quiet breathing is greater than 2000. For example,

$$Re = \frac{2 \times 1.5 \, cm \times 150 \, cm/sec \times 0.0012 \, g/mL}{1.83 \times 10^{-4} g/sec \cdot cm} = 2951$$

where 0.0012 g/mL is the density of air and 1.83×10^{-4} g/sec·cm is the viscosity of air. Airflow becomes less turbulent as airway radius and flow decrease.

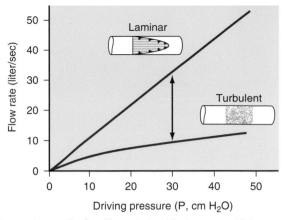

Figure Appendix C-2 The relationship between driving pressure and flow through a tube. Under laminar flow conditions, an increase in the driving pressure is associated with an increase in flow. In contrast, in turbulent flow, at any driving pressure, flow is less than under laminar conditions. The reason for this is that in turbulent flow some of the increase in driving pressure is expended by moving air in directions perpendicular to the airway axis. (Redrawn from Leff A, Schumacker P. *Respiratory Physiology: Basics and Applications.* Philadelphia: W.B. Saunders; 1993.)

In such a complicated system as the bronchial tree, with its many branches, changes in caliber, and irregular wall surfaces, fully developed laminar flow probably only occurs in the very small airways, whereas flow is transitional in most of the bronchial tree.

Turbulence is also promoted by the glottis and vocal cords that produce some "irregularity" and obstruction in the tubes. As gas flows more distally, the total cross-sectional area increases dramatically, and gas velocities decrease significantly. As a result, gas flow becomes more laminar in smaller airways even during maximal ventilation. The bottom line is that gas flow in the larger airways (nose, mouth, glottis, and bronchi) is turbulent, whereas gas flow in the smaller airways is laminar. Breath sounds heard with a stethoscope are due to turbulent airflow. Laminar flow is silent. This is one of the factors responsible for the difficulty in recognizing clinically small airway disease, which is said to be "silent."

Hemoglobin

Each gram of hemoglobin can store approximately 1.39 mL of O_2.

$$4 \, \frac{moles \, O_2}{mole \, Hgb} \times 22,400 \, \frac{ml \, O_2}{mole \, O_2} \times 1 \, \frac{mole \, Hb}{64,500 \, gm \, Hb}$$
$$= 1.39 \, \frac{ml \, O_2}{gm \, Hgb}$$

A small number of heme sites cannot bind oxygen because the iron on the site is in the ferric form. Thus, fully saturated Hgb carries approximately 1.34 mL of O_2/gm of Hgb.

INDEX

Note: Page numbers followed by "f" indicate figures and "t" indicate tables "b" indicate boxes.